Weightlifting Movement

Assessment & Optimization

WEIGHTLIFTING MOVEMENT ASSESSMENT & OPTIMIZATION

Mobility & Stability for
the Snatch and Clean & Jerk

Quinn Henoch, DPT

Copyright Page

ISBN 978-0-9907985-7-6

Catalyst Athletics, Inc.
www.catalystathletics.com

Anatomical illustrations by Glen Oomen

Contents

Acknowledgements vii

Introduction ix

Part I: Setting The Foundation 1

    Chapter 1: Terms, Concepts & Discussion 3

    Chapter 2: Trunk Stability & Weightlifting Posture 19

Part II: Screening & Assessment 43

    Chapter 3: Screening & Assessment: The Pull & Split 49

    Chapter 4: Screening & Assessment: Transition & Overhead 73

    Chapter 5: Screening & Assessment: The Squat 89

Part III: Building The Weightlifting Movements 121

    Chapter 6: Programming Considerations 123

    Chapter 7: Snatch Starting Position 137

    Chapter 8: Snatch First Pull 159

    Chapter 9: Snatch Finish/Extension 171

    Chapter 10: Snatch Third Pull 181

    Chapter 11: Snatch Receiving Position 191

    Chapter 12: Summary of The Snatch 245

    Chapter 13: Clean Receiving Position 247

    Chapter 14: Summary of The Clean 271

    Chapter 15: Jerk Front Rack 273

    Chapter 16: Jerk Dip 279

    Chapter 17: Jerk Drive 287

    Chapter 18: Jerk Split 295

    Chapter 19: Summary of The Jerk 319

    Chapter 20: Variations for Skill Transfer 321

    Chapter 21: Recovery 331

References 337

Acknowledgements

The content of this book has been taught to me, derived and/or adapted from individuals much smarter than myself. I want to thank all of my rehabilitation, strength & conditioning, and weightlifting heroes for filling my head with everything that I know.

To my weightlifting coaches: Ben Carter of Bluegrass Barbell, thank you for bringing me into the sport and staying with me while in physical therapy school. It is not easy coaching someone long distance who knows just enough to think he knows anything. Thank you for making me focus on the long term. Colin Burns of Ronin Weightlifting and Juggernaut Training Systems, thank you for trying to impart into my lifts the world-class technique that you have displayed on the international stage. You embody the rare combination of being a great lifter and a great coach.

To the ClinicalAthlete network and community: thank you for striving toward excellence in the rehabilitation and performance field. The public needs healthcare providers who understand athletes, and you all embody that mission. I have learned so much from you and grown immensely as a professional. I look forward to all of the positive changes that we'll be a part of together in our field.

Thank you to all of the lifting buddies, teams and various coaches I have trained with or had the pleasure of meeting over the past several years. Weightlifting may technically be an individual sport, but a team atmosphere can be an invaluable component of training. It certainly has been for me.

Thank you to Juggernaut Training Systems and Darkside Strength for allowing me to be a part of your team and giving me a professional platform that I would not have otherwise had. Traveling around the world and coaching the things that I love has been a dream come true.

To my classmates, professors, and colleagues from undergraduate and throughout the beginning of my career now, you have all had a significant impact on me in one way or the other. I am humbled to have worked with so many knowledgeable people in such a short amount of time. To the rest of my family and friends—thank you for your love, patience and support.

Finally, to Greg Everett and Catalyst Athletics, thank you for this opportunity. I remember when I was completing my last physical therapy student internship in San Francisco, it was always the highlight of my week to drive down the bay and train with your team. Now, to be creating something like this with you is an honor.

Introduction

My name is Quinn Henoch. I am a competitive weightlifter, but by no means a great one—pedestrian, really, when compared to the best in my class. I am a Doctor of Physical Therapy, but by no means the best or most knowledgeable therapist.

Nonetheless, I am a therapist and a competitive weightlifter, and from my experience in both fields, this is a rare combination: a health care professional who not only wants you to return to a grueling sport, but one that goes through the everyday grind himself, both in the clinic and on the platform.

My weightlifting background began from playing football. I was fortunate enough to be introduced to both the snatch and clean & jerk in my high school program. The lifts remained my favorite part of training through college, where I played defensive back for a small Division I-AA school in northwest Indiana, Valparaiso University.

The upside was that I was exposed to the lifts early and often, and had eight years to ingrain the movement patterns. The downside was that I had eight years to ingrain poor movement patterns. Perfecting the technicality of the snatch and clean & jerk was second fiddle to putting more weight on the bar.

After my football career was done, I desperately searched for something to replace it. I dabbled in competitive CrossFit for a short time until I realized that anything above a five-minute time cap scarred my soul. I competed in powerlifting until I was tired of being out-benched by women who were smaller than me. Weightlifting was the clear choice and where my passion lay all along.

I enrolled in physical therapy school around the time that I competed in my first weightlifting meet in 2010. This began my multi-year struggle of attempting to undo the wear and tear of twelve years of football and eight years of bastardizing the snatch and clean & jerk.

With the bulk of my competitive weightlifting career overlapping the beginning of my Doctoral education in physical therapy, I have been exposed to and experimented with countless strategies to improve movement and positioning related to weightlifting. I went through the *Two-Hour Warm-up* phase, where I hooked an apparatus to every joint in my body and made love to foam rollers like I was getting paid; the *Load the Barbell and Go* phase, where I thought I was immune to having to prepare my body for training; and everything in between. With this trial and error have come revelations, which will be discussed in this book.

Purpose & Disclaimers

Weightlifting is a challenging sport for not only the extreme technicality required to execute a full snatch and clean & jerk, but also the extreme body positions required to demonstrate such technique. Unlike a basketball player, for example, who can practice free throw shooting with little difficulty achieving the body position of a full shooting stroke, so many in the sport of weightlifting are limited in achieving the proper positions to perform the sporting skill. At that point, technical coaching of the lifts becomes very difficult.

I hate to be a Negative Nancy, but we must start with what this book is *NOT*. This book is *not* meant to coach the technicalities of the snatch or clean & jerk. Due to the fact that we are all humans, there are common truths for movement that will be discussed. However, referring to these common truths is not the same as referring to technical variations of executing the snatch and clean & jerk. There is certainly overlap, but I will do my best to leave that up to the weightlifting coaches.

This book is *not* meant to cure acute or chronic pain or rehabilitate current injuries or specific medical diagnoses. Now, that certainly does not preclude you from using the corrective strategies in the book if you have something going on, as optimizing your movement may very well help with some of those things. However, if you are hurt or injured, and it is affecting your training, I recommend you go see a qualified health care professional first, preferably one from the ClinicalAthlete network.

Having said that, weightlifting is a grueling sport. It does not take long to realize that if you are training seriously, aches and pains are just part of the game. Use your discretion or that of your coach or health care professional when differentiating between this and something that is more serious. It is my experience that the more proficient an athlete's movement, the fewer daily aches and pains they experience. The contents of this book will hopefully help with that.

Incorporating the contents of this book into your program does *not* guarantee an *immediate* increase in the amount of weight you can snatch or clean & jerk. Although this may happen, it is important to remember that training is a process, and the athlete needs time to learn and strengthen new positions and refine motor patterns. It is up to the coach or athlete to load progressively and appropriately.

Finally, this book is *not* meant to replace all of the great resources already available in regards to movement or mobility.

Enough of the negative talk—now for what this book *IS*. This book is meant to be a reference for weightlifters and weightlifting coaches of all levels, and is specific to the movements and body positions required of the snatch and clean & jerk—the two contested lifts in the sport of weightlifting.

For the beginner to intermediate level lifter, this book is meant to teach movement patterns and positions related to the two lifts. The goal is to increase the ease with which an individual can achieve a full overhead squat position, front squat position, back squat position, starting or pulling position, and overhead position in a power and split receiving stance—and to do so in a biomechanically conducive way to maximize stability and safety in said positions.

For the more advanced lifter, this book is a reference providing tools to maintain or enhance the motor patterns he or she likely already possesses related to the snatch and clean & jerk, without adding a lot of extra time to an already busy training schedule.

For the coach, this book is a reference to separate movement pattern issues from technique issues (understand that these two things are not always mutually exclusive), and provide guidance for addressing movement pattern issues in a time-efficient and safe manner, so that technique can become the coach's main focus once more.

This book is to be used in conjunction with all of the great resources that are already available pertaining to movement and the sport of weightlifting by providing a different perspective and adding to your knowledge repertoire. When I read a book or attend a continuing education course, I am looking to glean at least one piece of info that can be put into practice right away. If I can, the investment was worth it. I refer to these bits of knowledge as *golden nuggets*. It can be an exercise, cue, concept, perspective, etc. that resonates with you and is applicable. My hope is that the content of this book provides you with a golden nugget or two.

I have no apparent conflict of interest in regard to the book's content. I do not get paid by any movement system, school of thought, or alphabet soup governing body to push an agenda. I will do my best to distinguish what in this book is backed by scientific literature, and what is based on my own clinical experience (I'll try to be as unbiased as possible).

Above all, I simply want this book to be something that my weightlifting brethren can use for years to come to enhance their experience while participating in the greatest sport in the world.

One Last Disclaimer The information in this book is offered for educational purposes only. The reader should understand and be cautioned that there is an inherent risk assumed with any form of physical activity. Those participating in weightlifting or strength & conditioning programs should check with their physicians prior to initiating such activities, as these types of physical activities may not be appropriate for everyone. The author of this book is not a physician and assumes no liability for injury; this is purely an educational manual to guide those already proficient with the demands of such physical activity.

■ PART I

Setting The Foundation

In Part 1, we will define terms and discuss the rationale behind concepts in the context that they are used throughout the book. We will then begin a discussion regarding trunk stability, postural alignment and breathing patterns as they pertain to the snatch and clean & jerk.

Objectives

- Establish a common language between the author and the reader.
- Understand the relationship between weightlifting posture and core control along with the role they play in attaining the positions of the snatch and clean & jerk.
- Discuss proposed theories and mechanisms that govern human movement.
- Introduce basic drills that can be utilized as teaching tools for the abovementioned concepts.

■ CHAPTER 1

Terms, Concepts & Discussion

This chapter contains important terminology with related concepts and subsequent discussion.

Mobility

Mobility is the *potential* for motion of a body segment(s), joint system(s) or muscular system(s), and the ability to produce that motion through a full range. Simply put—the *potential* ability to produce wanted movement; or even more simply put, *mobility is movement potential*.

Mobility includes muscle extensibility, connective tissue flexibility and joint mechanics, all of which are defined below. In its purest form, mobility would be considered *without* influence from the nervous system. In other words, if you're put under anesthesia, mobility is how much range of motion your joint systems possess. However, in a real world scenario, we are obviously dealing with athletes that are awake—from this point forward, when referring to mobility and the physiological factors mentioned above, we will assume they *are* influenced by the nervous system to varying degrees, which is why sometimes demonstrating your full mobility potential is not always possible—especially under heavy load, stress, fatigue, etc.

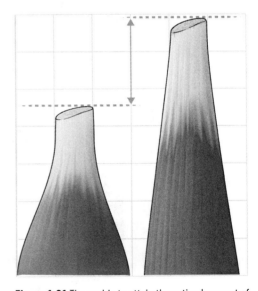

Figure 1.01 The goal is to attain the optimal amount of muscle extensibility and soft tissue flexibly to consistently achieve the desired positions of the snatch and clean & jerk. This does not mean you need to be able to do the splits.

Factors of Mobility

Flexibility The capacity of soft tissue structures (tendon, ligament, joint capsule) to be lengthened to allow the desired range of motion of a joint.

Muscle Extensibility The capacity of muscle fibers specifically to be elongated or stretched to allow the desired range of motion of a joint (Figure 1.01).

■ 3

Osteokinematics The movements of bones at joints in the three planes described below (sagittal, frontal and transverse).

Sagittal Plane Divides the body into left and right halves. Examples of osteokinematic movement in the sagittal plane: flexion/extension of the hip, shoulder, elbow and knee; forward and backward bending of the trunk; dorsiflexion and plantarflexion of the ankle (Figures 1.02 & 1.03).

Frontal Plane Divides the body into front and back halves. Examples of movements in the frontal plane: abduction and adduction of the hip or shoulder; eversion and inversion of ankle (Figure 1.04).

Transverse Plane Divides body into top and bottom. Examples of movement in the transverse plane: internal and external rotation of hip and shoulder; spinal rotation (Figure 1.05).

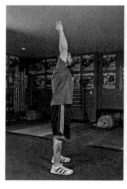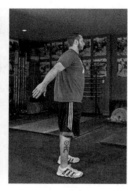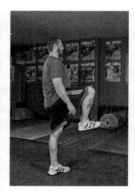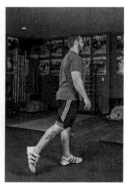

Figure 1.02 These photos demonstrate sagittal plane motion of the shoulder, hip, knee and ankle in an open chain (foot and hand are not fixed to a surface).

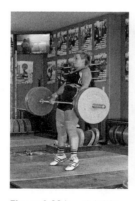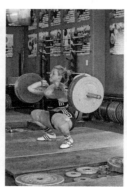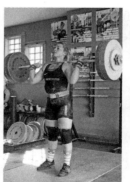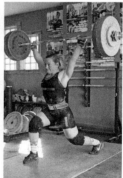

Figure 1.03 In weightlifting, movement in the sagittal plane is demonstrated with extension at the top of the pull (hip extension, knee extension and ankle plantarflexion) versus a deep squat position (hip flexion, knee flexion and ankle dorsiflexion) as well as in the split jerk with one hip in extension (back leg) and the other in flexion (front leg). In regard to the shoulders, sagittal plane movement is demonstrated when going from the rack position to fully overhead (a little less than 90 degrees of shoulder flexion to roughly 180 degrees of shoulder flexion), for example.

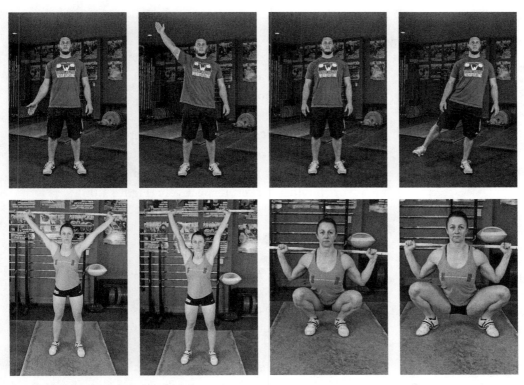

Figure 1.04 Frontal plane motion is demonstrated in the shoulders with a wider snatch grip (shoulder abduction) versus a narrower jerk grip (relative shoulder adduction), and in the hips when determining squat stance width from narrow (relative hip adduction) to wide (relative hip abduction).

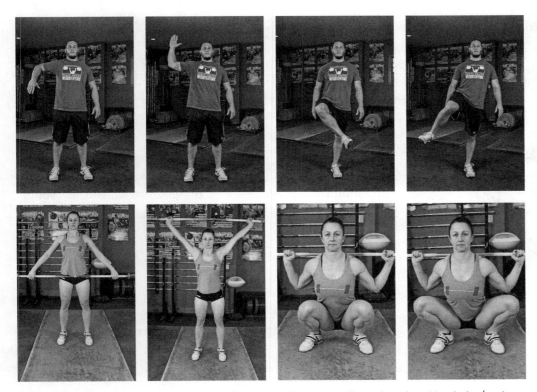

Figure 1.05 Transverse plane motion is demonstrated in the shoulders when pulling under and receiving the bar (moving from shoulder internal rotation to external rotation), as well as in the hip for lower body joint alignment during a full squat.

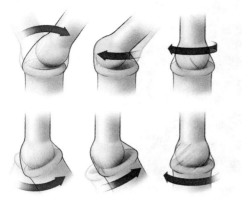

Figure 1.06 These subtle joint movements occur when moving a joint through a full range of motion. We will discuss specific joint arthrokinematics later, but it's important to understand that these movements are not necessarily under conscious control. They will happen naturally based on the alignment of the skeleton and the firing patterns of the muscles.

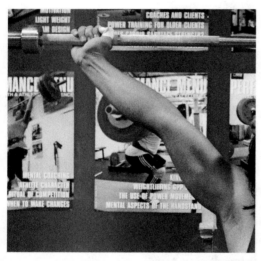

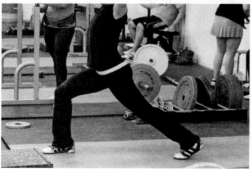

Figure 1.07 Some lifters possess more laxity in their joints than others and may utilize this as a passive restraint for stability (e.g. hyperextension of the elbow and lower back as pictured).

Important Note We must understand that during the weightlifting movements, the body is moving through all three of these cardinal planes simultaneously to various degrees. We are breaking them down in isolation here simply for teaching purposes.

Arthrokinematics Accessory movement of bones between joint surfaces. Examples: roll, slide and spin of the femur (thigh bone) or humeral head (upper arm bone) in the hip or shoulder socket, respectively (Figure 1.06).

Stability & Motor Control

Stability is the control of the abovementioned mobility factors. It's the ability to regulate the desired range of motion of a system, and the ability to resist undesired range of motion of a system. The literature defines it as follows:

Stability *"The ability to offset an external perturbation." (Stergiou 2011) "Inverse of the rate of divergence from the intended trajectory after a perturbation." (Stergiou 2011) "The degree to which a system can return to an orientation or movement trajectory after a perturbation." (McQuade 2016) "Instability—the inability to recover a position or trajectory after perturbation." (McQuade 2016)*

Passive Stability Control of a joint system using inert (non-contractile and non-neurological) tissues such as ligaments, joint capsules or bony structures ("Hanging on your ligaments") (Figure 1.07).

Active Stability The control of a joint structure using the neuromuscular system. Can occur under conscious (voluntary) or subconscious (reflexive) control.

Static Stability The ability of a joint system to *maintain* a desired position while resisting any change in that position.

Dynamic Stability The ability of a joint system to resist change or deviation from a desired range while *moving* through a desired range.

Stability & Motor Control in Weightlifting To put this all into weightlifting context, we'll use the snatch as an example. As the barbell moves from the floor toward the hip, the lifter is exhibiting active, dynamic stability through extension of the leg joints. At this point, the torso is exhibiting active, static stability as the muscles of the core fight to maintain spinal position and resist the forces of the external load.

After the lifter extends up and begins to pull under the barbell, the shoulders are now exhibiting active, dynamic stability in controlling the desired bar path. The shoulders then lock out and become one unit with the torso, resisting unwanted movement (static stability), while the legs dynamically finish the lift. This is all within the lifter's individual mobility capacity, and passive stability (using connective tissue for support) is occurring to some degree throughout all phases of the lift.

Important Notes As with the mobility factors described previously, we've defined these forms of stability separately, but it should be understood that for any movement or lift, we are simultaneously utilizing varying degrees of both active and passive stability means.

Also, we defined static stability as if it truly means a motionless system. In reality, static stability does not exist in the literal sense, because even a seemingly motionless joint system is performing countless, often imperceptibly small, dynamic corrections to maintain a general position—*static* is relative.

Movement

We'll define *movement* as the abovementioned mobility and stability factors combined with biomechanical principles to propel a body part(s) in the desired direction and/or achieve a desired position—such as a successful completion of the snatch or clean & jerk.

Motor Skill Acquisition (MSA) *"A process in which a performer learns to control and integrate posture, locomotion, and muscle activations that allow the individual to engage in a variety of motor behaviors that are constrained by a range of task requirements." (Newell 1991)*

Relating this concept to weightlifting, the snatch and clean & jerk are movement skills that must be developed over time through repeated sequencing via the neuromuscular system. Elements such as postural control and muscle activation become automatic, but it may be beneficial to break those elements down into components for motor learning purposes. MSA (specific to the motor skills of weightlifting) is the overall goal of this entire book, as we explore different strategies to facilitate it.

Movement Variability (MV) *"Allowing for desired adaptation to perturbations." (Harbourne 2009) "Increase the ability to adapt." (Glasgow 2013)*

MV is an important aspect for a weightlifter. It allows the athlete to have reflexive movement "options" within their joint systems' mobility-stability capacity. An optimal level of MV will facilitate the MSA process.

One example of movement variability would be a lifter adjusting his or her bottom position under a heavy snatch in order to successfully complete the lift. We have often seen lifters reposition themselves under load with what sometimes look like positions that would otherwise be dangerous—knees diving in or out, hips or shoulders shifting around, etc.—however, the lifter comes out of that movement unscathed. He or she was able to explore movement "options" in order to complete the task, utilizing the spectrum of mobility and stability that had already been established as within his or her capacity.

Muscle Contraction

Concentric Shortening of a muscle when contracted, overcoming an opposing force. *Example: The quadriceps perform a concentric contraction when standing up from a squat.*

Eccentric Lengthening of a muscle when contracted, succumbing to an opposing force. *Example: The quadriceps perform an eccentric contraction when lowering down into a squat.*

Posture

Posture is the skeletal alignment dictated by our interaction with gravity and the barbell. This term will *not* be used in regard to its role (or lack there of) with pain.

Neutral Spine Posture The spinal alignment that yields the optimal balance of passive and active stabilizers in order to perform a desired task safely and effectively (like walking, or say, the snatch and clean & jerk).

Unloaded Neutral Spine Posture Neutral spine when not lifting weights (Figure 1.08):

- Pelvis: Mild anterior tilt (pelvic bowl dumps forward slightly—8-15 degrees)
- Lumbar Spine (L1-L5): Mild lordosis (extension/arching—45 degrees)

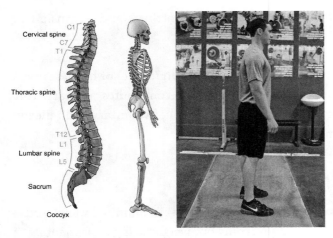

Figure 1.08 Example of a neutral spine posture at rest. Notice the natural rounding of the upper back to accommodate the ribcage with minimal rib flaring in the front. Also notice that the shoulders are stacked on top of the hips.

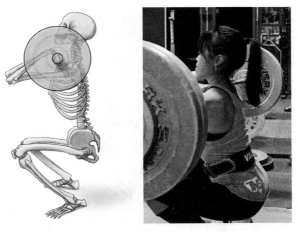

Figure 1.09 Example of a lifter demonstrating a load-supporting spinal posture. Notice the difference from unloaded posture is the slight relative extension of the upper back, creating a "tall" spine. In general, there may be a perceived increase in extension throughout the spine (versus hinging through only the lower back), and the shoulders remain stacked over the hips.

- Thoracic Spine (T1-T12): Mild kyphosis (flexion/rounding—40 degrees)
- Cervical Spine (C1-C7): Mild lordosis (extension/arching—35 degrees)

Load-Supporting Neutral Spine Posture Neutral spine when lifting weights—varies based on individual anatomy, technique, etc. (Figure 1.09).

The common thought is that an athlete will increase *extension* of the spine when under load to maintain lumbar lordosis and upright posture. The reality is that neutral spine under load is a *range* that can swing from *relative* amounts of spinal flexion and extension.

In general, we are striving to resist flexion forces through the spine, which may be perceived by the athlete as an increased amount of spinal extension. The upper thoracic spine may demonstrate slightly increased amounts of extension (relative lordosis) when overhead, pulling from the floor, and supporting load in the front rack—although, again, *resisting flexion* may be a more accurate description.

Thoracolumbar Junction The point in the spine where the thoracic vertebrae (T12) meet the lumbar vertebrae (L1) (Figure 1.10). This is a reference point that we will refer to frequently, usually as *T/L junction*.

Balance The combination of voluntary and reflexive control of the center of gravity (COG) and base of support (BOS) to maintain relative position

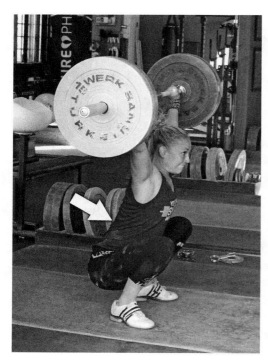

Figure 1.10 Learning to control position at the thoraco-lumbar (T/L) junction of the spine is an important step in maintaining load-supporting posture.

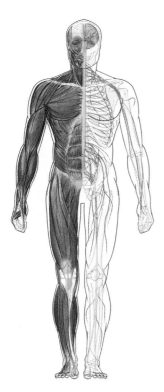

Figure 1.11 The nervous system is king. Everything that we have talked about so far and will talk about until the end of the book is ultimately controlled by this amazing network.

and postural stability against intrinsic and extrinsic (the barbell) forces.

Proprioception Self-perception (sense) of body/segment position and movement, which contributes accuracy, consistency and coordinative control of voluntary and reflexive movement.

The Nervous System

Central Nervous System (CNS) The brain and spinal cord—the mainframe governing our weightlifting movements.

Peripheral Nervous System (PNS) Made up of the *somatic* and *autonomic* systems, which work in sync to carry out the tasks of controlling our movement and dictating our readiness for training and recovering from it by transmitting signals to and from the CNS.

Somatic Nervous System (SNS) The branch of the PNS that directs the muscles that move our skeleton through the desired movement patterns. It is important to develop the appropriate combination of mobility and stability in the movements that we want, then to practice those positions and movement patterns (snatch, clean & jerk, back squat, etc.) to embed them in the CNS and make our somatic control as automatic as possible.

Autonomic Nervous System (ANS) Responsible for involuntary control of the internal body systems. Works with the SNS to determine our readiness to carry out desired movement that we have worked hard to develop, and also to recover from those movements. Consists of the *parasympathetic* and *sympathetic* systems.

Parasympathetic System Working in a harmonic balance with the *sympathetic* nervous system described below, the parasympathetic system is used to "throttle down" or "rest and digest." The parasympathetic system will slow heart rate and facilitate digestion, and is typically the primary autonomic driver in normal everyday life. Parasympathetic input is used for recovery and theorized to be involved to some extent during the learning of new skills, as it may be difficult to learn new motor patterns/skills or body positions if the individual is overly wired or trying too hard (Think of trying to replicate a skill that is not yet refined when you are nervous, tired, anxious, etc.). For low-load movement and mobility improvements, we will typically cue maintenance of a steady breathing cycle and for the athlete to stay relatively relaxed as he or she works through and attains new positions; then progressing qualities such as speed and load once the skill or movement pattern is obtained.

Sympathetic System This is the branch of the ANS that will ramp you up for strenuous, powerful movements and sustained bouts of training. We need the appropriate level of sympathetic drive and signaling to move heavy loads in the positions and movement patterns that you have *previously* dialed in. This system also must ramp down in order to recover from training.

Phases of the Snatch and Clean & Jerk

We can divide the movements of the snatch and clean & jerk into a series of phases to help with analysis and specific assessments and corrections.

Starting Position The position in which the athlete sets up prior to the barbell being lifted off of the floor. In this position, we typically see closed chain (foot in contact with ground) ankle dorsiflexion of 15-25 degrees— keep in mind this is typically with a weightlifting shoe that provides an elevated heel. We also utilize hip flexion (approximately 135 degrees) and hip rotational capacity to set the hips level with or just above the knees while maintaining a relatively neutral pelvis. A relative amount of thoracic extension is also common along with a certain degree of abduction and internal rotation of the shoulders. (Figure 1.12)

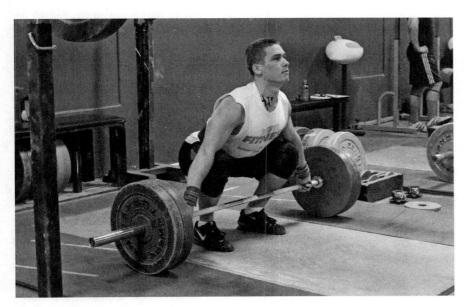

Figure 1.12 The starting position of the snatch

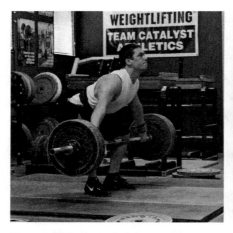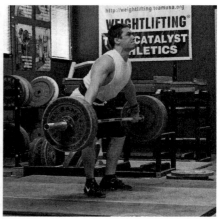

Figure 1.13 The first pull of the snatch

First Pull The movement from the point when the barbell breaks from the floor to the point where the bar passes the knee and approaches approximately mid-thigh. No rebending of the knees has occurred yet, and the knee is at approximately 140-150 degrees of extension, which demonstrates a certain amount of active control of a lengthened posterior chain. The hips and shoulders rise as one unit and the torso angle relative to the floor, along with the spinal curves, remain relatively unchanged from the starting position. The shins are roughly vertical by the end of the first pull. (Figure 1.13)

Transition (AKA *Scoop* or *double knee bend*) This is a transitional phase that begins the second pull (starting at approximately mid-thigh). The knees rebend slightly (10-15 degrees) and the hips and barbell meet in close proximity in order to realign the two bodies and provide leverage for the legs to push into the floor. The end of this phase is commonly referred to as the *power position*. During this transition, the speed of the barbell actually slows down slightly, but maintains an upward trajectory. (Figure 1.14)

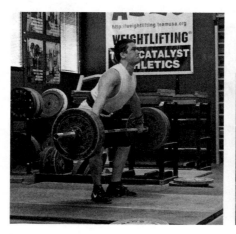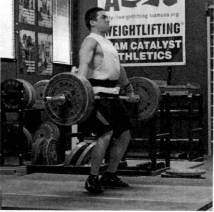

Figure 1.14 The transition of the snatch

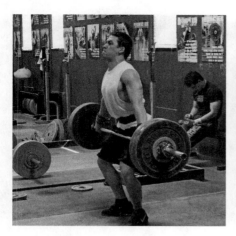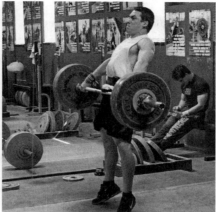

Figure 1.15 The finish of the second pull of the snatch

Second Pull (AKA *finish* or *explosion*) Starting directly after the first pull (approximately mid-thigh with the transition phase included) to full extension of the hips (approximately 180 degrees) and knees (170-180 degrees) and plantarflexion of the ankles (30-45 degrees). This is the moment before the lifter begins to pull under the bar. (Figure 1.15)

Third Pull (AKA *turnover*) Elbows bend, hips and knees rebend, and the athlete pulls under the bar to the point just prior to the elbows locking out overhead. The lifter's shoulders will transition from relative internal rotation to relative external rotation during this phase. For teaching purposes, it is common to think of the internally rotated position as a 90-90 *scarecrow*, although it is rare that a lifter actually achieves such a position in practice. However, that relative degree of shoulder internal rotation is important during the initial moments of the third pull in order to keep the barbell in close proximity to the lifter's body. Also of note is the trunk position, as the lifter may naturally exhibit a slight increase in spinal extension as he or she pulls under the bar. It is important to still maintain

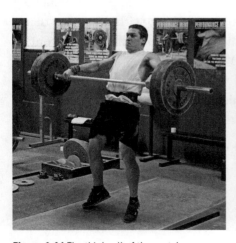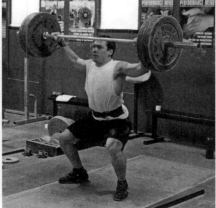

Figure 1.16 The third pull of the snatch

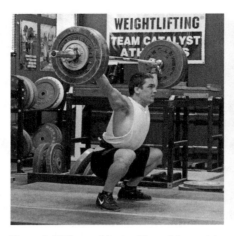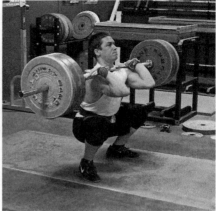

Figure 1.17 The receiving positions of the snatch and clean

a relatively parallel (stacked) relationship with the ribcage and pelvis in order to support the weight when it is received. (Figure 1.16)

Receiving Position The position of the athlete's body when the weight has been locked out overhead or received in the front rack. In the full versions of the lifts, this is an overhead squat or front squat. The wider grip (shoulder abduction) of the snatch provides some slack for most lifters in regard to overhead motion relative to the narrower grip of the jerk. Regardless, shoulder mobility is obviously a factor here. For the clean, the shoulder joint is flexed to 80-90 degrees, which is well within most athlete's comfortable ranges. Shoulder flexion is combined with external rotation and elbow flexion, however, which does add positional demand to soft tissue structures crossing the shoulder joint. Elbow flexion and wrist extension mobility are also factors for the front rack position. Elbow extension is utilized for the lockout of a snatch or jerk. For the lower body, mobility is necessary all down the kinetic chain with hip flexion (approximately 135-145 degrees) and varying amounts of rotation, knee flexion (approximately 135-145 degrees), and ankle dorsiflexion (approximately 20-30 degrees in weightlifting shoes). It should go without saying that a significant degree of stability is required throughout the body to control these ranges of motion. (Figure 1.17)

Jerk Dip The phase of the jerk in which the lifter flexes at the hips, knees and ankles with the bar in the front rack in order to store and generate energy for the drive up (Figure 1.18).

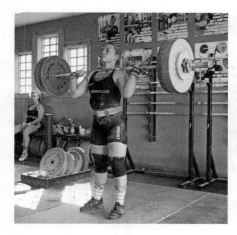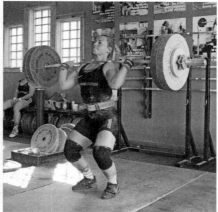

Figure 1.18 The dip phase of the jerk

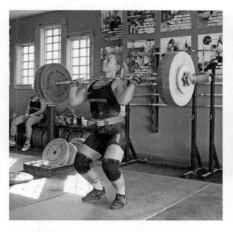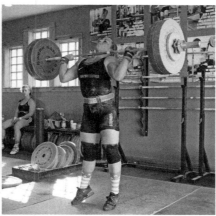

Figure 1.19 The drive phase of the jerk

Jerk Drive The phase of the jerk directly after the dip, in which the lifter extends through the legs to impart upward force on the barbell (Figure 1.19).

Jerk Receiving Position The phase of the jerk in which the lifter splits the hips after propelling the barbell off of the shoulders during the drive (Figure 1.20). This hip position allows the lifter to position him- or herself under the barbell with a stable base. Shoulder flexion mobility is demonstrated here, even more so than in the snatch due to the narrower grip width. Hip extension is demonstrated on the back leg to various degrees depending on torso angle and/or preferred split length. And, of course, trunk control to maintain the weight stacked over the ribcage and pelvis is important.

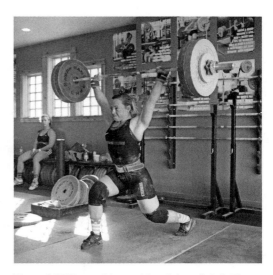

Figure 1.20 The receiving position of the split jerk. The most commonly missed lift in the sport requires an incredible combination of balance, speed, strength and timing.

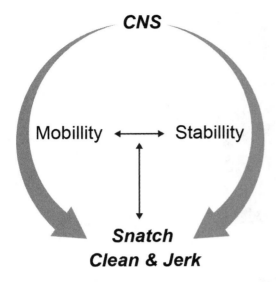

Figure 1.21 Movement is based on a mobility—stability continuum.

Discussion

There are countless descriptions of terms such as *mobility* and *stability* depending on whom you talk to, and I do not wish to make it black and white because I believe the definitions can be modified depending on context. But for the purposes of establishing a common language for this book, the preceding definitions are how we will refer to them.

With that being said, movement can be considered on a mobility-stability continuum (Figure 1.21). Everyone falls somewhere on this continuum, meaning that all athletes need individual combinations of both mobility and stability of their joint and muscular systems to move their bodies into the desired positions, and in this case, perform the weightlifting movements. Some fall further toward either end of the continuum in regard to the attributes that they possess. If a lifter is having difficulty achieving certain positions or supporting weight in certain positions during the snatch or clean & jerk, he or she may try to make an effort to move more toward the middle of the continuum.

Where one falls on this continuum is unique to the individual. For example, a 110lb female lifter who was a former gymnast and a 250lb male lifter who was a football player may fall near different ends of the continuum and may require different strategies to create the improvements in movement that they desire.

Stability and motor control are often used synonymously. When sufficient mobility is present, it should be controlled with the optimal combination of bony and ligamentous structures (passive stability) and the neuromuscular system (active stability). Although it's up for debate, stability does not necessarily mean strength—the ability to produce force—which is developed by progressive lifting of heavy barbells. Stability is more about *timing* of movement strategies. This is a skill that is developed over time with focused practice. Being able to maintain and move through the postures and positions that the weightlifting coach requires of the athlete can be thought of as stability or motor control, with the amount of weight that athlete is able to do this with being a measure of his or her strength.

Stability is an area that is often neglected by those attempting to improve their positions in the snatch and clean & jerk. It is common for lifters to spend significant amounts of time trying to improve mobility when the limiting factor may actually be stability/motor control. There are times when joints and muscles feel "tight," but mobility strategies are not effective or lasting. This chronic perception of tightness may actually be sent down from the CNS as a crude way to protect a lifter from a joint or body position where they lack stability (opinion-based assumption). (Figure 1.22)

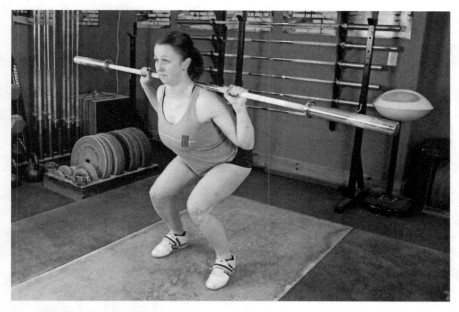

Figure 1.22 Mobility or stability issue?

We have probably all seen pictures on the internet of young children performing "perfect" squats. No, not every adult is meant to attain the same positions as those children, especially considering the fact that a young baby's immature hip structure is much different than that of an adult, and their big ol' heads act as useful counterbalances. However, there are takeaways from *how* children learn to move. They do not have squat coaches, nor do they stretch and mobilize to be able to perform those movements. They were born with the *mobility* and acquired *stability* by spending months exploring positions.

As adults, we can lose mobility due to various factors, so working to improve it may be necessary; but then time should be spent mastering prerequisite movement patterns and positions in order to develop the stability required to snatch and clean & jerk, and ultimately progress speed and load. Think of it as building yourself from the ground up, as we will detail with examples later. Jumping from the foam roller to the barbell works for some, but not all.

The concept of *neutral spine* is hotly debated. Here, we are making a distinction between the curvatures of the spine when external load (the barbell) is *not* present and when external load *is* present. The main difference is that the upper thoracic spine may be in a position of *increased relative* extension when external load *is* present. The actual excursion of motion that occurs with this increase in thoracic spine extension is small, and may be better conceptualized as resisting flexion or "anti-flexion" rather than an inordinate amount of extension range of motion. This will aid in maximizing passive and active spinal stabilizers to support the weight off the floor and overhead. As a basic guideline, we will recommend that most of

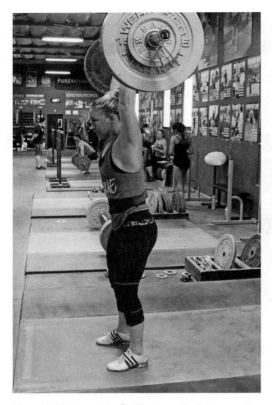

Figure 1.23 Lifter with a "tall" spine and relative upper thoracic extension while stacking the bottom of the ribcage over the top of the pelvis.

the *increased* spinal extension (AKA anti-flexion force) happen above the thoracolumbar junction in order to maintain a relatively parallel (stacked) relationship with the ribcage and pelvis. Such a torso position is conducive to supporting load and creating pressure and stability through the trunk. (Figure 1.23)

Ultimately, the goal when performing the snatch and clean & jerk is for the curvatures of the spine and orientation of your pelvis to remain *relatively* unchanged throughout the entirety of the movement—although, as we have mentioned, *neutral* is a range rather than a set position. The optimal spinal orientation will vary subtly from lifter to lifter, but we are looking to minimize *change*—where it starts is where it stays through the middle of the movement and to the end.

Our subsequent discussions of posture, breathing mechanics and core stability will be for the purpose of putting the trunk and pelvic musculature in the most advantageous position to work collectively as a unit, and the spine in the most advantageous position to support weight and transfer force to the barbell, during the snatch and clean & jerk.

CHAPTER 2

Trunk Stability & Weightlifting Posture

Motor Skill Acquisition (MSA)

Returning to the general goal of this book mentioned in Chapter 1, MSA is a *process*, not a single moment or event, and no one drill or mobility trick is going to make a permanent change in that specific moment in time—whether that's in regard to tissue structure or movement patterns. It takes repeated exposures and focused practice.

When an athlete attempts to learn a new skill, it is beneficial to find a starting point from which to acquire the new information. This starting point is the building block on which any subsequent learning, teaching, and cueing is layered. In the experience of this author, an effective starting point from which to teach a lifter the movement skills of the snatch and clean & jerk that yields a broad foundation is the mechanical and physiological basics of ribcage, pelvis and trunk positioning and stability.

Adaptability

A conducive environment for first learning *new* skills is one in which the overall stress level is decreased and effort level is submaximal. There are real world examples of this all over. In school, it's difficult for many individuals to soak up new information if they are lacking sleep or are mentally stressed. In a sport like basketball, first learning to shoot a free throw is typically done in a relatively quiet environment, with one or two cues to think about. If it's game seven of the NBA finals and the shooter is thinking about what position his elbow should be in during the shooting stroke, the outcome is not in his favor. MSA is in its early stages. In weightlifting, if you are unhappy with your overhead squat positioning and your answer is to continue snatching at 85%+ of your 1RM with little regard for focused practice with lighter weights or other corrective strategies, then you may be disappointed with your lack of progress.

This brings us back to the concept of Movement Variability (MV), in which an athlete has "options" to perform the task. With limited MV, we may have a lifter that seems stiff and robotic, as if they are fighting their own body. The system is rigid and has difficulty adapting. You'll often see this with beginner lifters who possess adequate strength to perform the lifts, but look like their head is going to pop when simply overhead squatting an empty barbell. This same lifter may also miss a lift in always the same way, always dumping it forward for example, in a slow, anti-climactic manner. Again, the system is rigid and predictable.

On the other side of the coin, an athlete with hypermobile joint tendencies may possess increased MV to a degree that makes their patterns/lifts inconsistent in nature. The system is unpredictable and "noisy." They miss forward, backward, side to side, wiggle all over the place, etc. There is no way to measure one's optimal amount of coordinative MV regarding the execution of the snatch and clean & jerk, as it will be individualized. However, we can teach trunk control with simple cues and/or positional drills that aid in finding an optimal range of MV to control the weightlifting positions. Essentially, you can ask yourself, *Am I able to consistently achieve the lifting positions that I desire (excluding injury and technical errors)*? If so, then MSA can occur. If not, we break the movement down to the most challenging variation with which the desired positions can be attained and build back up. Load, stress and fatigue can then be progressively layered on to train and reinforce those qualities for permanent adaptation and increased performance.

That is the progressive theme that will be followed in this book—some will benefit more from a bottom-up approach, in which beginning the MSA process will start in a "low-threat" environment (on the floor moving the shoulder joint and experimenting with range of motion, for example) using lower effort tension strategies to explore movement. For others, a top-down approach will be effective at creating the desired changes, as they primarily utilize barbell-specific variations for MSA, and only utilize lower-level corrective strategies for very specific needs. In both situations, the end goal is the same. This progression may span the course of weeks or months, or may simply be revisited during a warm-up or periodically throughout a training cycle, depending on the context and lifter.

Reflexive Lumbar & Pelvic Stability

The diaphragm is the primary inspiratory (breathing) muscle, performing about 70% of the work during the breathing process (we are all "diaphragmatic breathers"). It's a dome-shaped structure underneath your ribcage with the top of the dome at about the mid-thoracic level (T8-9) that separates the thorax above from the abdomen below. If your abdomen, commonly referred to as your *core*, were a soda can, the diaphragm would be the top of the can and the pelvic floor would be the bottom. Several other muscles make up the lattice that are the front, sides and back of the can. Think of this as your *can of stability*. (Figure 2.01)

When you inhale, the diaphragm contracts and descends toward your pelvis, creating a vacuum to draw air into your lungs. As it descends, it pushes down on the abdominal contents. The abdominal and pelvic floor musculature reflexively pushes back, performing an eccentric contraction to balance or oppose the pressure from the diaphragm. This reflexive contraction increases intra-abdominal pressure and contributes to lumbar spine stability—your *can of stability*.

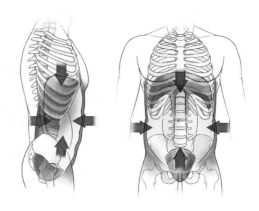

Figure 2.01 Here is your core at rest. Creating and maintaining opposing forces is a key to stabilizing this region under load.

We can see from Figure 2.01 that in resting neutral alignment, the diaphragm and pelvic floor face each other, more or less. This position gives those muscles leverage to counter one another, create pressure, and contribute to trunk stability. Under a heavy barbell, even with the slight increase in upper thoracic extension used to support load, we strive to maintain this ribcage-to-pelvis (top facing the bottom) relationship as much as possible (Figure 2.02).

Of course, successfully training and loading the weightlifting movements does not require a perfectly parallel relationship between the ribcage and pelvis, and there will be variance in an individual lifter's optimal torso position. However, it should be a torso position in which he or she can breathe into to create reflexive pressure in order to sustain it under load. We are looking to minimize "dents" in our can from sudden spinal hyperextension or flexion moments that destabilize our trunk and make it difficult to support the bar (Figure 2.03). This is why we use the parallel ribcage to pelvis as a starting point.

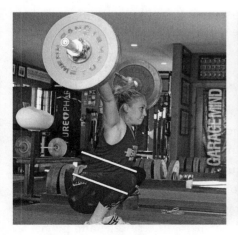 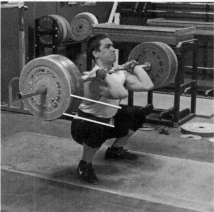

Figure 2.02 Again, these athletes exhibit tall and extended spines, but maintain a relatively neutral ribcage-to-pelvis and diaphragm-to-pelvic floor relationship (can of stability), where forces can oppose each other in balance.

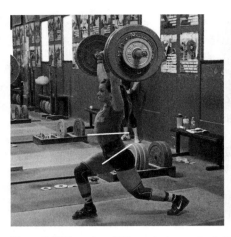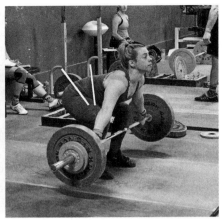

Figure 2.03 Examples of lifters who have potentially "dented" their cans of stability by extending (left) or flexing (right) at the T/L junction, losing the relationship of the diaphragm and pelvic floor. This is not necessarily a "good vs. bad" concept, but it's helpful for many lifters to learn to attain a neutral trunk position as a starting point in order to find what variation allows them the positions they desire.

The goal is to make the core's function automatic. Straining to get your air and putting deliberate mental focus on tightening your abs can be energy-costly and may inhibit fluid movement. Learning how to breathe under the bar in order to maintain posture and reflexively fire your abs can save you a lot of mental and physical energy. A lifter should not have to think about turning different muscles on or off when snatching or clean & jerking. Muscles should do this reflexively so all you have to hone is lifting technique.

Important Note Over the course of time, as motor skills become more finely tuned, a lifter's positions may deviate from neutral as he or she naturally gravitates to the positions that optimize performance. However, in the beginning stages of motor learning, it is beneficial to build competency through repetition of the more neutral trunk positions described above and throughout the rest of the book to maximize active neuromuscular control.

Demonstrating Potential Hip & Shoulder Mobility

Since the pelvis is where the hip joint resides, hip mobility and function are influenced by pelvic position. Since the ribcage is primarily where the shoulder joint is anchored, shoulder mobility and function are highly influenced by ribcage position. Consequently, pelvis and ribcage control can be considered a prerequisite to demonstrating your mobility potential in the hip and shoulder joints. If diaphragm and pelvic floor (manipulated by breathing patterns) position aids in stabilizing the ribcage and pelvis, as described above, then it also has a role in aiding the lifter to better demonstrate the hip and shoulder mobility that he or she possesses.

Thoracic Mobility

In regard to inhalation before a heavy lift, three hundred and sixty degrees of trunk expansion provides a broad, stout platform for the barbell to be supported in the front rack position, back squat position, or overhead. This makes intuitive sense, as you can imagine that widening your torso would provide more support for an external load versus being deflated and thin. More air = more control.

Anecdotally, lifters have reported to us that a robust inhalation in which they expand the ribcage 360 degrees (in particular the mid to upper *posterior* portion) affords them more perceived upper T-spine mobility—possibly by opening up the ribs and potentially the facet joints of the thoracic spine. Think of it as mobilizing your thoracic spine from the inside out. This is opposed to simply tilting the entire ribcage backwards in an effort to extend the thoracic spine, when in reality the motion is probably coming more from the T/L junction.

Scapular Stability

Many of us have heard the terms scapular *winging* or *tipping*, referring to when it appears that the shoulder blade is tilting off of the ribcage during resting posture or during arm movements (Figure 2.04). A common thought is that this indicates a lack of congruency between the shoulder blade and ribcage. A true diagnosis of scapular winging involves injury to the long thoracic nerve. If an injury like this is not present in the lifter's history (typically it is not—you would probably know), then *scapular winging* becomes a nebulous term, with limited ability to identify it, measure it, determine how much is too much, determine if it affects performance, etc.

As with anything in the realm of human movement, we cannot automatically deem scapular winging as "bad" without context, but I'll concede that if we have a choice, we'll pick a shoulder blade that's sitting flush on the ribcage, as that would demonstrate a stable anchor point for the shoulder.

The scapula is concave or curved inward on the side that rests on the ribcage. The natural kyphosis of the thoracic spine orients the ribcage so that it curves outward, creating a harmonious foundation for the concave shoulder blade to slide around the ribcage during shoulder movements (Figure 2.05).

Obviously, the shape of the shoulder blade bone does not change, but the orientation of the ribcage and thoracic spine can be altered. We can manipulate that to maximize the congruency with the shoulder blade in order to optimize

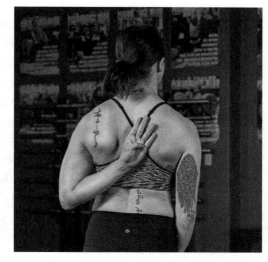

Figure 2.04 This is an example of a shoulder blade that does not seem to be sitting congruently on the ribcage, which may or may not affect shoulder mechanics and stability, but is probably not optimal.

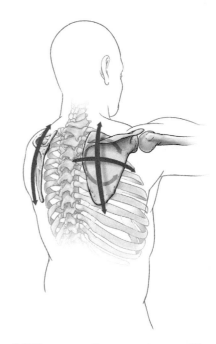

Figure 2.05 Here you see the congruent curves of the shoulder blade and ribcage creating a smooth sliding surface.

shoulder position, mechanics and stability when snatching and clean & jerking.

We'll talk much more on shoulder mechanics later.

Breathing Mechanics & Cueing

Breathing: a fundamental bodily function. Obviously, it's critical in regard to general performance, as gas exchange to our tissues is vital for their function. There's also the whole *staying alive* thing. From a safety standpoint, being able to create and release thoracic and abdominal pressure appropriately, through a well-timed breath, can help to mitigate bouts of dizziness or lightheadedness mid- or post-lift. It won't fix the instances when we put ourselves in the sleeper hold with the barbell, but anything that may increase safety while training and competing should be made a high priority.

However, not to be ignored is the role that breathing pattern cueing and positional teaching drills can play in teaching a lifter to position and stabilize the trunk. They are simple components to movement that any lifter can put some focus toward, and may help improve positioning in the snatch and clean & jerk without a ton of other "corrective" work—or at the very least, will augment or enhance whatever strategies you are using.

Initiating Inhalation through the Nose

There are numerous health benefits reported from breathing in through your nose. In regard to moving and stabilizing the trunk, however, beginning an inhalation through the nose preferentially facilitates the diaphragm and preloads the internal obliques and transverse abdominus more so than beginning an inhalation through the mouth, which preferentially facilitates accessory neck musculature. However, under heavy load, one may prefer to *finish* the inhalation through the mouth in order to maximize expansion and pressure.

Think about "pushing" the air down. This is important because the internal obliques and transverse abdominus have been shown to be the *first* called to action when stabilization and intra-abdominal pressure is needed. They are certainly not the strongest, but they seem to be the first. Recall that stability is about *timing*, and when discussing the deeper abdominal musculature, they probably do not function best in conscious isolation. Creating that downward pressure upon inhalation will drive their reflexive eccentric contraction.

360 Degrees of Trunk Expansion

Upon inhalation, there should be three-dimensional expansion of the abdominal and thoracic walls in all directions—front, back and sides. The trunk musculature opposes this expansion with an eccentric contraction facilitating stability, as we discussed earlier. Again, think about "pushing" the air down into the trunk and letting it fill like water from bottom to top.

Remember all that "draw your belly button into your spine" stuff? Gross. And wrong—at least in regard to weightlifting. Research has shown that bracing your core, as a whole, is superior for enhancing spinal stability compared to drawing the belly button in and attempting to isolate core musculature. The latter will make your can of stability skinnier and weaker. We want expansion, not shrinkage.

Exhalation through the Mouth

It may seem counterintuitive to even discuss exhalation as a means of core stability, since it's usually equated with losing core pressure. We certainly do not want to unexpectedly deflate under load, but while an inhalation increases intra-abdominal pressure, the exhalation has been shown to *increase* lumbar stiffness compared to the inhalation. This is because an exhalation contracts the abdominals and pelvic floor concentrically and pulls the lower ribs down—stacking them over the pelvis. It creates initial stiffness and *sets* position, while the 360-degree inhalation pressurizes and *reinforces* that stiffness and position.

Throughout the drills in this book, the intensity and duration of the exhalation will be manipulated to increase or decrease tension/stiffness based on the movement goal at hand. We cue an exhalation through the mouth to more effectively illicit the accompanying abdominal contraction.

Manipulating Tension

We can alter the amount of perceived tension and muscular effort utilized to attain a position or perform an exercise based on the goal, by exhaling/inhaling with more force, bracing the abdominal musculature to varying degrees of stiffness, etc.

For the stiff, robotic lifter that we described previously with decreased movement variability, it can be beneficial to cue and implement lower-tension strategies in which the athlete can relax, breathe calmly, sink into and explore ranges of motion.

For the wiggly, unpredictable lifter with increased movement variability, higher-tensioned strategies may be useful to improve positional stability. And, of course, either strategy may be appropriate depending on context. As we outline various recommendations in later chapters, we will modulate our threshold/tension strategies based on the goal at hand.

A Note on Belly Breathing

Simply pooching the belly forward when taking in a breath does not facilitate stability or mechanical advantage to the trunk. This pattern offers no abdominal resistance to the diaphragm and reduces the force of the diaphragm's contraction, because it has less leverage to push against. Remember, our lungs are in our chest, not our belly. I mention this because chest expansion has been demonized in the past, and based on the lengthy discussion that we just took part in, it should not be. Now, with the cue of *push the air down*, the belly button will undoubtedly move outward, but so will the rest of your torso circumferentially.

A Note on the Pelvic Floor

As important as it was to include a specific description of the diaphragm's function as it relates to trunk stabilization, it is equally important to discuss the role of the pelvic floor musculature. It is the base of our *can of stability*.

Pelvic floor dysfunction, more common in women, can be the result of medical issues that are far beyond the scope of this book. For lifters, the pelvic floor supports the weight of your organs plus internal and external pressures when performing the lifts. Reflexive pelvic floor control gives our abs and diaphragm a counterforce to push against when under that tremendous load. For some, a decrease in this reflexive control can result in incontinence when under load, also known as *stress incontinence*. This is more common in female lifters, especially those who have recently had children. *If you experience this, get evaluated by a qualified medical provider (preferably one from the ClinicalAthlete Network).*

A traditional set of exercises designed to strengthen the pelvic floor musculature are called Kegels. With these exercises, you are voluntarily contracting and relaxing the muscles that "hold in your pee" for a specified number of sets and reps.

The issue with this is that the function of the pelvic floor musculature is largely reflexive/subconscious by nature. We need those muscles to turn on at the right time when lifting weights, without having to think about it consciously. In other words, reflexive *timing* is more important than voluntary force. Skeletal posture is an important component in regard to the reflexive timing of the pelvic floor contraction, just as it was with the diaphragm. The two must work in sync. In fact, we can think of the pelvic floor as the diaphragm of the pelvis. Kegel exercises in isolation do not account for pelvic position, nor do they develop reflexive control of the pelvic floor musculature.

A quick demonstration of how position can affect our respiratory diaphragm and our pelvic diaphragm can be performed in quadruped. While on hands and knees, anteriorly tilt the pelvis, arch the lower back and flare

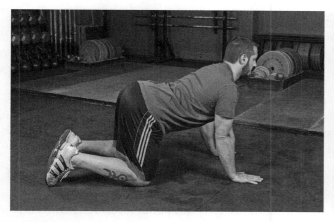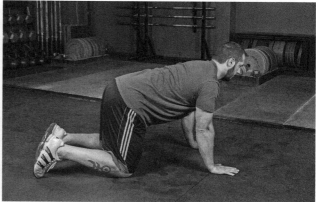

Figure 2.06 Compare the ease with which you can activate the two diaphragms of your core in both positions. The second picture depicts a position in which the respiratory and pelvic diaphragms face each other (parallel relationship).

the bottom ribs forward. Keeping the neck relaxed, take a deep breath in through your nose and push the air down as low as it can go, as if you were pushing against a weightlifting belt. Then exhale through your mouth fully as if you were blowing up a balloon.

Now posteriorly tilt your pelvis to attain a flatter spine (maybe even slightly rounded). Again, take a deep breath in through your nose, trying to push the air down deep into your lower lungs and back, and then exhale fully. Compare the ease with which you were able to breathe in and out in both positions and create circumferential pressure. Now compare the same two positions, but perform a Kegel contraction where you "hold in your pee" or "close your holes" for three seconds in each. Compare the ease with which you can do this in both pelvic positions. Lastly, perform both a deep breath in and out through your nose and mouth, and a Kegel simultaneously. Compare how it feels in both pelvic positions. Try this in seated or standing as well. (Figure 2.06)

For many of you, it was probably easier to take more air into your lower abdomen without straining with a pelvis that was slightly posteriorly tilted and a low/mid back that was flatter. The same was probably true for the Kegel. This position puts the top and bottom of your "can" in parallel, so that their forces can easily oppose one another. It's a very advantageous position for unloaded, reflexive core function.

This is simply a demonstration that position matters in regard to muscle function. Obviously we will not be lifting heavy weights with a posteriorly tilted pelvis and completely flat or slightly rounded spine, but we can use these types of demonstrations as teaching tools to find the proper balance of position and core function that will provide natural carryover to the lifts.

I will not be prescribing specific pelvic floor strengthening exercises in this book, because all of the drills will aid in reflexive pelvic floor strengthening when we keep core stabilization patterns in mind. Having said that, if you have position already dialed in and you want to throw in some "hold in your pee" reps for added strengthening, then that has merit because you have taken care of the prerequisites first.

Fundamental Drills

The following exercises will begin the process of developing reflexive control of the respiratory, trunk and pelvic floor musculature. The positions of these drills are designed to put your "can of stability" in a mechanically advantageous position in order to maximize the benefits of a full inhalation and exhalation. They are *teaching tools*. It is understood that the body positions necessary for weightlifting may put the trunk and "can of stability" in positions different than this. However, by practicing these drills, we can begin to reap the benefits described in this chapter with the goal of having a natural carryover to our weightlifting movements.

Supine Squatting

This position affords us the most external support from the ground to allow the athlete to relax and feel the subtle positions and cues. Having the feet up on a wall aids in maintaining a nice relationship between the pelvis and ribcage. Having the knees and hips bent mimics a squatting pattern.

Starting Position

- Place your feet flat on a wall. The foot angle can mimic your normal squatting stance, but try to maintain three points of contact on each foot: big toe, little toe and heel.
- Bend the hips and knees to 90 degrees.
- Place the hands on the ground or on the lower ribs.
- Keep the shoulders and neck relaxed.

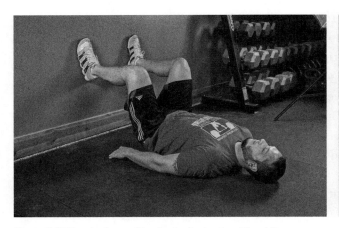 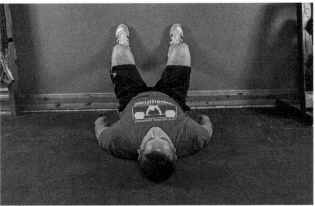

Figure 2.07 The starting position for the Supine Squatting drill

- Keep the chin tucked slightly so that the back of the neck is long. Have something under your head if needed to keep from straining your neck backward. (Figure 2.07)

Execution

- Inhale through the nose, and then perform a *FULL EXHALATION* through your mouth to pull the bottom ribs down so that they are flush with your abdomen.
- Upon exhalation, lightly dig your heels down into the wall, pulling your tailbone off the floor slightly (Figure 2.08). This will recruit the hamstrings and position your pelvis such that your pelvic floor and diaphragm face each other (mechanically advantageous for the diaphragm and pelvic floor).
- When you think you have exhaled fully, exhale more, even if you think you have run out of air. Then pause for 2 seconds before your next inhalation.
- Maintaining your pelvic position, slowly inhale through your nose, expanding your abdomen and low back, then chest and upper back. Let the air "fall in like water"—think about it filling your torso like a bucket of water from bottom to top.
- Exhale *fully* through your mouth like you are blowing up a balloon and *pause for 2 seconds* before your next inhalation. This is a teaching technique for the abdominals.
- Perform 2-4 sets of 5 breath cycles (1 cycle = 1 inhalation + 1 exhalation).

Important Points

- When we refer to *fully* exhaling, it is during *unloaded* mobility and movement drills. By no means am I suggesting any lifter

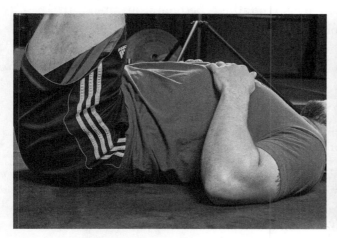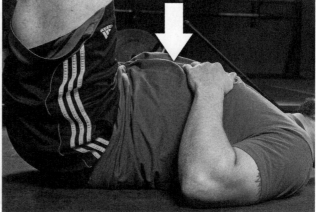

Figure 2.08 Tailbone slightly raised by pulling down the wall with the hamstrings to bring the bottom (pelvic floor) of the "can of stability" in line with the top (diaphragm) in the Supine Squatting drill. Remember, this is simply our initial starting/teaching position.

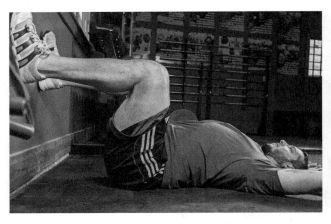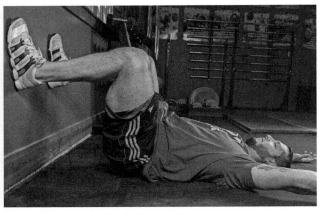

Figure 2.09 The lower ribs should be gently pulled down and disappear after a full exhalation. This is "setting neutral."

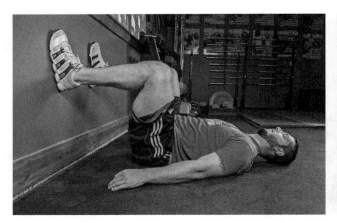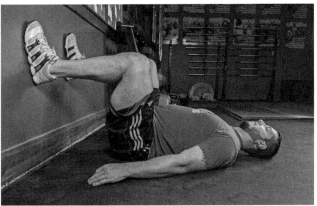

Figure 2.10 On the left, you see the ribcage after a full exhalation. On the right, you see the ribcage expanded after a full inhalation. Notice that the low back position stays constant, so we are assured true ribcage expansion.

completely deflate themselves when they are about to lift the bar or under heavy load. Breathing techniques when lifting are described in later chapters. Here we are exaggerating a full exhalation to help the athlete become acquainted with his/her abdominals. It's a teaching tool that will allow for a full, robust inhalation—getting all of the air out will make it easier to get it in.

> You may experience an "ab shake" at the end of the complete exhalation. This is a good thing.
> You should feel the lower ribs "disappear" or flatten into the abdomen and the abs turn on (Figure 2.09).
> When exhaling, try not to strain like you are lifting 200 kilos—let it occur smoothly—relatively low effort/tension.

- Inhale slowly through your nose and let the air keep flowing in like water filling the trunk from bottom to top (Figure 2.10).

- ❯ Release ab tension enough to allow for maximal inhalation.
- ❯ The abdomen and low back should expand first, followed by the chest and upper back.
- ❯ Maintain the pelvic lift throughout and keep your low back from arching away from the ground when you breathe in. Remember, your lungs are in your chest, not your low back. You shouldn't have to arch your lower back in order to get a full, expansive breath of air.
- ❯ The neck should remain relatively relaxed and the head position does not change. Think "long neck."

Variations

Heel Dig into Bench Putting a bench under the heels may give the athlete more leverage to recruit the hamstrings and pull the hips underneath (Figure 2.11). This can also be beneficial for the athlete in terms of stabilizing and maintaining the drill position while he or she practices full breath cycles. Feeling a little hamstring muscle burn is normal here, and this extra bit of posterior chain neural drive is typically reported by the athlete as a beneficial way to warm up that area. Maintain the active "heel dig" throughout the set.

Depth We can change the depth of the supine squat for more carryover into a standing squat by scooting closer to the wall (Figure 2.12). It's recommended that you literally inch your way down after each set so that your hips have time to adjust to a deeper position. With each full exhalation, you may feel the tension in the hip joints subside. Use the breath to dictate what depth you are comfortable performing this drill in, as opposed to jamming into ranges that you do not have access to just yet. As a rule of thumb, if the current depth is not completely comfortable after five full breath cycles, scoot away from the wall a tad to give yourself a little bit more slack.

In this deeper supine squat position, you should really be able to feel your lower abdomen expand into your thighs during the inhalation, when you "push the air down." This can also be combined with the bench under the heels and hamstring recruitment.

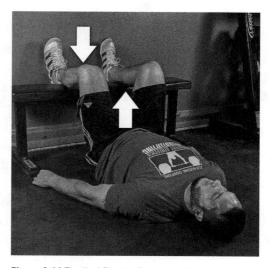

Figure 2.11 The Heel Dig into Bench variation of the Supine Squatting drill. Lightly dig the heels down into the bench, engaging the hamstrings and stabilizing the position.

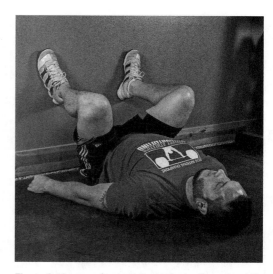

Figure 2.12 Increasing depth in the Supine Squatting drill. Practicing the breathing and bracing technique in a deeper supine squat position can help athletes develop comfort in their bottom positions.

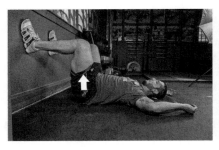 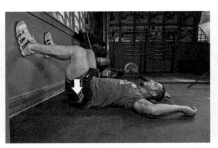 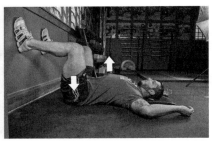

Figure 2.13 Pelvic tilt variation of the Supine Squatting drill. Exhaling through the mouth as you lower the pelvis to the ground will ensure that the ribs stay flush with the abdomen and spinal extension is distributed at multiple segments (what we want). The second picture demonstrates this, while the third picture demonstrates an athlete who has disengaged the anterior abdominal musculature and allowed the ribs to flare.

Pelvic Tilt As mentioned previously, the posterior pelvic tilt and small amount of subsequent lumbar flexion that has been cued in the previous drills is simply a starting point for an athlete to learn control of his or her "can of stability." To support external loads during the weightlifting movements, we understand that anterior pelvic tilt and lumbar lordosis will be beneficial for spinal stability.

During the Supine Squatting drill, the athlete can practice allowing the pelvis to drop back down to the ground into a relative amount of anterior pelvic tilt (Figure 2.13). Begin the drill the same exact way as outlined above. During the second full exhalation, allow the pelvis to lower back down to the ground slowly. Exhale as you are lowering the pelvis so that the ribs stay flush with the abdomen. This will allow for the necessary spinal extension to occur without simply hinging at the T/L junction. After lowering back down to the ground, complete the full breath cycles as outlined. This can be combined with increasing depth and/or a bench under the heels for hamstring recruitment.

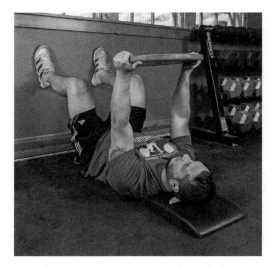

Figure 2.14 Increasing abdominal tension in the Supine Squatting drill with a plate press to aid in increasing core pressure.

Tension Utilizing increased abdominal tension during any of the abovementioned positional variations can also be beneficial to teach a lifter to create and maintain pressure while breathing. If the brain has to choose between breathing and maintaining core tension, it will most likely pick breathing— it's a useful skill to be able to do both.

Simply experiment with increasing forcefulness of the exhalation, which should yield increasing abdominal tension, and then try to inhale and expand the torso while maintaining that tension. Breathe into the tension.

You can utilize a plate press to provide even more leverage for the abdominals and diaphragm to create pressure (Figure 2.14). Exhale forcefully and slightly reach a plate up to the ceiling. Maintain that position and tension while inhaling, and repeat.

Quadruped Squatting

With this drill, we can now focus on driving air into our upper back for posterior ribcage expansion. The benefits of this were explained previously in this chapter with regard to thoracic mobility, and again, we utilize a position that mimics a squat for carryover to the weightlifting movements. During an inhalation in this quadruped squatting position, your abdomen presses against your thighs and drives pressure up. During the exhalation, your pelvic floor musculature will contract and lift, which may allow you to sink into a deeper squat position.

Starting Position

- Rest on the hands and knees, positioning the knees and feet in a way that will yield a comfortable amount of hip flexion. For many, this will mean the knees are slightly wider than the feet.
- The tops of the feet can be flat on the floor (although make note that we will be revisiting this position later in the book for screening and correcting purposes, with instructions to dorsiflex the ankle and pull the toes underneath the feet).
- Spread your fingers, creating as much ground contact as possible.
- Keep your head and neck relaxed in mid-range. (Figure 2.15)

Execution

- Inhale through your nose with a relaxed neck while maintaining position.
- Exhale *fully* through your mouth, pushing lightly through your elbows and forearms, protracting your shoulder blades and rounding your upper back slightly.
- Rock the hips back past 90 degrees.
- Maintain this new position as you inhale again, filling the upper back with air. "Push the air down" and fill from bottom to top.
- Exhale and repeat, maintaining the scapular "reach."
- As you rock back to a deeper and deeper squat, you can reposition the hands to be underneath the shoulders.
- Perform 2-4 sets of 5 breath cycles. (Figure 2.16)

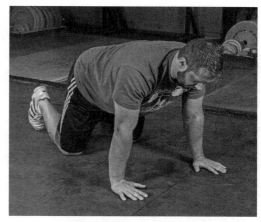

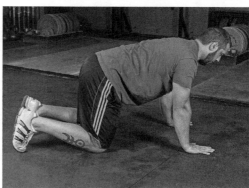

Figure 2.15 The starting position for the Quadruped Squatting drill

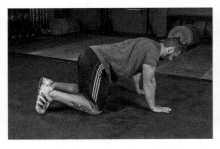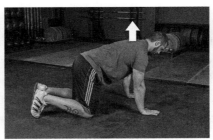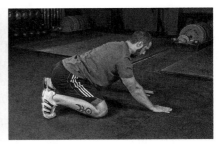

Figure 2.16 Quadruped Squatting drill. In the first picture, an athlete is in a relaxed quadruped squat starting position. In the second picture is the athlete reaching through the shoulder blades (protraction) and lightly pressing into the ground during the exhalation. Notice how the shoulder blades spread apart (protracting, not shrugging), and the upper back is raised to the ceiling slightly. Maintain this position throughout the set. In the third picture, the athlete is rocked back into the "squat" position.

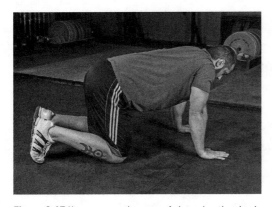

Figure 2.17 Here you see the error of shrugging the shoulders toward the ears. Keep your shoulders out of your ears and push straight down to stabilize the scapula.

Important Points

- Be sure not to shrug your shoulders up toward your ears (Figure 2.17).
- For some, breathing in this position may be difficult, as it forces the athlete to expand his or her ribs. If this is you, the tendency may be to come out of the quadruped squat position (rock forward) as you breath in. Don't let this happen. Stay rocked back and let the air flow in as it may, without straining—low tension.

Movement Tip "Reaching" with the shoulder complex (specifically referring to the glenohumeral joint and scapulothoracic joint) will be a common cue used in many of the drills throughout the book. This action restores congruency between the shoulder complex and ribcage by preferentially facilitating muscles that assist with scapular protraction and upward rotation. These scapular motions are utilized for the front rack and overhead positions, and aid in clearing space for the shoulder complex to move freely against depressive forces that muscles like the lats can produce. You can also think of this action as "moving the ribcage backward" toward the shoulder blades. Either way, the result is a nice flush relationship between the shoulder blade and ribcage that we will use as a starting point for shoulder movement and thoracic spine extension.

Variations

On Forearms To better mimic the torso angle of a squat, drop your chest so that your forearms rest on the ground with your elbows underneath the shoulders or slightly flared out. Spread the fingers to create maximal ground contact and sensory feedback to the brain. You may need to reposition the hips to accommodate the increased hip flexion range of motion.

Similar to the Supine Squatting drill, allow your hips to accept the positions by utilizing full breath cycles.

Remember to maintain the squatting position when you inhale, and work to attain 360-degree trunk expansion—especially your side chest walls and upper back. Push the air down and out. This is a great remedial position for the front rack. (Figure 2.18)

Overhead Piggybacking off of the previous variation, the lifter can begin to incorporate shoulder flexion while maintaining ribcage position and using 360-degree expansion to oppose muscles such as the lats that tend to inhibit full overhead mobility.

After every 2-3 breath cycles, begin to inch your hands farther and farther forward. Pause after each incremental change and reinforce it with a couple of breaths. This is not meant to be a stretch in the traditional sense of forcing length, but rather, just as we have done previously, use full breath cycles to sink into new range. You may still feel some mild stretching sensation in the lats and between the shoulder blades, but many of you will be amazed at how much range of motion you can gain without having to force things. If you feel pinching (see the impingement discussion in Chapter 7) on the tops of your shoulders, bring the forearms back to the previous position. (Figure 2.19)

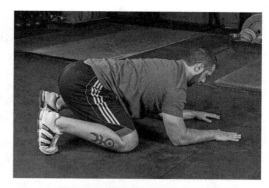

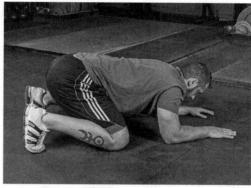

Figure 2.18 On Forearms variation of the Quadruped Squatting drill. In the first picture, the lifter performs a scapular reach that restores the normal kyphotic curve of the upper back and scapular congruency. In second picture, the athlete demonstrates a passive scapular position that will not yield posterior upper back expansion.

Tension As was true in the Supine Squatting drill, utilizing increasingly forceful exhalations can strengthen your stabilization pattern in this position. As you exhale with slightly more force, push into the ground with your forearms with slightly more force, and push your knees and feet into the ground with slightly more force. This will basically elicit a total body contraction while you are reinforcing it with full breath cycles. You may

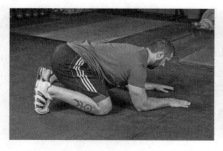 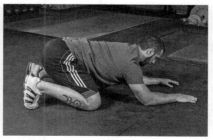 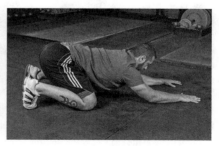

Figure 2.19 Overhead variation of the Quadruped Squatting drill. After every 2-3 breath cycles, you can begin incrementally positioning your shoulders into more flexion. All other positions and cues described previously should remain constant. If you're able to inch your arms up high enough, your upper thoracic spine will begin to extend naturally, which is beneficial for the front squat/rack positions. Maintain that light scapular reach.

find that when you relax your muscles, you are able to sink into a deeper squat position, which is likely a response from your nervous system allowing you to access more range.

Supine Overhead Wall Press

We now incorporate concepts from the Supine and Quadruped Squat drills into a drill that requires a bit more active control through the core than the previous. This one can be manipulated to mimic an overhead squat, front rack or jerk, all while teaching the athlete to create trunk stability in those positions. Think of this as an anti-hyperextension activity, as you are resisting forces that would create hinging at the T/L junction just as you would when holding weight overhead.

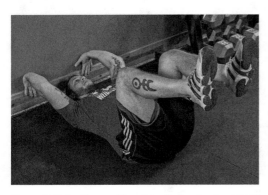

Figure 2.20 Starting position of the Supine Overhead Wall Press. This drill will act as our supine version of an overhead squat. The overhead position will further challenge the trunk musculature to maintain position.

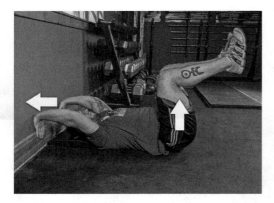

Figure 2.21 Pressing into the wall in the Supine Overhead Wall Press provides leverage for the athlete to create reflexive tension in the trunk musculature. The slight tailbone lift stacks the pelvis and ribcage, creating a nice environment for 360 degrees of expansion. Be sure that the pelvis lifts straight up as opposed to simply rolling backwards.

Starting Position

- Lie supine with head support about 6 inches away from a wall.
- Place the arms overhead with the hands flat on the wall (or fists against the wall if there is some type of wrist issue preventing the flat hand).
- Bend the hips and knees past 90 degrees with the knees slightly wider than the feet. (Figure 2.20)

Execution

- Begin with an inhalation through the nose.
- Exhale through the mouth while simultaneously pressing into the wall with the arms. During this exhalation and wall press, the tailbone should lift straight up off of the floor slightly.
- Maintain this pelvic position and inhale through the nose again. Exhale and press into the wall. As with previous drills, be sure to exhale fully and pull the lower ribs flush with the abdomen. This should yield a bit of that "ab shake" that we like so much.
- Perform 3-4 sets of 5 full breath cycles, maintaining the pelvis-ribcage relationship. (Figure 2.21)

Variations

Increased Shoulder Flexion By scooting further away from the wall, the demand for core stability is increased to maintain the pelvic-ribcage relationship and to resist a hyperextension moment through the lumbar spine. The increased shoulder flexion also provides beneficial opposition to all soft tissue structures that oppose overhead mobility. Increase the intensity/force of the exhalation and wall press to increase your leverage and keep your rib position set. (Figure 2.22)

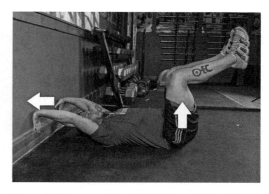

Figure 2.22 Increased Shoulder Flexion variation of the Supine Overhead Wall Press drill. After each set of 5 breaths, move a few inches farther away from the wall.

Pelvic Tilt As we did with the Supine Squatting drill, we can use this slightly more advanced exercise to teach a lifter how to control pelvic tilt using the abdominals. Begin this version the same way as before, by lifting the tailbone slightly during the first exhalation. Then, during the next exhalation, allow the tailbone to slowly lower down toward the ground, but keep the lower ribs pulled down flush with the abdomen. This will allow for segmental spinal extension to occur without simply hinging at the T/L junction. After lowering the pelvis to the ground, complete the full breath cycles as outlined above. (Figure 2.23)

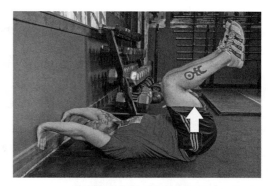

Standing Overhead Wall Press

Up to this point, we have been relying on the ground to provide support. This is great as an initial teaching tool for learning new movement patterns and positions, but obviously things need to be integrated into a standing position to create carryover to the weightlifting movements.

In the following drill, we use a wall to cue our position and focus on incorporating the trunk and bracing control that we've practiced into a standing, overhead position.

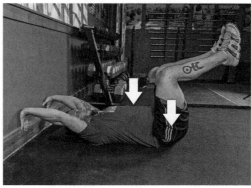

Figure 2.23 Pelvic Tilt variation of the Supine Overhead Wall Press drill. Exhaling through the mouth as you lower the pelvis to the ground will ensure that the ribs stay flush with the abdomen, and spinal extension is distributed at multiple segments (what we want).

Start Position

- Stand about 8 inches away from the wall with the knees slightly bent and forearms against the wall.
- Inhale through the nose to begin the drill. Exhale through the mouth while simultaneously performing a slight posterior pelvic tilt to pull the pelvis underneath the ribcage. The lumbar spine should still be slightly lordotic.
- Protract the shoulder blades (spread them apart) by pushing the forearms into the wall. This will move the ribcage

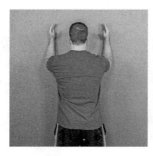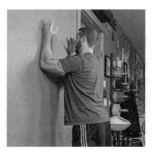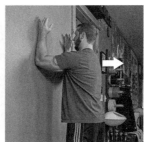

Figure 2.24 Starting position for the Standing Overhead Wall Press drill

backward relative to the shoulder blades, just like we did with the quadruped squatting drill—it's the scapular reach.

- Your shoulders should be stacked directly over your hips, or even slightly in front of the hips. If the shoulders are behind the hips, simply scoot the feet back a bit. (Figure 2.24)

Execution

- Maintaining the pelvis-ribcage relationship, slowly slide the forearms up the wall as you perform a full exhalation, moving 3-4 inches at a time. At the end of the exhalation, pause in whatever overhead position you are in and inhale through the nose to create 360 degrees of trunk expansion, attempting to drive air into your upper back between your shoulder blades.
- Exhale again and attempt to slide up the wall farther. Do not sacrifice trunk position to attain more shoulder flexion—allow the range to come naturally.
- Perform 3-4 sets of 5 breaths. (Figure 2.25)

If you are monitoring the athlete performing this drill, notice how the scapulae will become fixated to the ribcage as soon as the athlete actively

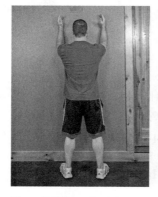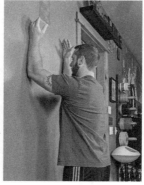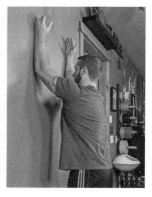

Figure 2.25 By maintaining a constant trunk position in the Standing Overhead Wall Press drill, the athlete learns how to dissociate shoulder movement from spinal movement and attain overhead mobility with a stable trunk.

presses the forearms into the wall and pushes the ribcage back slightly. Going back to our discussion on scapular winging, this exercise shows you how a simple low-load strategy can alter a pseudo-diagnosis that gets so much attention (many times not warranted). You'll see a similar response in our loading strategies later in the book, in which shoulder blade position and mechanics all just take care of themselves naturally in a response to external load.

This drill is also an option to include when prepping the front rack position of a clean, front squat or jerk. It will teach the athlete how to drive air into the upper back and expand the torso under the barbell.

Belt Breathing

The following concept can be used as a very effective and quick teaching tool for athletes to learn what it feels like to create circumferential expansion of their trunks.

Execution

- Stand comfortably with the feet about hip width apart and a weightlifting belt *lightly* strapped around the lower torso.
- With your hands on the lower ribs, exhale *fully* through the mouth, making the lower ribs disappear, *without* rounding the shoulders or slouching the spine. Stay tall through the spine.
- *Lightly* tighten the belt around the lower torso after the exhalation.
- Inhale *fully* through the nose, "filling the belt" 360 degrees without extending or flexing the spine.
- Repeat for sets of 3-5 breath cycles. (Figure 2.26)

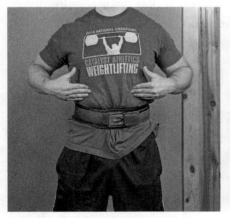 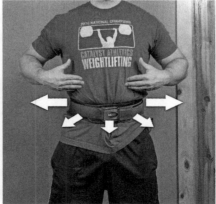

Figure 2.26 Belt Breathing drill to practice expanding the trunk 360 degrees with inhalation.

Cues

- When exhaling, the athlete should feel the lower front ribs go down.
- After tightening the belt, the athlete should feel him- or herself *pushing* the air down into the belt. Think of the belly button moving forward and down as you inhale.
- The athlete should feel tension around the belt 360 degrees during and after a full inhalation.
- The athlete, coach or lifting partner can test this expansion by trying to fit their fingers between the belt and various places around the athlete's torso during or after the inhalation.

Variations This drill can be performed with any of the fundamental drills we outlined previously, and in any position relevant to the snatch and clean & jerk—pulling position, squat, split jerk stance, etc. The main objectives are using an exhalation (doesn't have to be full) to set the ribcage position, and feeling anterior, lateral and posterior tension around the belt when inhaling. This is the type of expansion that should be happening with or without a belt, but the belt provides a nice cue.

A Note On The Utilization of A Weightlifting Belt

For the majority of lifters, it is my opinion that *if* a weightlifting belt is being used, it should be used as an overload/performance tool, *not* as a crutch or protective mechanism. There is little supportive evidence that a belt prevents or reduces injury, and if a lifter feels the psychological or physical need to wear a belt to protect them from injury or just to be able to train, than perhaps there is an issue that needs to be evaluated by a healthcare professional (preferably from the ClinicalAthlete Network). Of course, there are exceptions to this—one being that the lifter's livelihood depends on his or her weightlifting performance, and he or she feels that the belt allows them to train and/or compete. This scenario does not apply to most of us.

We'd rather beginner lifters first learn to "create their own belt" using their very own abdominal musculature, and then later experiment with a lifting belt for overload and performance enhancement as they or the coach see fit. Remember, using a weightlifting belt does not automatically equal more weight lifted, although there is certainly evidence that it can improve lifting performance—many lifters feel benefit, some don't. Experimentation and discretion is required to figure this out.

If you have a medical issue pertaining to blood pressure or sensitivities to the Valsalva maneuver, consult your physician before using a weightlifting belt.

Summary

You either just had the best geek-out session of your life reading all about trunk stability and weightlifting posture, or you stuck a pen in your eye. However, now the foundation is set and we will be on the same page in regard to position and stabilization patterns for the remainder of our journey. What was outlined in this chapter are incredibly simple but powerful tools that can augment whatever movement or training strategies you are already implementing.

PART II

Screening & Assessment

This section of the book will discuss screening and assessment of various movement qualities related to the snatch and clean & jerk. The three protocols will be:

1. Pull & Split
2. Transition/Overhead
3. Squat

Objectives

- To understand the utility and limitations of movement screening.
- To identify painful movement that may require referral to the appropriate professional.
- To implement basic screening and assessment protocols with understanding of how findings may guide movement and corrective strategies.

What Is A Screen?

A screen gauges risk. It does *not* diagnose or predict outcomes. From a medical standpoint, for example, if an individual's blood pressure is elevated, it does not mean you can diagnose the patient with arterial disease or predict the occurrence. However, he or she may in fact be *at risk* for cardiovascular dysfunction based on the blood pressure screen.

In regard to weightlifting, the ability or inability to overhead squat to a depth comfortably below parallel, or the ability or inability to lock the arms out fully overhead does *not* predict what that athlete's performance will be on the competition platform, nor does it predict injury or longevity—it simply gives you a picture of relative risk.

For example, if an athlete can squat comfortably below parallel without pain or apprehension and with positioning that meets coaching and athlete standards, then the screen did the job of showing that the joint systems can achieve the positions that we plan to progressively overload. If the athlete was not able to achieve the desired depth and/or positioning was not to the desired standard, you do not have enough information to deem *tight hips*, *tight ankles*, *weak core*, etc. as the cause. All that you know is the movement standard was not achieved, which may or may not respond favorably to speed or load.

The screen did the job of identifying a potential route of investigation. Compared to many other sports, the positions and patterns of weightlifting are relatively predictable. In general, you already have an idea of a movement standard. A simple question that you can ask yourself as you implement a movement screen is *Can the joints get into the positions that you plan to load without pain or apprehension?*

If the answer is *yes*, then we layer on speed and load to reinforce and strengthen those positions for MSA, as any well-planned, progressive program would. If the answer is *no*, perhaps we assess a bit deeper to find a possible *why* or an alternate path.

If there is pain present that is beyond the realm of common soreness associated with training, it's recommended to consider a health care professional's advice (preferably one from the ClinicalAthlete Network).

Limitations of Movement Screening

- They are poor *predictors* of performance or injury (discussed above).
- Unloaded or lightly loaded movements may not always detect painful situations, which sometimes do not rear their heads until there is more weight on the bar. This is why your day-to-day training is as much a screen and assessment as the protocols that will be laid out here.
- Some athletes' movement capacity actually gets *better* with a little bit of load—meaning a lifter's overhead squat with a weightless dowel rod may not meet your standard; but if you throw a little weight on the bar (30-60% of 1RM for example), all of a sudden movement competency improves. We don't know exactly why this is. Perhaps the added load sends some proprioceptive input from the joint systems to the nervous system for improved positional awareness. Perhaps the added muscular recruitment needed to support the load creates an optimal level of stability. Based on clinical experience, this scenario makes up the minority, which is why we still include unloaded movement testing, but it reiterates the

previous point that day-to-day training is probably your most useful screen.

- There's no *standard* for "good" or "bad" movement. Stated a different way, there may be no such thing as "good" or "bad" movement. This is why you can have 5 difference coaches or clinicians look at a movement and get 5 different opinions as to whether it's good, bad, optimal, injurious, etc. (this is a research concept called *reliability)*. A more accurate description could be that there are body positions that our tissues/systems are less adapted to, and there are body positions that likely allow for better leverage to lift weights from a biomechanical standpoint. The latter is mostly what we are looking for in an unloaded movement screen. Remember, *Can the joints get into the positions that we plan to load?*

- Evidence has shown that athletes can improve their "score" during standardized movement screening if they are coached through the tests. What are we really screening then? Are we truly testing movement capacity, or are we simply testing the athlete's ability to follow directions? (*Is the test testing what it is supposed to test?* is a research concept known as *validity)*. It is for this reason that the protocols to follow will not have a standardized score and should not be considered a "system." They are simple movements or positions that require little cueing in order to provide the coach or athlete with a general sense of what they are working with, and to rule out any obvious issues before loading those positions.

What is an Assessment?

An assessment is commonly used to identify specific impairments related to the findings of a screen. Returning to the blood pressure example: after a blood pressure screen reveals elevated numbers, an assessment may include a battery of tests to identify specific conditions related to the cardiovascular system.

For the weightlifter, following an overhead squat screen, for example, in which the lifter or coach desires a different movement strategy than the lifter was able to demonstrate, we can break the pattern down to regressed positions and/or look at the function of specific joint systems to identify a potential source of limitation or to identify and suggest alternative paths.

How We Will Blend the Two

Since we are generally only concerned with *non-painful* movement function, the protocols to follow are outlined in a way that does not require the assessor to have manual skills or be a healthcare professional. We are also attempting to limit the subjectivity or the need to interpret the findings of the tests. Many times, a screen or assessment will lead to more questions than answers due to confusion about what is observed. The goal is to prevent that from occurring here. We want to spend only the necessary amount of time determining whether the athlete's joints can get into the positions specific to the sport of weightlifting: *Can the joints get into the positions or not?* The screens and assessments can be lead by a coach or used by the athlete as self-administered tests. We will screen basic, general movement patterns first, then, if necessary, assess to further differentiate between mobility and stability needs.

A couple of points to think about as you go:

1. Not everything is a problem. *Don't chase ghosts,* as they say. If a joint doesn't go in a certain place, perhaps it's just a matter of anatomy and simple alternatives can be used with respect to that. These protocols are more about learning a bit about your body's individualities—how it works, how it moves, etc.—than they are about finding things that are dysfunctional or "wrong" with you. Just because you are performing a screen does not mean there *has* to be an issue.

2. Perhaps you find a thing or two that you thought *was* a problem or the cause of your perceived limitation, but turns out it's not actually a big deal and a simple tweak or cue can correct it. Happens a lot. In fact, a big goal with our screens/ assessments is not necessarily telling you exactly what to correct or how to correct it, but rather what not to waste your time on.

Mobility-Stability Continuum

Let's revisit this concept before diving into the tests. I used an example of a 250lb football player and a 110lb gymnast earlier in the book. These two athletes may come to you with identical looking overhead squats (unable to squat below parallel, unable to keep the bar overhead, etc.), but could fall on vastly different points within the mobility-stability continuum, meaning the corrective strategies used to address these perceived limitations may be much different for the two athletes despite the issues appearing similar.

If the movement is not broken down further, it is difficult to differentiate between mobility and stability needs and recommend the appropriate corrections or barbell variations. In the medical field, prescribing the same medicine for two different diseases just because they have the same symptoms would be a risky course of action and probably considered malpractice. It's a similar concept for athletic movement. At that point, you are simply throwing shit against the wall and seeing what sticks. This is also commonly where it takes an athlete 45 minutes to warm up before getting on the barbell because he or she is trying to stretch and mobilize every possible thing that could be holding back his or her movement. Ain't no one got time for that.

You may find that an athlete who appeared inflexible or immobile when overhead squatting has more than enough joint motion when the movement is broken down. For someone who is already *hyper*mobile, stretching muscles and mobilizing joints may be ineffective at best, and in some cases, may exacerbate his or her issues.

The goal is to *expedite* the process of optimizing the movement and/or position with the *appropriate* corrective strategies based on your findings. Stability problems can masquerade as mobility problems and vice versa. Use what is found in the screening and assessment to guide your preparation and barbell skill practice to keep it concise and effective based on your individual needs. Minimize the guesswork: *Screen and Assess—Don't Guess*.

■ CHAPTER 3

Screening & Assessment: The Pull & Split

This section will discuss testing for the pulling phase of the lift, from the floor to the top of the second pull (the finish) of the snatch and clean, as well as the split position of the hips for the most common jerk variation (the split jerk). The tests for these two movement patterns are combined because of the similar requirements of flexion and extension of the hips. Remember, we are simply interested in whether or not the athlete's joints can get into the positions that they will be training. Reinforcing those positions will be a matter of coaching and correcting later.

The screen will consist of these basic tests:

- Forward Bending
- Backward Bending
- Active Straight Leg Raise
- Hip Hinging (alternative test)
- Thomas Test

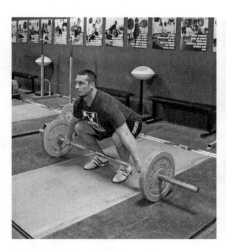 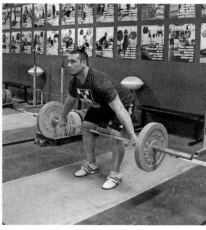 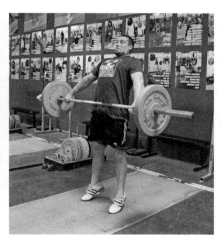

Figure 3.01 The pull of the snatch

If you are a coach screening a lifter, make sure the lifter lets you know if something hurts. You do not have to ask them at the end of every movement, as long as it is understood that he or she should tell you any time pain is present. If painful movement is identified, use discretion and refer out to a medical professional appropriately.

If necessary, the assessment will consist of these additional tests:

- Quadruped Lumbar ROM
- Active Straight Leg Raise Correction Differentiation Positional Hack

These tests will give us a sense of the lifter's capacity to move through the hips in the sagittal plane and gauge tolerance to movement through the spine in the sagittal plane. When going through the tests, we will continuously bring it back to the relevance they have to the pull and split position.

Pull Screens

Forward Bending

The purpose here is merely to ensure the lifter can naturally bend the spine without pain or apprehension, and can be used as a simple *Does it hurt or not?* and *Can he or she do it or not?* type of test. We want to make sure there are no glaring issues with the spine, and the test can also give a general idea of how much tension the athlete is holding. It's a "clearing" test.

Most coaches and athletes are aware of the fact that there is research suggesting a certain degree of lumbar flexion under load may increase the risk for acute back injury. But hey, things happen sometimes during training or competition. In fact, there is also research that suggests a *relative* amount of lumbar flexion or "butt wink" (more on this later) is inherent and unavoidable during the movements required for weightlifting, such as hip hinging and squatting. If *some* amount of lumbar flexion is probably going to happen, and considering that there will likely be reps at some point in a lifter's career where position is lost to an even larger degree, let's make sure there is a buffer zone of apprehension/pain-free range of motion.

Starting Position

- Stand with the feet hip-width apart and toes facing forward.
- Keep the knees *slightly* unlocked.
- Let your arms hang at your sides.

Execution

- Bend forward and reach for your toes with your arms straight and chin slightly tucked.
- Do not bend your knees any more than in the starting position.
- Let your spine comfortably round from the base of the neck to the tailbone. (Figure 3.02)

Key Points

- Does it hurt?
  - › If yes, proceed with caution or get checked out (Find a ClinicalAthlete Provider). Caution should be taken with regard to programming the full lifts from the floor. Perhaps block pulls and power variations are a better option to train for the time being to allow the athlete to move within a range in which he or she is confident.
- Make note of hyper- or hypomobility. Don't try to pinpoint muscles, just make note. This can give general ideas of whether you're dealing with a tense individual or a spaghetti noodle.
  - › Hypermobility: athlete can palm the floor (Figure 3.03).
  - › Hypomobility: athlete cannot reach the crease of the ankle (Figure 3.04).
- Clear test: No pain and range somewhere within the two extremes described above—able to reach the crease of the ankle, but unable to palm the floor, with no pain or apprehension.

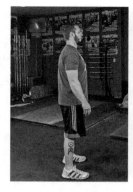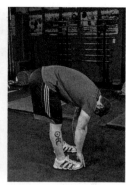

Figure 3.02 The Forward Bending screen

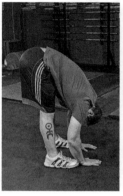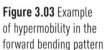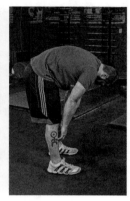

Figure 3.03 Example of hypermobility in the forward bending pattern

Figure 3.04 Example of hypomobility in the forward bending pattern

Variation If the athlete demonstrated hypomobility, allow him or her to space the feet out slightly wider, turn the toes out 20-30 degrees, or both, and retest. In some cases, an increase in range of motion may be seen. This could indicate that the athlete may be more comfortable utilizing a slightly wider stance and/or some external rotation of the toes/hips for the start and pull positions. This is not an inherently "bad" thing, contrary to popular belief.

Backward Bending

This screen is simply to determine if the athlete tolerates global spinal extension, which is what he or she will be facing during overhead movements and at the top of the pull. Also, a quick hyperextension moment through the low back happens sometimes under a jerk, so let's just make sure that the athlete has a buffer zone to tolerate such a position.

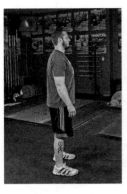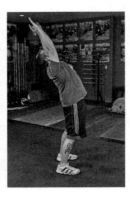

Figure 3.06 The Backward Bending screen

Starting Position

- Place the feet hip width apart with your toes facing forward.
- Keep the knees slightly unlocked (soft bend).
- Let your arms hang at your sides.

Execution

- Lift both of your arms overhead.
- Reach and bend back as far as possible, comfortably, without losing balance (Figure 3.06).

Key Points

- Does it hurt?
  - > If yes, proceed with caution or get checked out.
  - > As stated earlier, a lifter can lose position during a split jerk and hyperextend the lower back. As with the pull and forward bending, we want the athlete to have a buffer zone. If unloaded extension is uncomfortable, it is more likely that loss of position in a split jerk will not feel great either. Progress overhead lifting cautiously with strict press variations to push press to jerk variations. Behind the neck variations can also be a great option for an extension-sensitive athlete, as they can simply work on driving the barbell straight off the back and keep the torso neutral rather than having to move the face out of the way of the barbell from the front rack.
  - > It's important to note that general spinal hyperextension may be an uncomfortable position for many people. General tightness across the low back is a relatively common finding and not necessarily abnormal. It's shooting pain and apprehension to the movement that we are looking out for.

Variation As with the forward bending test, if the athlete reported discomfort in the lower back or felt that the front of the hips were the limiting factor to the movement, allow him or her to space the feet out slightly wider, turn the toes out 20-30 degrees, or both, and retest.

In some cases, an increase in range of motion or perceived ease of the movement may be reported. This could indicate that the athlete may be more comfortable utilizing a slightly wider stance and/or some external rotation of the toes/hips for the pull positions in order to maximize hip extension at the finish, and also in the jerk stance to maximize hip extension during the drive phase. This will just be something to take note of and experiment with during barbell training.

Active Straight Leg Raise (ASLR)

Also known as a Supine Hip Hinging screen, this is not simply a hamstring length test. This is a test to determine the hips' capacity to hinge independently of one another, and there are a lot of tissues involved. Although the pulls of the snatch and clean require us to hinge from both hips simultaneously, this test is looking to identify symmetry from side to side. Also, this test identifies whether an athlete can actively flex one hip while keeping the other in extension, similar to what is required in the split jerk, without the need to move through the lower back.

The ability to flex and extend the hips is also tested during the pull when we are going from the flexed starting position to the extended finish position with straight knees. So again, there is way more going on with this test than just hamstring length. Yes, it shows active hamstring length in the moment, but more importantly, it will demonstrate the athlete's ability to stabilize his or her trunk in order to effectively *demonstrate* his or her hamstring length.

Also, for many, it can quickly eliminate the notion that it is the hamstrings that are the limiting factor, which is a common thought, but less commonly the reality.

Starting Position

- Lie on your back with your legs extended and ankles flexed up to point the toes toward the ceiling.
- Keep your arms out to the sides and head neutral with support.

Execution

- Keeping both legs locked straight, *slowly* lift one leg as high as you can while pressing the down leg against the floor.
- Avoid bending the knee of the lifted leg.
- Keep your toes facing straight ahead and avoid rotation of either foot outward.

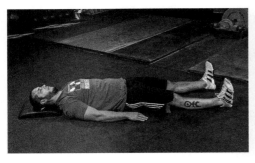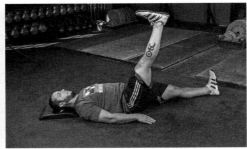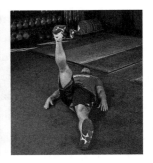

Figure 3.08 ASLR test start and finish positions. The photos show a finding of about 70 degrees of range, which is typically adequate for the positions of the pull. Notice the athlete keeps the toes facing the ceiling and knees straight.

- Maintain the same lower back and ribcage position from start to finish.
- If the testing leg bends, the bottom leg comes off the floor, correct and retest. (Figure 3.08)

Key Points

- We are looking for the athlete to be able to achieve around 70 degrees of hip flexion.
- We standardized the test with ankles dorsiflexed and knees locked straight for a reason, which is to increase the sensitivity of the test, which allows us to rule things out. For example, if a lifter can keep the knees locked, ankles flexed up, and lift the leg to 70-90 degrees (straight up to the ceiling) with no pain or apprehension, that is adequate mobility for the pull considering first that the lifter will likely have even more range passively, and second, even at the most lengthened position of the posterior chain during the pull, the knees are bent about 35 degrees, which will create even more slack (Figure 3.09). In this case, we can effectively rule out posterior chain tightness or tension as a *primary* limiting factor to achieving the desired pull positions. This is helpful information, because now you know you do not have to spend time stretching and mobilizing the hamstrings or posterior chain tissue in an effort to create a true structural length change (light stretching is totally fine if it makes you feel good). You already have plenty of length. You can simply work on stabilizing, reinforcing and strengthening the mobility you have in the desired positions.
- Is the athlete *unable* to achieve the standard on *either* side?
  - › This doesn't necessarily mean you need to go cranking on the hammies. We can dig a bit deeper in the assessment to determine if the athlete has adequate mobility for the pull position right above the knee (end of the first pull)

with respect to individual anatomy. That's ultimately what we are concerned with.

- Is there a noticeable asymmetry (20 degrees or
  more)? Make note of this, as significant asymmetry
  in the hips and pelvis may lead to subtle compensation when pulling from the floor. For example,
  if one leg can achieve the above position and one
  cannot, that can be one of the many causes of the
  twist or lateral shift that is observed in some lifters
  when pulling from the floor. An asymmetry in
  this test may not affect a lifter at all (don't chase
  ghosts); however, if you have noticed said twisting
  or shifting in the pull before, perhaps this needs
  to be a focus. This is a key point in any test—try to
  match findings with things that have been happening in training to provide the most evidence for the
  necessity of intervention.

- Combine the findings of this test with the forward
  bending test for greater context. If an athlete
  can palm the floor in a forward bend and has 70+
  degrees of strict ASLR, there is relative confidence that
  adequate posterior chain mobility is present. If you have an
  athlete with limited toe touch and limited straight leg raise,
  simply take caution with the full lifts. It certainly does not
  exclude them from pulling from the floor, especially if there's
  been no issue with it in the past (don't chase ghosts), but we
  may work to increase that range of motion in the meantime
  for a buffer zone.

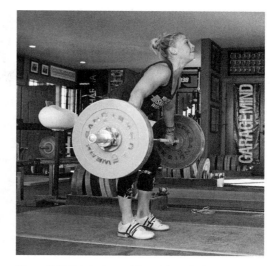

Figure 3.09 This is the position of the pull that requires
the most posterior chain flexibility. The knees are slightly
unlocked to about 35 degrees, the hips are flexed to about
90 degrees, the low back is slightly lordotic, and the
shoulders are over the bar.

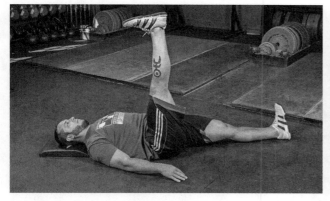 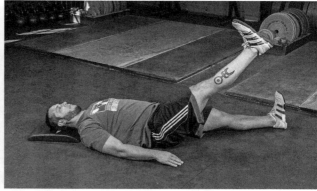

Figure 3.10 In the first picture, you see a lifter who has more than adequate mobility to achieve the desired position of the end of the second pull. In
the second picture, you see an athlete with a more limited straight leg raise. He still may have adequate mobility for the end of the second pull, but
we'll do more digging.

An Alternative Test Option: Hip Hinging

It makes intuitive sense to test a lifter's ability to flex forward while keeping a neutral spine (flat back) when screening to determine whether or not they can pull from the floor. This type of movement pattern is commonly referred to as a *hip hinge*.

Here is the rationale for using this as an optional test, as opposed to including it outright in the screen: Frequently, less experienced lifters will struggle performing a pure hip hinge regardless of how mobile or stable they are. It's simply a new pattern and often requires a bit of coaching, which is not really what we are after during a screen or assessment. What we are interested in is simply seeing if the joints can get into the positions that they are going to be loaded in. If an athlete has a full toe touch and around 70 degrees of Active Straight Leg Raise, we can surmise that he or she possesses adequate joint mobility and soft tissue flexibility to perform an adequate hip hinge. Whether or not that athlete possesses the adequate stability/motor control/competence for optimal technique is a different story, but again, I see that as a coaching issue, which can be developed in the warm-up and general programming.

Having said all of that, going from a toe touch straight to a hip hinge test may save you a little time from having to get on the floor for the ASLR. Again, hip hinging is simply flexing at the hips without changing the curve of the spine—looks a lot like the top of the first pull (Figure 3.11). The ability to perform this movement pattern is important for pulling weights off of the floor safely and effectively.

Starting Position

- Stand with your feet hip-width apart and toes forward OR in your established pulling stance.
- Have a coach or lifting partner hold a PVC pipe against your back with three points of contact: the back of your head,

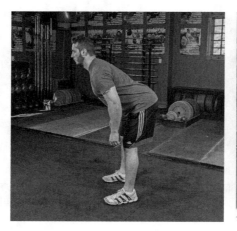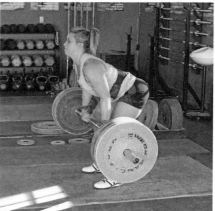

Figure 3.11 The Hip Hinge Screen and the hip hinge pattern in weightlifting

upper back and tailbone (alternatively, you can hold the PVC pipe yourself).

- Slightly bend your knees.

Execution

- Bend your trunk forward at the hips while pushing your hips back slightly to remain balanced.
- Keep your shins vertical and do not bend the knees more than in the starting position.
- Maintain the three points of contact with the PVC pipe and hinge as far as your range will allow. (Figure 3.12)

Key Points

- The athlete should be able to reach a full hand length below the bottom of the kneecap without a significant/observable change in the lumbar spine, as this will ensure adequate range during the end of the first pull when the shins are vertical.

Positional Hack Exhale with moderate force through the mouth to flatten the front ribs and engage the abs (approximately 30% of max contraction), then slightly tilt the pelvis so that the low back is extended just enough to fit a hand between the PVC pipe and spine, but not an entire forearm. Perform a hip hinge as described above while maintaining this neutral spine position. Now flare the lower ribs and arch the low back so that an entire arm can fit between the PVC and low back (Figure 3.13). Perform a hip hinge maintaining this hyperextended position.

Does hyperextending decrease the range of motion? Most likely it did for many due to the pre-stretch of the hamstrings from the anterior pelvic tilt. If an athlete has a limited hip hinge or rounds the low back when pulling, do not be so quick to condemn the hamstrings as being tight before you have addressed the position of the pelvis.

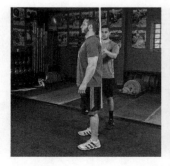 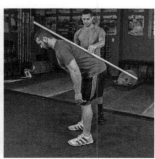 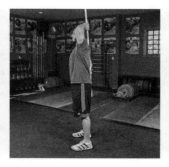 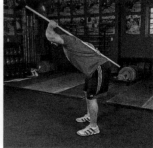

Figure 3.12 The Hip Hinge screen can be performed with a partner holding the PVC pipe, or the pipe can be held by the athlete. Note that in the latter case, limited shoulder mobility can make this position difficult or skew the results of the hip hinge.

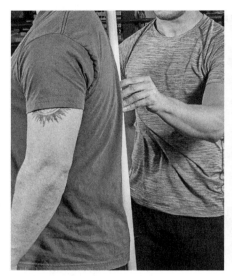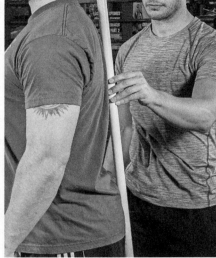

Figure 3.13 In the first picture is the relationship between the spinal curves and PVC pipe after positioning the ribcage and pelvis. In the second picture is the relationship between the spinal curves and PVC pipe after hyperextending the spine and anteriorly tilting the pelvis. Test the hip hinge pattern in both positions and compare movement differences.

This is not to deem extension bad—we need it. It's simply a demonstration that pelvic position has an effect.

Thomas Test

This is a common test used by therapists, athletic trainers and others to assess hip extension mobility. It can be performed with the help of another person or as a self-assessment (a mirror is handy in this case).

In the pull, hip extension range of motion is greatest at the end of the second pull/finish (165-185 degrees); in the jerk, hip extension is used to finish the drive phase and to "split" the pelvis/hips during the receiving position of the split jerk (Figure 3.14). This means putting one hip into extension while the other one is flexed. Obviously a certain amount of hip mobility is required for this, as well as a significant amount of stability through the trunk and pelvis in order for most of the motion to come from the hip joints as opposed to the low back or pelvis. Add to this the fact that the arms are overhead supporting load, and we have a pretty complex movement pattern to deal with. Don't worry—we keep it simple with this test. Stability and integration overhead will be coached later. Let's just look at the mobility capacity of the joints first—*movement potential*.

Starting Position

- Sit on the edge of a table or bench with the crease of the back of your hip near the edge.

- Make sure the surface is high enough so that the ground doesn't limit the range of motion.
- Grab both knees and lie on your back, flexing your hips past 90 degrees.

Execution

- Put your hands around one knee only, keeping that hip flexed past 90 degrees.
- Let your other leg slowly drop toward the ground in the pure sagittal plane.
- Keep the knee of the down leg flexed to 90 degrees.
- Keep the lower back and pelvis motionless as the leg lowers. This is important to isolate true hip extension. (Figure 3.15)

Key Points

- We are looking for the drop leg to reach the table or bench (parallel with the ground) with the knee bent to about 90 degrees.
- Does the athlete achieve this?
  - > If yes, the athlete likely possesses adequate hip extension mobility to achieve full hip lockout during the finish and split. Having the knee bent increases the sensitivity of the test by increasing the stretch on the quad muscles, which means we can rule out truly short hip flexors as being the primary limiting factor to achieving active hip extension.

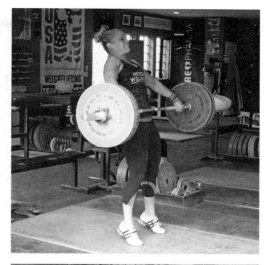

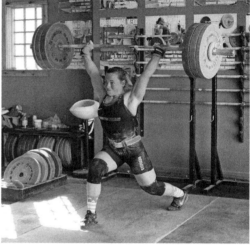

Figure 3.14 We use hip extension to generate power in the finish of the pull and in the jerk drive, and for the split position of the back leg in the jerk.

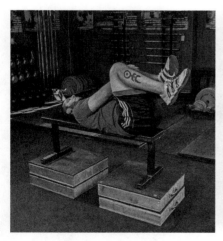 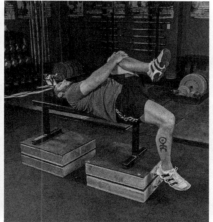 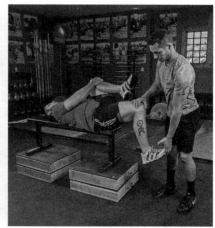

Figure 3.15 The Thomas Test start position, the test performed as a self-assessment, and testing using a partner.

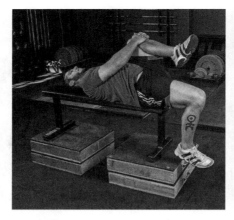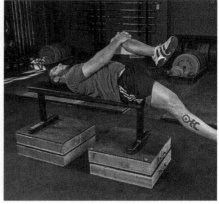

Figure 3.16 By altering knee flexion/extension, one can get a sense of hip extension in a position that mimics the pull or jerk. For some, a straight knee will allow for slightly more hip extension mobility.

> > If no, allow the knee of the down leg to relax/straighten a bit (Figure 3.16). That will slack the quad musculature and for some allow for increased range. For an athlete who experiences this increase in mobility with a straight knee, it may indicate that he or she should spend a little more time during warm-ups making sure that that back hip of the jerk is locked out to the best of his or her capacity.

- Now perform both bent and straight knee tests by allowing the leg to fall out to the side into slight abduction (Figure 3.17). Note any differences in range of motion when you allow this to happen. If hip extension was limited in the straight sagittal plane, but the hip falls freely into full extension if you allow a bit of abduction, this again may be an indication that experimenting with a slightly wider pull stance or jerk stance may afford you a bit of hip extension range. Letting the leg fall out to the side during this test has

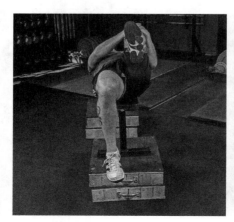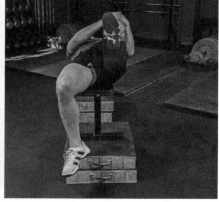

Figure 3.17 A way for a lifter to determine the position that allows for maximal hip extension is by experimenting with various degrees of abduction in the Thomas Test.

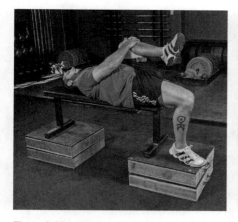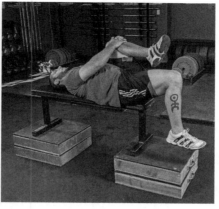

Figure 3.18 In the first picture is an example of full hip extension capacity in the Thomas Test. In the second picture is a test showing more limited hip extension.

often been seen as an unwanted compensation. However, we will view it as simply respecting anatomy. Remember our goals for screening—don't chase ghosts, and use the tests to learn a bit about your body.

- This test does not have predictive power. For example, if an athlete demonstrates full range of motion during the test, that does not guarantee that they will utilize full hip lockout at the top of the pull or drive of the jerk, but it does demonstrate his or her capacity to do so.

- If the lifter has an apparent hip extension limitation and also has tendencies to cut the finish of the pull short of full extension, or relies on spinal hyperextension in the jerk, which affects trunk stability, then we will work to improve the lifter's ability to express hip extension within ranges that they can control.

If the Toe Touch and Hip Hinge were clear, but ASLR was limited, hip extension (the down leg) may be a player on one or both sides. To be clear, this is not because there is a muscle that crosses the hips from side to side. It is more that limitations in hip extension make controlling movement at the hips more challenging in general. This can be subtle, but if your hips do not extend completely when lying supine, many times that puts the pelvis in a bit more anterior pelvic tilt and lumbar spine in a bit more lordosis. We know from our positional hack test earlier that anterior pelvic tilt pre-stretches the hamstrings, which is the possible explanation of how restricted hip extension on one side could affect the active straight leg raise (flexion) on the opposite side. You'll see this during more positional hacks in the assessment. It's relevant to the finish position of the pull and the finish of the jerk drive, because depending on if the extension is coming from the hips or lower back, that may affect the fluidity with which you can flex the hips pulling under the bar, or push the front leg forward into hip flexion during the jerk. It's also relevant for the trajectory of the barbell, as we are looking for the hips and back to extend simultaneously for upward propulsion.

In this scenario, since our goal with movement screening is simply to determine if the *joints can get into the positions that we want to load*, the *active* straight leg raise can be modified to a *passive* straight leg raise, in which the lifter uses a band to bring the leg into the straight leg raise, or a partner helps. If the leg reaches the standard of 70-90 degrees, then we can surmise that the joint *can* get into the position, and the *active* straight leg raise is limited by pelvic position and/or motor control.

Pull & Split Assessment

The lifter or coach can come here for further testing to have a clearer idea of what issues to address (if any), or to determine whether to refer to another professional.

Quadruped Lumbar Flexion

The idea with the following lumbar tests is to differentiate between the spine and soft tissue from the pelvis and below. If the range of motion during the toe touch was limited, you can come here to at least determine that the athlete can comfortably move through the spinal segments with no issue by taking any posterior chain limitation out of the equation.

Starting Position
- Rest on the hands and knees with the shoulders over the hands and the hips over the knees.

Execution
- Tuck the tailbone, which will posteriorly tilt the pelvis and flex the lumbar spine.
- Flex slowly, one spinal segment at a time, until there is a global flexion curve in the spine.
- For added sensitivity to the test, rock the hips back toward the heels slightly, then bring the forearms to the ground, all while maintaining lumbar flexion. (Figure 3.19)

Key Points
- We are simply looking for pain/apprehension-free motion here.
- If the toe touch was pain-free as well as this drill, then we have done a decent job of ruling out flexion or forward

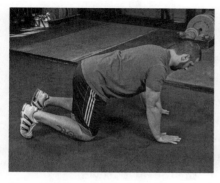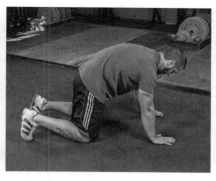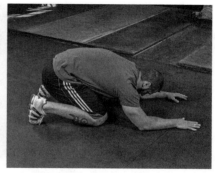

Figure 3.19 Quadruped Flexion test for the lumbar spine. This unloaded, flexed position should not be a scary or painful thing for a healthy spine. Focus on moving one spinal segment at a time.

bending of the spine as a primary point of concern in regard to something that needs to be sent out to a health care professional. The toe touch may have still been limited in terms of range of motion, which will be further teased out in the straight leg raise series.

- If there is pinpoint or radiating pain (different than just a general stretching sensation) with this drill, consider consulting the appropriate professional before performing the lifts from the floor, especially if this is coupled with a painful toe touch. This won't be the case for most. Rest assured that the spine is a robust structure and not some fragile piece of glass, which seems to be the common misconception. Don't chase ghosts. We are simply ruling things out.

Quadruped & Prone Lumbar Extension

Starting Position

- Rest on hands and knees with the shoulders over the hands and the hips over the knees.

Execution

- Arch the lower back or "dump the hips forward" as far as you can comfortably, which will anteriorly tilt the pelvis and extend the lumbar spine.
- Extend slowly, one segment at a time, until there is a global extension curve in the spine.
- For added sensitivity to the test, lie prone and press up to the forearms, and then to the hands (if comfortable range of motion allows), and push down and forward into the floor with the forearms or hands. This will add a little bit of compression force. (Figure 3.20)

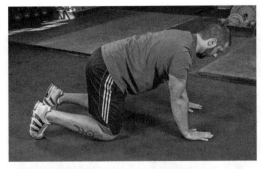
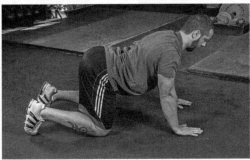
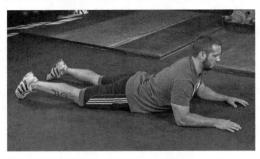
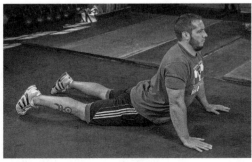

Figure 3.20 Quadruped & Prone Lumbar Extension tests

Key Points

- You may notice, especially with the quadruped test, that most athletes possess more than enough lumbar spine extension mobility and are able to hyperextend past where most coaches cue the spine to be under load. If an athlete struggles with maintaining a neutral lumbar lordosis in the starting position of the lift or the bottom of the squat ("butt wink" even with light weights), but demonstrates the ability to hyperextend the lumbar spine in quadruped or prone, then focus may need to be somewhere other than the spine in terms of attaining a flatter back position. We will address this in detail later. In this case, simply cueing the athlete to "arch harder" may not be effective without coupling that with some positional tweaking of the pelvis and hips.

- As with the flexion testing, we are simply trying to confirm that the lifter does not have some sort of sensitivity to lumbar extension. If a lifter often complains of tightness or achiness in the lower back when going overhead, and those feelings were recreated during these tests, time may need to be spent teaching that athlete how to attain overhead positions without hyperextending the lower back.

Active Straight Leg Raise Differentiation Series

If the Active Straight Leg Raise was limited and you also find it difficult to attain the position at the top of the first pull in which you are in a hip hinge position, come here for a breakdown. Retest your ASLR to first remind you of where you were if time has passed in between tests.

Starting Position

- Lie supine with one leg locked straight and the ankle flexed up (toes toward the shin).
- You can bend the other knee slightly to plant the foot flat on the floor.

Execution

- Exhale through your mouth as if you are blowing up a balloon to make the lower ribs disappear down into the abdomen and to activate abdominals.
- Do not deviate from this spinal position.
- Slowly lift your straight leg as far as possible without moving the pelvis or low back (Figure 3.21). Make note of the range.
- Perform the same test reaching an approximately 10-15kg plate up to the ceiling (Figure 3.22).
- Perform the same test with the toes pointed away (ankle plantar flexed), and note any changes in range of motion (Figure 3.22).

Key Points

- If the ASLR improves with these modifications, we may not have a true structural shortness in hamstring length, and this athlete will likely benefit from focusing on trunk position and stability during our corrective strategies; or we may have limited hip extension on the opposite side, which would have been determined with the Thomas Test.
  - › What we did was give the athlete extra stability by cueing an exhalation (and possibly holding a plate) to set a neutral spine position and facilitate the abs. Flexing the opposite knee slightly decreases the lever of the torso and makes it easier for the athlete to avoid arching the low back when he or she lifts the leg. We did not stretch anything, nor did we manipulate the pelvis or low back in a way that would not carry over to

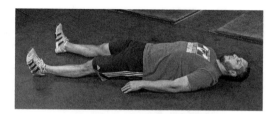
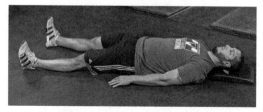
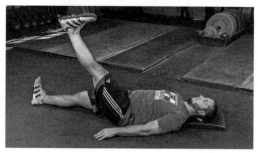

Figure 3.21 Starting position for the Active Straight Leg Raise Differentiation Series. The first picture shows the starting position before an exhalation to set the ribs. The second picture shows the starting position after an exhalation to set the ribs down. The third picture shows the athlete performing the test.

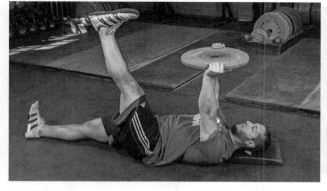
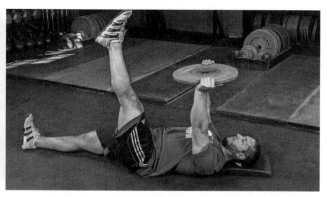

Figure 3.22 In the first picture, the athlete is reaching a plate toward the ceiling during the test to give a reflexive cue for even more abdominal control. The second picture shows the athlete plantarflexing the ankle to differentiate the calf from the hamstrings.

weightlifting. We simply gave the athlete stability, and he or she was able to better demonstrate the mobility already possessed.

> Additionally, flexing the opposite knee decreases the need for hip extension on that side. If that was a limiting factor in the Thomas Test, it is now taken out of the equation.

> Plantarflexion of the ankle shortens the calf musculature and gives a bit of slack to the neural structures of the posterior chain. If your Active Straight Leg Raise improves with ankle plantarflexion, we can say that it certainly wasn't a hamstring limitation. Remember one of our goals is to rule out things that you have potentially been spending significant amount of time on attempting to correct.

Door Frame/Rack Variation Using the upright frame of a squat rack or door frame provides us some leverage with which to explore our supine hip hinging ability, and will hopefully be the start of improving our positions during the pull.

Starting Position

- Lie supine with head support.
- Place one leg against the base of a rack or doorframe, and the other slightly bent at the knee with the foot flat on the floor.
- Keep a soft bend in the up knee. (Figure 3.23)

Execution

- Begin with a full, mildly forceful exhalation through the mouth to pull the lower ribs down. The lower back should have a minimal amount of lordosis. This spinal position will be maintained throughout.

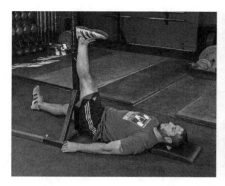 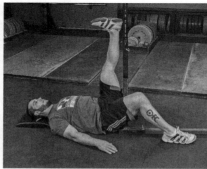 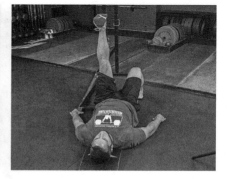

Figure 3.23 Setting up on a rack to assess supine hip hinging ability with the Door Frame/Rack variation of the ASLR.

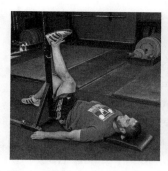 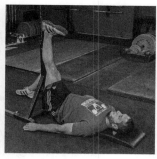 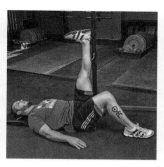 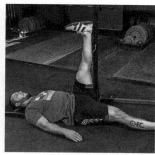

Figure 3.24 Execution of the Door Frame/Rack variation of the ASLR test. The athlete flattens the leg to the wall, demonstrating a 90-degree supine hip hinge, which is adequate for the pull. To differentiate between hip extension and flexion limitations, attempt to flatten the down leg, all while maintaining the same spinal/pelvic position as the start.

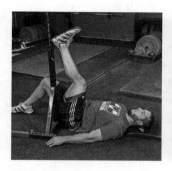 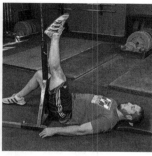 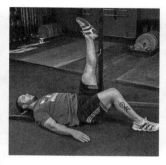 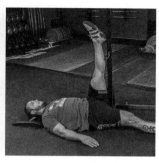

Figure 3.25 The athlete flattens the leg to the wall with a plantarflexed ankle, demonstrating that the hamstring actually has the extensibility adequate for the positions of the pull. To differentiate between a hip extension limitation on the opposite side, attempt to flatten the down leg, all while maintaining the same spinal/pelvic position as from the start.

- We begin by manipulating the up leg. Keeping the top ankle dorsiflexed, attempt to straighten the top knee. If you can do this with no change in lumbar position, you have adequate posterior chain mobility on that side for the positions of the pull.
- From here, attempt to straighten the down leg by sliding the heel forward. If you can flatten the top leg but are unable to flatten the down leg, then you have identified a hip extension mobility limitation on the down side, which may be relevant for the finish of the pull and jerk drive. (Figure 3.24)
- If you are unable to flatten the top knee with a dorsiflexed ankle, try the same test with a plantarflexed ankle, which slacks the neural tissue of the posterior chain, along with the calf musculature (Figure 3.25).
- Then perform the heel slide with the down leg to differentiate between opposite side hip extension (Figure 3.25).

Key Points

- This may seem like some tedious work, but in reality, it will take only a couple of minutes to progress through this series of tests, and if it ends up saving you hours of time from unnecessarily stretching your hamstrings, then it's well worth it.

- The point here is simply to create a little more awareness regarding where limitations in mobility and movement are actually coming from and whether or not you even have true mobility restriction to begin with. Remember that our goal for screening and assessment is simply answering the question *Can the joints get into the positions that we want to load*? Some of you may find that you can attain a full supine hip hinge position with the down leg flat, but you need to unlock the top knee slightly. That's totally fine, as your knees will also be unlocked during the top of the first pull. If you felt like tissues in the backs of your legs were going to rip off, and you also have trouble staying over the bar and keeping your shins vertical at the top of the first pull, then we'll likely spend some time here as a corrective strategy. But now you know, because you took the time to test.

- There will be many athletes who have no trouble flattening either leg with dorsiflexed ankles. Passive stretching will be a *do it if it feels good* rule of thumb, but no need to crank on muscles in an effort to try and create structural length. You have enough for what we need to do. If this is you, and you also demonstrated an original ASLR that made you look like a very *inflexible* person, we likely have some motor control patterns to tighten up.

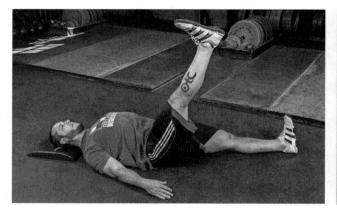 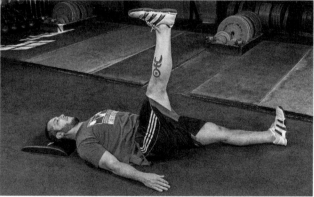

Figure 3.26 In the first picture, the athlete is demonstrating his or her maximum range of motion with an excessively tilted pelvis. In the second picture, the athlete is demonstrating his or her maximum range of motion with a neutral pelvis (but still with a relative amount of lumbar lordosis and anterior pelvic tilt). Note the range of motion difference.

Positional Hack—Pelvic Tilt's Effect on Supine Hip Hinging Using either of the Active Straight Leg Raise screening or assessment test positions, and with or without a weight, perform the test with a hyperextended lower back and flared ribs versus a slightly braced neutral position using a full exhalation to set yourself (Figure 3.26). Note the difference in how it feels. Again, position can affect mobility—positively or negatively.

Pull Screening & Assessment Example Cases

Here are four different examples of what you might see when taking a lifter through these tests. Each case reveals slightly different placement in regard to the Mobility-Stability Continuum, and in turn slightly different strategies are used to correct.

Example Case 1

Findings

- Screen
  › Hypermobile or normal toe touch
  › Limited hinge
  › Normal ASLR
  › Normal Thomas Test
- Assessment
  › No need to test

Correctives Implemented

- Simply coaching the athlete in a proper hip hinge pattern. The athlete possesses adequate mobility for the hinge.

Example Case 2

Findings

- Screen
  › Hypermobile or normal toe touch
  › Restricted ASLR
  › Limited hinge
  › Normal Thomas Test
- Assessment
  › Full ASLR mobility with top leg support from rack or wall

Correctives Implemented

- Trunk and pelvis stability and positional coaching
- Hip Hinge coaching

Example Case 3

Findings

- Screen
  - › Hypermobile or normal toe touch
  - › Normal hip hinge
  - › Restricted ASLR on one or both sides
  - › Restricted Thomas Test on one or both sides
- Assessment
  - › Able to flatten the up leg to the wall or rack
  - › Unable to extend and flatten the bottom leg

Correctives Implemented

- Hip extension range of motion and control
- Trunk and pelvis stability
- The athlete possesses adequate posterior chain mobility based on toe touch and hip hinge, yet demonstrates restriction with ASLR. A positive Thomas Test with an improvement in the ASLR if the opposite leg is bent indicates a possible hip extension range of motion limitation.

Note

- With this case, if we changed the hip hinge from *normal* to *restricted*, the correction would simply be coaching. This is because the toe touch range of motion was adequate, as was the ASLR during assessment.

Example Case 4

Findings

- Screen
  - › Hypomobile toe touch
  - › Limited hip hinge
  - › Restricted ASLR on one or both sides
  - › Full range on Thomas Test on both sides
- Assessment
  - › Quadruped screening clear of pain or apprehension
  - › Unable to extend the up knee to the wall or rack
  - › Able to extend and flatten the bottom leg

Correctives Implemented

- We may consider using block pulls for this athlete if he or she is having difficulty maintaining neutral lumbar lordosis during the pull.

- Work combinations of mobility and static stability near the end ranges that the athlete possesses in an effort to work them back down to the floor.

Summary of Screening & Assessing The Pull & Split

If no range of motion restrictions were present in the four (five including Hip Hinge) screening tests, it is likely that the athlete does not need to spend much time lengthening the posterior chain or hip flexors with the focus of creating permanent structural change, and instead should work to better control the range of motion that they possess. Be sure to always address trunk and pelvic position before deeming a specific area *tight*. Further assessment is likely not necessary in this case.

Some may wonder why some type of lunging pattern was not included in testing for the split jerk, such as an overhead lunge, for example. That would be totally appropriate and feasible as a screen for the split pattern. However, it was not included here because the lunge pattern often times becomes more an issue of practice and coaching, which is included later in the motor control section of this book. The Thomas Test lets us know whether the joints can get into the position for a split, which will guide our coaching and corrections later.

The order of these tests can be manipulated as the athlete or coach sees fit for time efficiency. For example, the assessment test can be conducted immediately following the related screen.

1. Backward Bend → Toe Touch → Toe Touch with exhalation and pelvic squeeze → Quadruped lumbar mobility
2. Active Straight Leg Raise → Active Straight Leg Raise Differentiation Series
3. Hip Hinge
4. Thomas Test

■ CHAPTER 4

Screening & Assessment: Transition & Overhead

This section will address testing for the transition (third pull) phase of the snatch and clean, as well as shoulder elevation. If the lifter plans on training with weights overhead (every weightlifter ever), than the upper extremities and mechanics of the thorax should be looked at.

The screen will consist of these basic movements:

- Upright Row with Snatch Grip
- Apley Scratch Test
- Standing Back to Wall Shoulder Flexion
- Wrist Extension

If needed, the assessment will consist of two additional tests:

- Supine Shoulder Flexion
- Supine Shoulder Internal & External Rotation

Transition-Overhead Screen

Upright Row with Snatch Grip

This screen is to *exaggerate* the third pull of the snatch, in which the shoulder must be internally rotated and elevated. It will be performed with a nearly weightless object such as a PVC pipe, dowel or an empty barbell for lifters with some experience.

We highlight the term *exaggerated* as this elbow position (elbows way up and out at 90-90) is rarely achieved during the execution of the snatch. However, the shoulders certainly go through a transition of internal to external rotation during the turnover, so we exaggerate the position as a screen. Also, during a movement such as a muscle snatch, the shoulder internal rotation and elbow

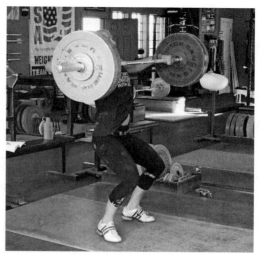

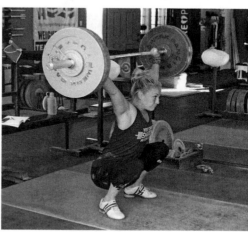

Figure 4.01 The shoulders require a significant amount of both mobility and stability during these lifts.

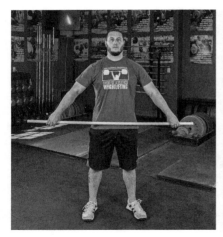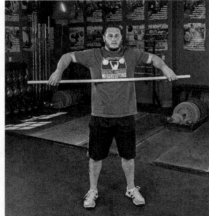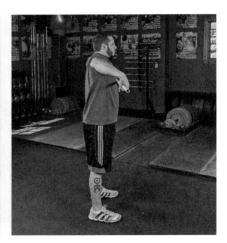

Figure 4.02 The Upright Row with Snatch Grip

position may be more exaggerated than in a full snatch lift, as the muscle snatch is a teaching tool for bar path.

Starting Position

- Stand with your feet hip-width apart.
- Take a wide grip on a PVC pipe or dowel so that it rests at the crease of your hips with your arms hanging straight.

Execution

- Perform an upright row by pulling elbows up and out as high as you can comfortably.
- Keep the PVC as close to your body as possible. (Figure 4.02)

Key Points

- Resist the urge to coach movement here. Remember, it's just a screen to help rule out any glaring shoulder issues. Use only the two cues above.
- We are looking for the PVC to reach the bottom of the sternum while keeping it within an inch of the body.
- Does it hurt or is there a range of motion limitation?
  - › If yes, make a note and monitor during the subsequent tests. Another common report during this test is that it's easier for the athlete to perform that movement on one side of the body than the other. There may even be a noticeable twist in the bar path, or different shoulder and elbow positions from left to right (as seen in Figure 4.02). An asymmetry does not automatically mean a problem, but it is something to note, especially if it is also seen in subsequent tests and has been affecting the lifter during training in the past.

> Re-test with various grip widths to increase the sensitivity of the screen, and further confirm that the shoulder is fine in this position. Most should not have a problem.

> For experienced lifters, an empty barbell can then be used. Experiment with grip widths but also shoulder blade position. Protract the shoulders and upright row the bar, retract the shoulders and upright row the bar, etc. There is no right or wrong here. Find a position that allows the most comfortable range of motion while keeping the barbell close to the body.

Apley Scratch Test

This is a common test for the shoulder complex. It is *not* simply a shoulder internal or external rotation test. In fact, it is a poor test in that regard because there is way more going on than that. Yes, there is shoulder rotation, but there is also shoulder flexion/extension, shoulder adduction/abduction, scapular upward/downward rotation, thoracic spine extension/rotation, etc. This is why it is included as a general screen to look at shoulder girdle function and side-to-side asymmetry. We like the correspondence as a test for the snatch because of the similarity of shoulder position during the test and also during the transition from the third pull to the receiving position of the snatch.

As was the case with the previous upright row test (shoulder internal rotation and elevation), we are gaining a general sense of shoulder function and ruling out any glaring sensitivities to such positions. Although the shoulder does not cross the body's midline during the weightlifting movements, demonstrating the ability to do so without issue is again the expression of a movement "buffer zone" that we described with the Toe Touch screen for the pull.

Starting Position

- Stand tall with your feet hip-width apart.
- Let your arms hang down at your sides.

Test 1 Execution

- In *one* smooth motion, raise one arm up overhead maximally and then reach the hand down toward the opposite shoulder blade or down the spine with fingers straight.
- Do not move the low back or rotate the torso.
- Do not strain, and do not try to "snake" your hand any further down than it wants to go.
- Repeat with the opposite arm. (Figure 4.03)

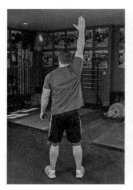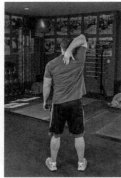

Figure 4.03 Apley Scratch Test 1

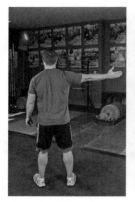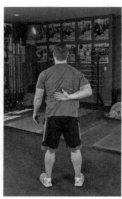

Figure 4.04 Apley Scratch Test 2

Test 2 Execution

- In *one* smooth motion, reach one arm behind your back toward the opposite shoulder blade or up the spine.
- Do not move the low back or rotate the torso.
- Repeat with the opposite arm. (Figure 4.04)

Key Points

- Does this hurt?
  - › If yes, make note. It certainly does not automatically preclude the lifter from training, but proceed with caution and/or consider a formal assessment outside of this book.
- For Test 1, we are looking for the athlete to at least touch the top/inside corner of the opposite shoulder blade. A coach or lifting partner can mark how far down the spine the arm goes.
  - › Make note of bilateral restriction or an asymmetry more than fingers' length.
- For Test 2, we are looking for the athlete to be able to touch the bottom of the opposite shoulder blade. This will be difficult for thicker builds, so a coach or lifting partner can mark how far up the spine the arm goes.
  - › Make note of bilateral restriction or an asymmetry more than fingers' length.

Asymmetries are the main focus here, but are only relevant when considering the athlete's training habits. For example, has the lifter had a noticeable twist upon receiving the bar in a snatch? These types of quirks are common and the causes can be multi-factorial. However, this test can at least clue you in on a route. Think of it this way—applying force to a symmetrical barbell with an asymmetrical thorax can prove difficult, and in some cases can relate to the twist that we are referring to.

Test 2 can also be a way to observe, in some athletes, the shoulder blade winging that we alluded to earlier. As the lifter reaches behind his or her back, you may see that shoulder blade on that side "flop" off of the ribcage. I mention this strictly for observational purposes, because unless there is some history of long thoracic nerve injury (not likely), it can easily be taken away. More on that to come.

Standing Back to Wall Shoulder Flexion

Now we take a look at pure overhead movement at angles most closely related to the snatch and jerk. We use a wall to aid in positioning to minimize movement compensation by the lifter, and consequently minimize the need to coach through the test.

Starting Position

- Stand with the back against a wall, feet roughly shoulder-width apart and 8-12 inches away from the wall, and the knees slightly bent.
- Establish two points of contact on the wall: tailbone and upper back.
- Exhale slightly to pull the ribs down. The low back should be in a state of slight lordosis to mimic the normal curves of the spine. This will mean maintaining enough space between the

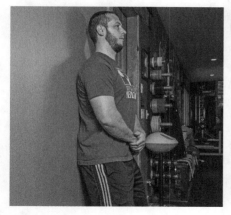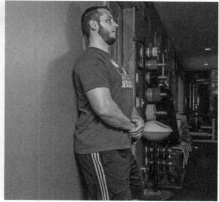

Figure 4.05 We are looking for the lifter to maintain a neutral lumbar spine (first picture) during the test rather than hyperextending through the lower back (second picture) as a means of attaining full shoulder range since we are, after all, trying to determine shoulder mobility.

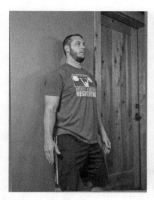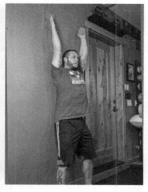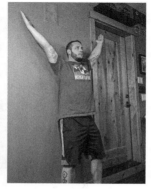

Figure 4.06 Test your overhead range using different arm angles, mimicking that of the snatch and jerk. Be sure to remain motionless through the low back and pelvis and keep the elbows locked.

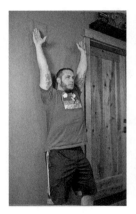
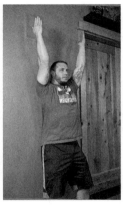
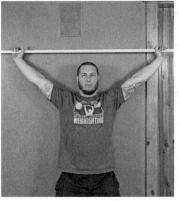
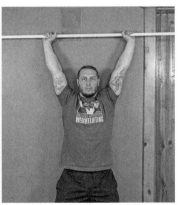
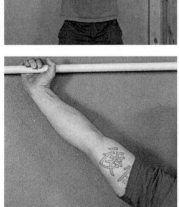
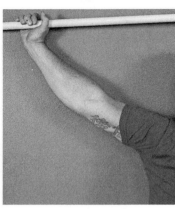

Figure 4.07 Experiment with different amounts of internal and external shoulder rotation, gauging which position affords you the most range of motion and/or comfort. Be sure to remain motionless through the low back and pelvis and keep the elbows locked. Explore combinations of various amounts of rotation and abduction.

Figure 4.08 Holding a dowel or PVC pipe, experiment with various grip widths and relative amounts of shoulder internal (bottom left) or external (bottom right) rotation.

low back and wall to fit a hand in between, but not an entire forearm. Maintain this exact position while testing shoulder range of motion. (Figure 4.05)

Execution

- Slowly raise your arms overhead as high as you can at various angles with elbows straight while maintaining the two points of contact on the wall and without altering your low back or ribcage position (Figure 4.06).
- Test with palms away and palms facing each other (Figure 4.07).
- You can also use a dowel or PVC pipe here to simulate holding a bar overhead (Figure 4.08).

Key Points

- We are looking for the athlete to attain 170-180 degrees of shoulder elevation (flexion) to indicate full mobility of that joint system (Figure 4.09).

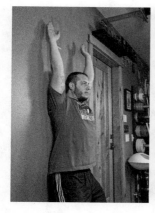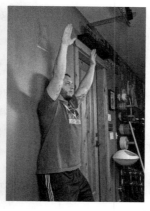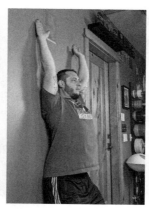

Figure 4.09 Full versus partial shoulder elevation. In the last picture, you see the athlete attain a full overhead position, but doing so by moving through the lower back. This may be corrected simply by verbally cueing the athlete to maintain a consistent back/wall position, or could be an indication that the athlete lacks full shoulder mobility and is compensating through the spine.

> In standing, this will mean reaching the wall with the full length of the arms without altering the trunk's relationship with the wall.

> For many lifters going through this series of tests, you may have found that certain amounts of internal or external rotation and abduction/adduction afforded you a greater overhead range than other positions.

> If the athlete cannot attain this, then we may have identified a shoulder joint mobility restriction. Move on to the Supine Shoulder Flexion test to follow.

Wrist Extension

This test is to clear the wrist to be able to tolerate extension with loading, as in the overhead position (and front rack of the clean). This will be appropriate for someone who is completely new to loading the wrists in such a manner or someone who is coming back to training with a history of wrist injury. If you have training experience and have never experienced wrist issues, the findings of this test may be insignificant for you. There are two tests: one performed in a seated or standing position, and one in quadruped position.

Test 1 Starting Position
- Seated or standing with hands together.

Test 1 Execution
- Use one hand to maximally extend the opposite wrist with the elbow bent and fingers straight.

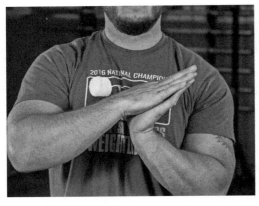

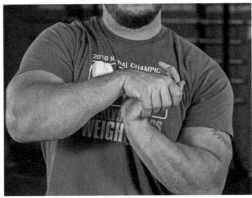

Figure 4.10 Wrist Screen 1. Straight fingers will take into account soft tissue, and flexed fingers will test end range of the wrist joint. Pictured are examples of normal ranges of motion.

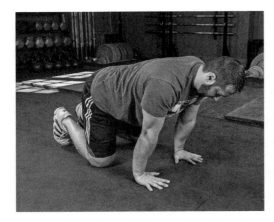

Figure 4.11 Wrist Screen 2. This test will load the wrist similarly to when a bar is overhead. The athlete pictured is demonstrating a test clear of range of motion restriction.

> Hang out at the end range and gently oscillate there for 5 seconds.

> Make note of asymmetry or pain.

- Repeat with your fingers bent. This tests the wrist joint at increased range of motion since the finger tendons are slacked. (Figure 4.10)

Test 2 Starting Position

- Quadruped with the hands underneath the shoulders and the fingers relaxed and pointing forward.

Test 2 Execution

- Rock your shoulders forward so that they are slightly in front of the wrists.

- Oscillate gently up and down, periodically increasing your pressure and deliberately creating load through the wrist. (Figure 4.11)

Key Points

- In the standing or seated test, with over pressure from the opposite hand, we are looking for the back of the wrist to achieve about 70-90 degrees of extension with the fingers straight. With the fingers bent, closer to 90 degrees is what we would expect with little to no discomfort in the joint line.

- In the quadruped test, close to 90 degrees or more of wrist extension when the athlete rocks forward is what we would expect.

- Is the lifter is able to achieve these positions without shooting pain in the wrists?

  > If yes, we have cleared the wrist from being a *primary* mobility limitation.

  > If there is an asymmetry or range of motion restriction in these tests, the wrist may be a mobility emphasis. Refer Chapter 13 for wrist mobility drills.

Important Note The wrist is an inherently weak but mobile joint. Most people, barring some type of injury history or true structural issue, possess adequate wrist mobility to perform the weightlifting movements. Often discomfort or restriction felt at the wrist joint can be addressed by altering shoulder and trunk positions during the lifts to stack the joints and distribute forces more effectively. In these cases, the wrist is simply the victim of a larger issue.

Transition-Overhead Assessment

Supine Shoulder Flexion

Come here for further testing of the shoulder complex if perceived limitations were experienced in previous testing. This will be very similar to the back to wall testing, but gravity is taken out of the equation and the athlete is fully supported by the floor, giving a purer sense of overhead mobility.

Starting Position

- Lie supine with your hips and knees bent to place the feet flat on the floor.
- Place your arms at your sides and keep your head neutral with support.

Execution

- Exhale through your mouth to get the front/bottom ribs down. This will help limit compensatory movement through the back and ribcage. The lower back can have a slight lordosis (enough to get fingers between the back and floor). Breathe comfortably in this set position, but do not deviate from it.
- Lift your arms toward the ceiling with palms facing away. Slowly raise them overhead without changing the position of the low back or letting the ribcage pop up significantly. Gauge range of motion.
- Return to the starting position.
- Now slowly raise the arms overhead with the palms facing each other without changing the position of the low back, letting the lower ribcage pop up, or letting your hands rotate from where they started. Gauge range of motion.
- Finally, raise the arms overhead with the palms facing toward your face without changing the position of the low back, letting the lower ribcage pop up, or letting your hands rotate from where they started.

- Now, just as you did against the wall, explore the above testing with various amounts of shoulder abduction (simulated grip widths from narrower to wider). This may clue you in to what position will afford your shoulder the most overhead range when supporting the barbell overhead. (Figure 4.12)
- You can use a PVC pipe or dowel with various grips to simulate holding a bar overhead (Figure 4.13).

Key Points

- We are looking for the athlete to comfortably reach the ground overhead with some combination of shoulder rotation and/or abduction. Individual positions will vary.
  - › If the supine overhead testing is demonstrating full range of motion overhead, but the wall test was much more

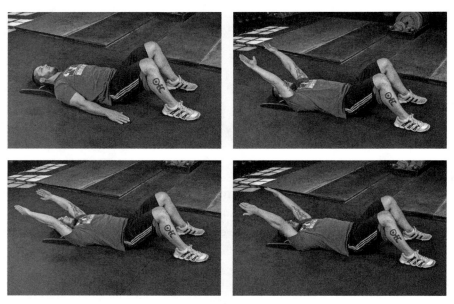

Figure 4.12 Supine Shoulder Flexion tests: With the palms facing away, much of the musculature that would restrict overhead motion is slacked. With the palms facing each other, the shoulder is in mid-range rotation and joint congruency is high. With the palms rotated towards the athlete's face, the soft tissues that limit elevation and facilitate internal rotation are put on stretch.

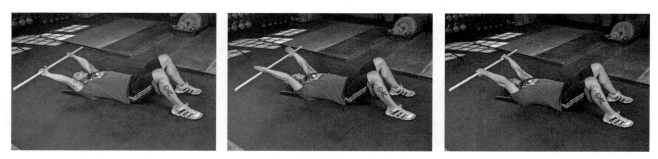

Figure 4.13 You can use a dowel or PVC pipe during the Supine Shoulder Flexion tests to simulate holding a bar overhead.

limited in nature, then we may be addressing a motor control issue with that athlete. He or she is demonstrating the potential for full overhead range (the joints go there), but do not use it in the standing position. We can use pressing variations or simple corrective drills to teach the lifter to dissociate shoulder range of motion from the trunk and integrate it into the lifts.

> If not, we may have a shoulder mobility limitation and will work to increase mobility while integrating it into use as described above.

- With the palms facing toward the athlete's face, we are looking to reach within 6 inches of the ground without changing the position of the ribcage or low back. Because large muscles such as the lats and pecs are on stretch here, we expect the range of motion to be less than in the two previous positions. For some, mobility will be significantly limited with this subtle change in arm position, and a difference of more than 6 inches in range of motion is enough to potentially affect the athlete's ability to attain a comfortable front rack position and overhead jerk position, especially for those who tend to jerk with a relatively narrow grip. The lats and other shoulder depressors along the chest wall may be a mobility focus. We can mobilize those in a way that does not over-stretch the shoulder capsule if we have already deemed that the joint itself is mobile enough with palms facing each other.

> If the athlete was within 6 inches of the ground, then again a large focus will be on stabilizing the overhead position rather than mobilizing it.

> Refer to Chapter 18 for mobility of the lats and chest wall.

Supine Shoulder External & Internal Rotation

Come here if there was limitation or asymmetry in the Apley Scratch or Upright Row with Snatch Grip tests.

Starting Position

- Lie supine with your hips and knees bent to place the feet flat on the floor.
- Place something under your head for support.
- Place your shoulders and elbows in a 90-90 position with your forearms perpendicular to the ground and plates or small towel rolls under the upper arm to line up the elbow with the shoulder.

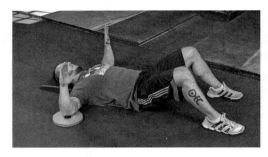

Figure 4.14 Starting position of Supine Shoulder External & Internal Rotation tests

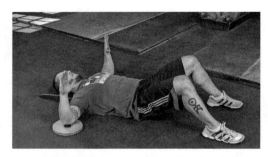

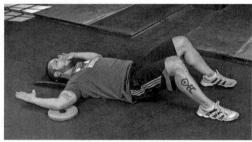

Figure 4.15 The Supine Shoulder External Rotation test

- Exhale through your mouth to set your rib position to neutral with a slight lordosis in lower back (enough to get a hand between the back and floor).
- Breathe comfortably in this set position, but do not deviate from it. (Figure 4.14)

External Rotation Test Execution

- Slowly rotate your hands back toward the floor, maintaining the 90-90 position (Figure 4.15).

Key Points

- We are looking for both hands to reach the floor (90+ degrees of external rotation).
- Full range of motion here aids in a comfortable front rack position, as well as reaching back for the barbell during a back squat.
- LIMITATION: Obviously in the front rack the elbows are pointed forward rather than out to the sides. The above test is simply easier to standardize. The front rack itself can be a screen, which we will discuss in a subsequent chapter.
- If an athlete has no restriction when performing this test but feels shoulder tightness in the front rack of the clean or jerk, we may still address soft tissue structures such as the lats, but optimizing shoulder and thoracic spine position will be a primary focus.

Internal Rotation Test Execution

- Slowly rotate one hand forward toward the floor, maintaining the 90-90 position (Figure 4.16).
- Monitor the shoulder with the opposite hand. Simply allow it to rotate through its axis rather than popping it upwards or allowing the elbow to slide down. (Figure 4.17)

Key Points

- We are looking for about 70 degrees of internal rotation and side-to-side symmetry with the arm abducted 90 degrees.
- This range of motion aids with a comfortable transition phase (third pull) of the snatch. Now, we discussed above that this pure form of shoulder internal rotation does not typically occur during the snatch, but if one or more of your shoulders is limited in internal rotation, and you have had

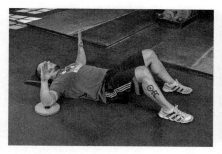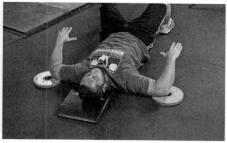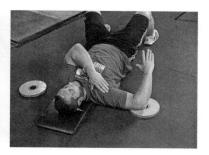

Figure 4.16 Supine Shoulder Internal Rotation test being performed with one and two arms.

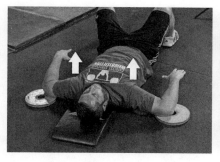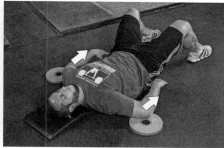

Figure 4.17 In the Supine Shoulder Internal Rotation test, do not allow the front of the shoulder to pop up. Keep the shoulder rotation through the same axis—pretend there is a rod from the shoulder through the elbow. We also want to maintain our high elbow position and not allow it to slide down. With the single-arm test, use the free arm to monitor the position of the shoulder being tested.

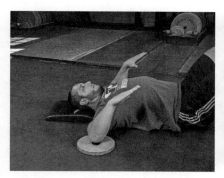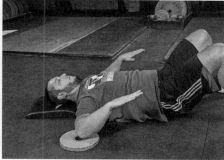

Figure 4.18 Test to see if your shoulder internal rotation range of motion is affected by a change in ribcage position. The first picture shows range with the ribs up and back arched, and the second picture shows range with the ribs and back set properly.

difficulty maintaining a close body-barbell relationship during the transition, this is a potential contributing factor (excluding general technical errors, of course).

Positional Hack Allow your ribs to pop up toward the ceiling in the starting position of the internal rotation test. Attempt to internally rotate your shoulders by pulling your palms down to the ground like a scarecrow. Make note of how this feels. Now exhale to get the ribs down and brace that position as you repeat the test. (Figure 4.18)

Feel a difference? For many, it was likely more comfortable the second time, and possibly more range of motion was achieved. Just as hip mobility can be affected by pelvic position, shoulder mobility can be affected by ribcage position. In the third pull, our bar path may be dictated not only by the shoulder joint itself, but by the position of the ribcage. This is why we recommend maintaining a stacked ribcage-over-pelvis position as much as possible, even during the transition.

Transition-Overhead Screening & Assessment Example Cases

Here are two different examples of what you might see when taking a lifter through these tests. Both cases reveal slightly different placement in regard to the Mobility-Stability Continuum, and in turn, slightly different strategies are used to correct.

Example Case 1

Findings

- Screen
  > Limited Upright Row with Snatch Grip test
  > Limited Apley Scratch test on one or both sides
- Assessment
  > Normal supine range of motion testing in all planes

Correctives Implemented

- Ribcage positioning and core control. The athlete has the range of motion, but needs to learn to control it in standing.
- Scapular stability and mechanics

Example Case 2

Findings

- Screen
  > Normal range of motion during Upright Row with Snatch Grip, but reports tightness on right side
  > Restricted Apley Scratch test with right arm reaching behind back
- Assessment
  > Restricted Supine Flexion with palms turned toward the face on both sides
  > Restricted Internal Rotation on right side

Correctives Implemented

- Ribcage positioning and thoracic spine mobility
- Mobility work to soft tissue structures limiting shoulder flexion
- Scapular retraining to attain internal rotation on right, and overhead pressing variations to integrate mobility work

Summary of Screening & Assessing The Overhead-Transition

The shoulder is an inherently mobile structure. With that being the case, it is very important that the mobility work you do is actually of benefit in allowing you more ease in positioning for the snatch and clean & jerk, as opposed to arbitrarily tugging on something that does not have a lot holding it together in the first place. Practice with stabilizing and positioning the shoulder will likely be the priority for most.

Be mindful that you are not *chasing ghosts* during the shoulder screening process. *Can the joints get into the positions that we plan to load?* That's the focus. You will likely see many subtle asymmetries here and there on most athletes with regard to resting posture and position of the shoulder blades. The scientific evidence tells us that subtle asymmetries are inherent in being a human. Take a big picture approach and try to connect dots of things you see in the screen to things you see in training before make conclusions or assumptions.

CHAPTER 5

Screening & Assessment: The Squat

_____

This section will address testing for the overhead squat and front squat positions. The difference in the two movements from an unloaded perspective is that the clean requires only about half of the shoulder flexion that the snatch requires. However, the clean adds an element of elbow flexion, which lengthens tissue crossing both joints (shoulder and elbow). Also, the front rack position, with the shoulder positioned in more of the straight sagittal plane of flexion along with external rotation, tensions the tissues that oppose those planes, such as the lat.

From a weighted perspective, having the load anterior to the midline of the body during the front squat increases the challenge of achieving and maintaining an upright torso (and relative amount of thoracic spine extension). Obviously the snatch requires an upright torso as well, but sometimes lifters can get away with a more inclined torso or save a lift even if they dive the chest/torso forward a little. With the clean, it's more difficult to overcome such a position and still successfully complete the lift. For the pelvis and lower body, the two squatting patterns are very similar. The screen will consist of three basic movements:

- Ankle Dorsiflexion
- Overhead Squat
- Front Squat

If needed, the assessment will consist of additional tests:

- Overhead or Front Squat with Elevated Heels
- Air Squat without & with Elevated Heels
- Counterbalance Squat without & with Elevated Heels

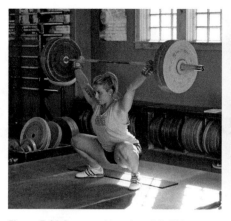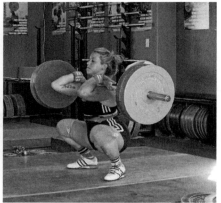

Figure 5.01 Squat positions in weightlifting

We then move on to specific testing of hip structure to determine individual squatting stance:

- Supine Passive Hip Flexion with External & Internal Rotation
- Supine Wall Hip Internal Rotation
- Quadruped Rockback with Neutral Spine
- Counterbalance Squat with Varied Stances

Squat Screen

Ankle Dorsiflexion

Ah, the ankle… This is a joint that can be the bane of squatting existence. It's absolutely true that limited ankle dorsiflexion can have an effect on squatting mechanics and even muscle activation at the hip. However, it's also a bit of a scapegoat, as we are quick to blame tight ankles as the primary cause of poor squats. So let's screen it right off the bat to see if it actually is a significant issue. We are concerned primarily with closed chain ankle dorsiflexion with the foot fixed to the ground and the knee bent, as this resembles squatting and the set up position of the lifts.

Starting Position

- Half-kneeling or standing facing a wall
  > Half kneeling will better simulate the squatting pattern with the hip flexion component. I have also found that in standing, athletes can use their bodyweight to leverage forward and jam into range that they wouldn't normally have access to. This is fine as a mobilization, but for an assessment, we want to see the lifter's true range, and half kneeling does a better job of this. Sometimes, however, standing is more feasible. If this is the case, just make sure to adhere to the cueing below.

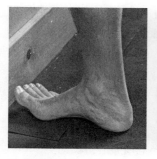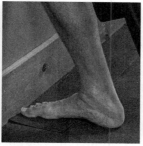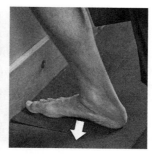

Figure 5.02 Lifting the toes creates a stable midfoot arch. Spread the toes and place them back down flat. Be sure to maintain three points of contact at all times—the big toe, little toe and heel. Do not allow the midfoot to collapse (last picture).

- Place your bare foot flat on the ground with three points of contact—the big toe, little toe and heel, and with your big toe touching the wall. Keeping the balls of the feet down, lift the toes up. This will create a stable midfoot arch. Spread the toes as well as you can and place them back down *flat* (not scrunched), while maintaining that arch in the midfoot. This will ensure that the movement truly comes from the ankle joint and not through mid-foot collapse. (Figure 5.02)
- Hold a PVC pipe or the wall for balance if needed.

Execution

- Shift your weight forward, bringing your knee toward the wall and flexing your ankle while maintaining three points of contact on your foot—big toe, little toe and heel.
- Your knee should travel forward over your second toe or roughly the middle of your foot.
- If you are able to touch the wall without collapsing through the midfoot or allowing the heel to lift up, scoot the foot back a half-inch and retest. Reset the toes/arch each time. Repeat this sequence until you have found the maximum distance your foot can be from the wall while still maintaining the abovementioned foot position. (Figures 5.03 & 5.04)

Key Points

- Make a note whether you feel a stretch in the back or a pinch in the front. A stretch in the back (achilles, calf) is a normal sensation since we are lengthening that area. A pinching sensation in the front may indicate what we generally term

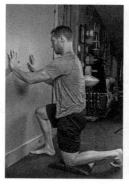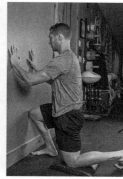

Figure 5.03 The ankle dorsiflexion screen in half kneeling position

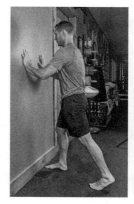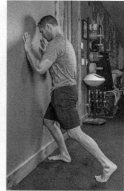

Figure 5.04 The ankle dorsiflexion screen in standing position

as *impingement* (sounds way worse than it usually is), and will be an indication for us to alter joint position in some way. We will talk more about the significance of this later.

- Can *both* knees reach the wall comfortably with the toes roughly 3-4 inches away (a fist's distance) without your heel coming off the ground?
  - > If yes, then rule out the ankle as the *primary* source of limitation during a squat. It does not mean you are not allowed to mobilize or stretch it as part of your routine, but it means that it's not our primary concern. Being able to reach the wall approximately 3-4 inches away from your toes gives you roughly 20 degrees of closed chain dorsiflexion. This is adequate to reach full depth in a squat, especially when you add weightlifting shoes into the equation. Some may find that they can touch the wall with much more than 3-4 inches of distance from the wall, further cementing the fact that you should put your focus elsewhere to improve your movement.
- Is there a difference from side to side of more than 1 inch?
  - > Make a note, as this may be an area of mobility focus for the athlete.
  - > If one ankle cannot dorsiflex as well as the other, then the shin cannot translate forward as well during a squat. Depending on the lifter's stance and amount of asymmetry, this could lead to subtle compensations in one's squatting movement, perhaps one of the many causes of a shift or twist in one's squat. But again, correlating the finding in the screen with something that's been happening in the athlete's training is better evidence to spend time intervening than discovering an asymmetry in range of motion without any perceived limitation in training.
  - > Refer to Chapter 7 for ankle mobility.
- Are you unable to reach the 3-4-inch mark (roughly a fist's distance) on *either* side?
  - > Make a note.
  - > Intuitively, this may seem like an obvious place to start mobilizing. However, if the lifter is symmetrically short of the 3-4-inch mark and has no history of ankle injury, maybe it just is not in his or her cards to have Gumby ankles, and other movement strategies will yield more bang for the buck. It's still a point of mobility emphasis, just not *as* concerning as the asymmetry described above.

- Having said this, if there is a history of bilateral ankle or foot injury, or history of wearing restrictive footwear for long periods of time (military personnel, for example), then this will likely be a mobilization emphasis. Refer to Chapter 7.
- As a side note, one can also start the test at a fist-distance between the foot and the wall, or measure 4 inches between the big toe and the wall, instead of starting with the big toe against the wall. If you can reach the wall on the first shot, then the test is done.

Overhead Squat

The unicorn. The White Buffalo. The overhead squat. Everyone wants theirs to be beautiful, and there is a sense of shame when one cannot perform said movement. Just kidding. Kind of. (Side note: weightlifters can be very judgmental.) Obviously, to some degree, the ability to perform a reasonable semblance of an overhead squat has an impact on the lifter's ability to perform a full snatch, so looking at it is important if you plan on loading up some snatches. For a beginner, use a dowel or PVC pipe. For a lifter with any experience, a barbell works.

Starting Position

- Barefoot (we will elevate heels later if need be).
- Place your feet roughly shoulder-width apart. If you're an experienced lifter, your normal squat stance is what we will use.
- Turning your toes out is absolutely fine as long as it is symmetrical (Figure 5.05). Experienced lifters should use their normal amount of toe-out.
- Use a grip wide enough for the dowel to rest in your hip crease at arms' length.
- Lock your arms out overhead so that the dowel is over the back of your head and upper back.

Execution

- Keeping the elbows locked straight and the bar overhead, squat down as deeply as possible while maintenance the feet flat on the ground (Figure 5.06).

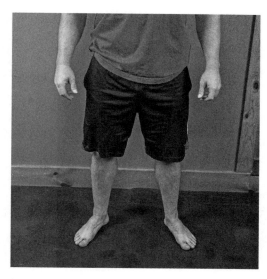

Figure 5.05 This is what approximately 30 degrees of toe-out looks like. Anything up to this range is a perfectly reasonable position to squat from. Some lifters may even require more, and if other principles are followed (discussed later), there is nothing wrong with it.

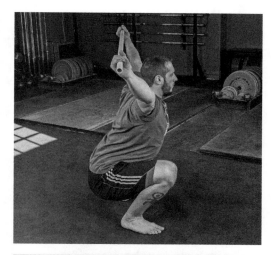

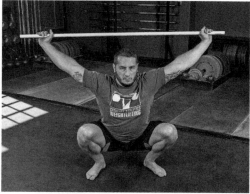

Figure 5.06 Example of an overhead squat that meets all criteria to pass the screen

Key Points

- Does it hurt (ankles, knees, hips, back, shoulders)?
  - > If yes, make a note and proceed with caution. Use discretion if possible referral to a professional is needed.
- You are looking for the following movement criteria:
  - > The dowel stays directly over the back of the head/upper back throughout the entire movement rather than shifting forward (Figure 5.07).
  - > There is minimal change in the spinal curves from the beginning to end of the squat (The torso is allowed to be inclined forward, as this is not the same as changing the spinal curves). Also, some degree of "butt wink" (posterior pelvic tilt/lumbar flexion at bottom of squat) is very common, and not necessarily problematic. In fact, a subtle degree of this has actually been shown to be a normal component of the deep squat. How much is too much? Great question, and it certainly depends on context. Have the lifter pause at the bottom of the squat, and if the low back is still lordotic or flat, it is likely not a concern. In many cases, if you see a butt wink, it is an athlete moving from hyperextension of the lumbar spine to a more neutral position, and not actually going into a position of true lumbar flexion. If it's a case where the athlete is clearly flexing the spine at the bottom of the squat, then it can be an area of correction. (Figure 5.08)
  - > The squat depth places the hip crease below the crease of the knee (Figure 5.09).
  - > The knees track in the same plane throughout the squat—over the middle of the foot, as opposed to *excessive* inward or outward movement of the knees. You know it when you see it. (Figure 5.10)
  - > There is no change in foot position of any kind during the movement. Where the feet start is where they should stay from beginning to end. The feet are our anchor and we want them stable. (Figure 5.11)
- For a beginner or someone new to the overhead squat, you may have to repeat the cues and give them multiple attempts.
- Is the athlete able to meet *all* of the above criteria?
  - > If yes, then the athlete has demonstrated the ability to put his or her joints in the positions that will be trained. You have essentially cleared the requisite mobility requirements to be able to progressively load an overhead squat.
- Does the lifter fail to meet *any* one of the five criteria?
  - > If yes, move on to the assessment portion below.

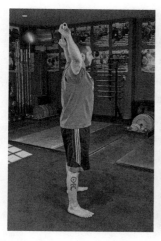
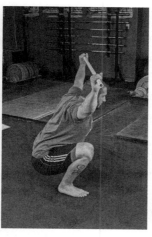

Figure 5.07 This overhead squat does not meet the criterion of the bar staying in the same overhead position. Here the athlete has allowed the bar to shift forward.

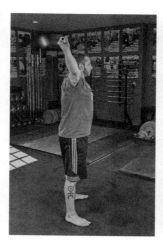
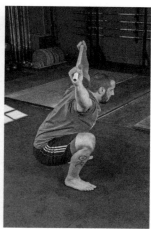

Figure 5.08 This overhead squat does not meet criterion of keeping the spinal curves constant. Here the athlete has deviated by flexing the spine.

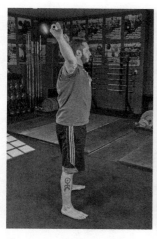
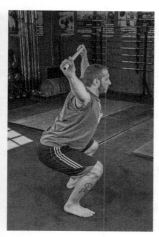

Figure 5.09 This overhead squat does not meet the depth criterion of the hip crease below the knee.

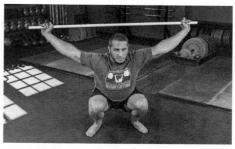
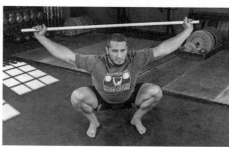

Figure 5.10 These overhead squats do not meet the criterion of the knees tracking in the plane of the foot. Pictured are knees inside and outside this proper path.

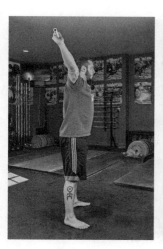
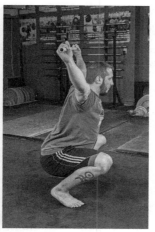

Figure 5.11 (left) This overhead squat does not meet the criterion of keeping the foot position constant throughout the movement, as the heels are coming up off the floor. The toes coming up, rolling to the inside of the foot, rolling to the outside of the foot, or one or both feet spinning on the floor are all criteria-breakers as well. Use your discretion here, as a simple cue to correct these things may be all that is necessary, such as, "Only squat as low as you can without moving your feet."

Other Important Notes

- If the criteria are not met, you still do not have enough information to truly distinguish between a mobility or stability problem or start deeming things as "tight" regardless of the results of the ankle screening. All you know is the athlete cannot overhead squat barefoot.
- If an athlete is able to perform an effortless barefoot overhead squat, and gives you that *What's so hard about this?* look, make note. This individual will likely not need to spend much time stretching or mobilizing body parts in an effort to create actual structural change. The mobility is there already.

Front Squat

Just as we examined the overhead squat for the snatch, we will do the same for the clean by looking at the front squat. For an athlete with weight-lifting experience, use a barbell. For someone that has never performed a front squat before, simply have him or her lightly put the thumbs on the shoulders to mimic the front rack position, or use a lighter object like a training bar or PVC pipe (*if* the athlete can achieve a decent rack position with such a light object).

Starting Position

- Barefoot (we will elevate heels later if need be).
- Place your feet shoulder-width apart. If you're an experienced lifter, your normal squat stance is fine.
- Toe-out is allowed as long as it is symmetrical. If you're an experienced lifter, use your normal amount of toe-out.
- Place your grip on the bar or PVC pipe about 1-3 inches outside the shoulders, or use your normal front squat grip width if you're an experienced lifter.
- Lift your elbows and get your upper arms parallel to the ground or as close as possible.
- Keep your whole hand around the bar as best you can.

Execution

- Squat down as deeply as possible while keeping the feet flat.
- Maintain the elbow and upper arm position. (Figure 5.12)

Key Points

- You are looking for the following movement criteria:
  - › There is minimal to no change in the elbow/upper arm position throughout the movement (Figure 5.13).

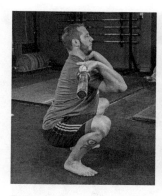 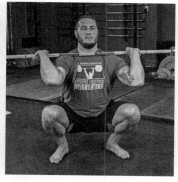 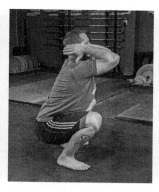 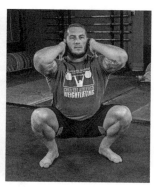

Figure 5.12 Front squats that meet all criteria to pass the screen

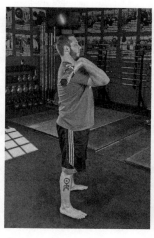 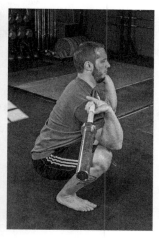

Figure 5.13 This front squat does not meet the criterion of maintaining the elbow/upper arm position.

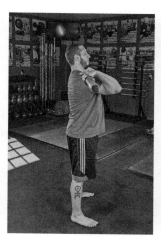 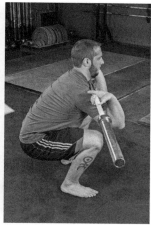

Figure 5.14 This front squat does not meet criterion of keeping the spinal curves constant. Here the athlete has deviated by noticeably flexing the spine.

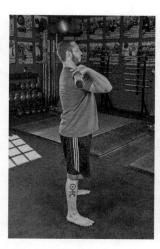 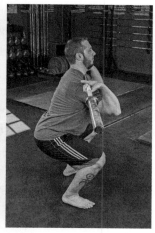

Figure 5.15 This front squat does not meet criterion of hip crease below knee.

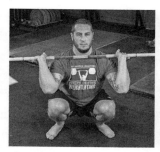 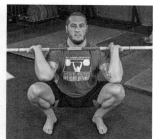

Figure 5.16 This front squat does not meet the criterion of the knees tracking through the plane of the foot.

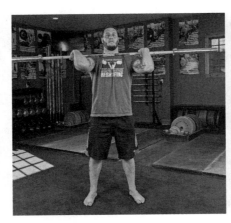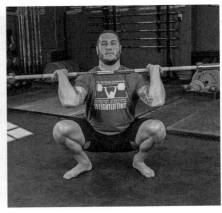

Figure 5.17 This front squat does not meet the criterion of keeping the foot position constant throughout the movement, as the feet are spinning during the squat. The toes or heels coming up off the floor, rolling to the inside of the foot, or rolling to the outside of foot are all criteria-breakers as well. Use your discretion here, as a simple cue to correct these things may be all that is necessary.

> There is minimal change in spinal curves from beginning to end of the movement (Figure 5.14).

> The hip crease is below the crease of the knee in the bottom of the squat (Figure 5.15).

> The knees track over the middle of the foot (Figure 5.16). We are concerned with *excessive* inward or outward movement of the knees.

> There is no change in foot position from beginning to end of movement (Figure 5.17).

- For a beginner or someone new to the front squat, you may have to repeat the cues and give them multiple attempts.

- Is the athlete able to meet *all* of the above criteria with no apprehension or pain?

  > If yes, then it's safe to start progressively loading the front squat, as you have essentially cleared the requisite mobility to perform this movement.

- Does the lifter fail to meet *any* one of the criteria?

  > If yes, move on to the assessment portion below.

  > Keep in mind that just because an athlete does not pass all criteria, it does not mean they are banished from loading the front squat. It just means there may be some things we can clean up that make the pattern more comfortable and sustainable for supporting load. Many lifters will have trouble maintaining a whole hand grip on an empty barbell, for example. For these lifters, adding 40-50kg may aid in allowing them to attain the test position. And maybe they never attain a full hand grip on the bar when front squatting. For the screen, we are interested in what we consider ideals.

Other Important Notes

- Remember, if the criteria are not met, you still do not have enough information to truly distinguish between a mobility or stability problem, regardless of the results of the wrist and ankle screening. All you know is the athlete has difficulty front squatting barefoot.
- If an athlete is able to perform an effortless barefoot front squat, make note. This individual will likely not need to spend much time stretching or mobilizing body parts in an effort to create actual structural change. The mobility is there already.

Movement Tip For an athlete performing a self-assessment, a full-length mirror is beneficial for observing your own patterns and posture. I recommend every gym have a portable mirror for athletes and coaches to assess and correct positions. Being able to simultaneously *see* and *feel* the correct positions, patterns, etc., works wonders for the athlete's brain connections. See it, feel it, practice it, then put the mirror away in the closet once you are comfortable.

Squat Assessment

We have screened the squatting pattern. Nothing was painful, but the athlete was unable to perform a barefoot overhead or front squat to your standard. Do we stop here and hope weightlifting shoes fix the issue? Do we try stretching and mobilizing whatever we can think of? Do we do front and side planks or other ab exercises to increase core strength? Maybe yes, maybe no, to all of that. Let's dive a little deeper to clear the muddy water and determine a better place to start. Remember, screen and assess—don't guess.

Overhead or Front Squat with Elevated Heels

Weightlifting shoes, small plates, or other flat, stable objects can be used to elevate the heels. If shoes are not used, try to make the height no more than 1.5-2 inches. The same protocol is used for the overhead squat and front squat. Elevating the heels does two things: First, it places the ankle joints into relative plantarflexion, allowing the shins to travel further forward—essentially taking an ankle dorsiflexion limitation out of the equation. Second, it provides the athlete with an anterior (forward) weight shift, which makes it much easier to sit the hips down without falling on his or her butt. It's a counterbalance.

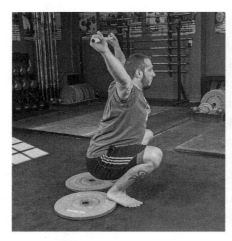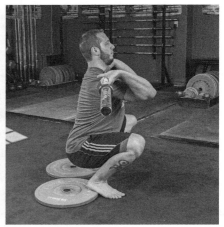

Figure 5.18 Elevating the heels can give you a better idea of the athlete's potential for the squatting movement.

Starting Position

- Start in the same position you did for the overhead or front squat, but with your heels elevated.

Execution

- Same as outlined previously for the overhead or front squat.

Key Points

- Is the lifter able to perform the movement meeting *all* of the criteria described previously for the overhead or front squat with the heels now elevated?
  - › If yes:
    - If ankle mobility was limited during the screen, that may be a factor and will likely be an area of mobility focus.
    - If the ankle screen was clear, but the lifter still benefitted from an elevated heel, then it was likely not the increased dorsiflexion that helped him or her. It was most likely the anterior weight shift. They needed a counterbalance. Ideally your core is your counterbalance. In this case, the lifter has cleared the requisite mobility, but would likely benefit from overhead and front squat stabilization drills. Refer to Chapters 11 and 13.
  - › If no, move to the next regression below.

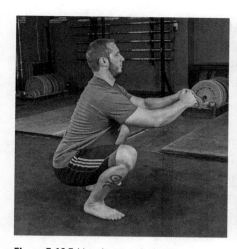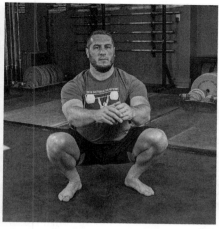

Figure 5.19 Taking the upper body component out of the movement by performing a simple air squat can further tease out what is going on in the squatting pattern.

Air Squat without & with Elevated Heels

The air squat is an easier movement to perform than the overhead or front squat because of the decreased demands of the upper thorax and shoulder girdle to support a very upright/overhead position. The overhead position lengthens the lever that your core must stabilize. There is more slack in the system for the athlete in which to move when the arms are not overhead or in the front rack. It also takes any shoulder limitation off the table, which you would have already identified in the previous chapter.

Starting Position 1

- The position will be the same as the previous squatting tests, but with the arms in front near the ribs or outstretched forward.

Execution

- Squat down as deeply as possible while keeping your feet flat (Figure 5.19).

Key Points

- You are looking for the following criteria:
  - › Minimal change in spinal position from the beginning to the end of the squat.
  - › The hip crease is below the crease of the knee in the bottom of the squat.
  - › The knees track over the middle of the foot (We are looking for *excessive* inward or outward movement of the knees).
  - › There is no change in the foot position.

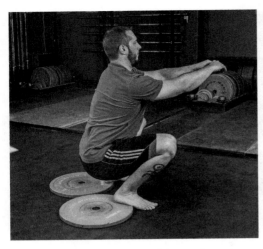

Figure 5.20 Taking the arms out of the equation and elevating the heels gives a more isolated look at the hips' ability to attain a full squat position.

- Is the lifter able to meet *all* of the above criteria?
  - › If yes, and the ankle screen was clear, you have cleared mobility for the lower body. So why was the lifter not able to achieve the overhead or front squat? Perhaps there is a mobility restriction in the shoulder or thoracic region (see upper body screening and assessment previously), or a motor control error when the athlete has to coordinate the position of the ribcage and shoulders along with the pelvis and hips.
    - Refer to Chapters 11 and 13 for overhead and front squat stabilization drills.
  - › If no, move to the next regression.

Starting Position 2

- The position will be the same as Starting Position 1, but with your heels elevated 1.5-2 inches.

Execution

- Squat down as deeply as possible without allowing the feet to move (Figure 5.20).

Key Points

- We are looking for the same criteria as for the air squat.
- Is the athlete able to meet *all* of the criteria when the heels are elevated?
  - › If yes, and the ankle screen was clear, you have cleared mobility of the lower body. However, focused time should be spent finding the lifter's preferred squatting stance and teaching them to create stability within that position. There may still be upper body mobility issues, or lack of motor control when integrating the upper and lower body together, as we discussed with the air squat previously.
    - Refer to squat bottom position drills in Chapter 11.
  - › If no, and the ankle screen was clear, we'll dig deeper into hip mobility.

Counterbalance Squat without & with Elevated Heels

We now move on to a test that involves holding a weight. This may seem counterintuitive, as this would appear to be a progression as opposed to a regression. However, a counterbalance squat can be an extremely useful

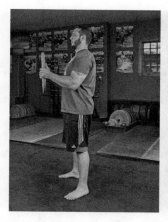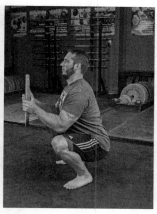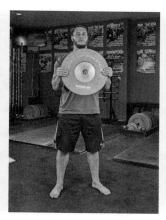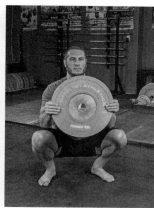

Figure 5.21 Counterbalance Squat Test 1

teaching and assessment tool—holding a weight in front of the body gives the athlete a substantial counterbalance and elicits reflexive abdominal contraction. This allows the athlete to reflexively organize his or her trunk and hip position more effectively without having to be coached on it.

Starting Position 1

- Same as for the air squat, but holding a light kettlebell, dumbbell or plate anywhere from 6-12 inches away from chest (whatever is most comfortable).

Execution

- Squat down as deeply as possible. For this, the cue to "Sit straight down and upright" works well.
- Keep the feet flat.
- Hold the weight in the same position throughout the movement. (Figure 5.21)

Key Points

- We are looking to meet the same criteria as for the air squat.
- Is the lifter able to meet *all* of the criteria?
    > If yes, and the ankle screen was clear, you have cleared mobility for the lower body, and further validated the idea that this athlete will benefit from trunk and pelvis stability work.
        - Refer to squat corrective drills in Chapter 11.
    > If no, and the ankle screen was clear, we may have a hip mobility problem or deeper core stability problem. Move on to the counterbalance squat with elevated heels.

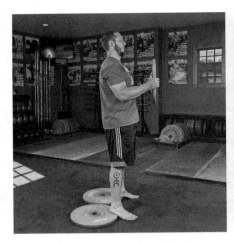
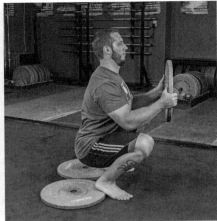

Figure 5.22 Counterbalance Squat Test 2

Starting Position 2

- Same as for the counterbalance squat, but with the heels elevated 1.5-2 inches.
- This one is about as "counterbalancy" as it gets. We are giving the lifter all the help we can to be able to sit down into a full squat.

Execution

- Squat down as deeply as possible. For this, the cue to "Sit straight down and upright" works well.
- Keep the feet flat.
- Hold the weight in the same position throughout the movement. (Figure 5.22)

Key Points

- Is the lifter able to meet *all* of the criteria?
  - ❯ If yes, and the ankle screen was clear, then you have cleared mobility of the lower body and can be relatively certain that this athlete will benefit from things that focus on stabilizing the trunk and pelvis.
    - Be mindful, however, that the athlete is utilizing squatting mechanics that demonstrate realistic carryover to the snatch and clean. For example, with the counterbalance squat, it is possible for a lifter to exhibit a squat in which the shins and torso remain very close to vertical. However, this position is not reminiscent of the squatting mechanics that a weightlifter uses, as the torso and shins need to be inclined forward to some degree to maintain balanced levers.

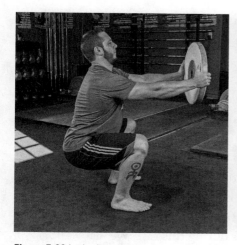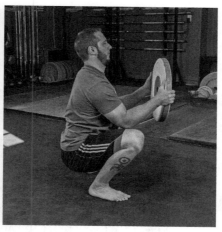

Figure 5.23 In the first picture, you see the athlete performing a squat in which the shins and torso are nearly vertical. This is not a realistic squatting position for a weightlifter and does not allow the assessor or athlete to get a sense of the hip, knee and ankle integration needed for a weightlifting-style deep squat. In the second picture, the athlete is hinging naturally at the hips, knees and ankles. If he or she is able to do this with a counterbalance comfortably and pain-free, then theoretically he or she possess the mobility to attain this position without the counterbalance.

A squat with nearly vertical shins and torso does not give an accurate depiction of ankle and hip mobility as it pertains to the squatting positions most conducive for weightlifting. (Figure 5.23)

- Refer to squat corrective drills in Chapter 11.

> If no, and the ankle screen was clear, move on to Finding Your Squat Stance below.

Finding *Your* Squat Stance

This section will be beneficial for lifters of all levels. For the athlete who went through all of the previous squat tests and still experienced difficulty performing the movement to the standard deemed fit for loading, we shall dig deeper to determine a starting point in building your squatting pattern. For the lifter who is comfortable squatting, these tests can be great reinforcement to your movement, and you may even find a more optimal squatting position than you previously had.

What we are going to do is perform a series of tests and movements that will provide the lifter with insight into to the individual structure of his or her hips and how that will determine individual squatting stance preference.

Supine Passive Hip Flexion with External & Internal Rotation

Here we are assessing global hip mobility. We are lying on our backs and moving the hips passively, so there is little to no stability required. The goal here is to determine an initial understanding of individual hip and pelvis structure.

Starting Position

- Lie supine on the floor with your hips and knees straight, ankles lightly dorsiflexed, and toes pointed up to the ceiling.

Execution

- Exhale through your mouth to get the front/bottom ribs down; you may feel your low back flatten against the floor slightly, but maintain a slight amount of lordosis. You do not need to actively brace the abs during this test. We just want to eliminate any excessive low back arch in order to get a true feel for hip mobility. Maintain the same relationship between your back and the floor throughout this test.
- Pull one knee to your chest with the foot in line with the knee. Make a note of how this feels in your hip joint. Is the motion comfortable and free? Or does your hip feel crowded and/or pinchy in the crease or outside?
  - › Now move the knee up and around more toward the outside. Slowly and gently test different abduction angles of the hip joint relative to the straight plane that we tested initially. Did you find an angle that was most comfortable, i.e. your hip felt mobile and free without feelings of pinching in the joint? You have begun the process of identifying your optimal squat stance.
  - › Perform the same test on the opposite leg. Find the most comfortable and mobile position for your hip.
- Now we add components of hip rotation into the same test, further determining the structural makeup of our hips. For hip flexion plus internal and external rotation (Figure 5.24):
  - › Keeping one leg straight with the ankles flexed up and toes facing the ceiling, flex the other hip by bringing the knee toward the chest and stop at about 90 degrees.
    - Rotate the test hip into external rotation, then into internal rotation. Slowly and gently move back and forth between the two testing end ranges.
    - Then, gently explore different ranges of flexion the way that we did previously by moving up and around and out to the side with the hip. This time, test internal and external rotation in the various angles.
    - It's important to keep the other leg relatively straight and motionless to limit accessory motions.

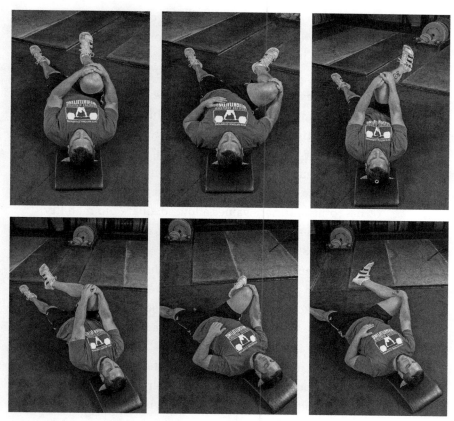

Figure 5.24 In this series of pictures, we are exploring hip range of motion in an effort to determine squatting stance for an individual lifter. We begin by exploring relative amounts of hip flexion and abduction, which will give insight into how wide a lifter is comfortable squatting. We then explore hip internal and external rotation, which will give insight into what angle the feet will point.

- Monitor the pelvis and low back, and keep those areas motionless as well.

Key Points

- Is the athlete able to comfortably flex both hips well past 90 degrees with both external and internal rotation bias with no feelings of restrictions, asymmetries or impingement?
  - › If yes, then hip joint mobility, as a stand alone, may not be of primary concern, and any perceived movement limitations in previous testing may have been based on motor control deficits.
- Was there side-to-side asymmetry, restriction or feeling of impingement (pinching) noted?
  - › If yes, restoring hip mobility/congruency to the restricted plane of motion may be an appropriate strategy in the movement program. These things will inherently be addressed in our corrections.

- The position of the hip that felt the most comfortable in regard to the various combinations of flexion and rotation that were tested will likely closely mimic the position of your hips when squatting.
  - › Most athletes will have slightly more external hip rotation mobility than internal hip rotation. This makes intuitive sense, as sitting cross-legged is more comfortable than W-sitting for most. The exact "normal" ranges of motion vary from source to source but we'll put them at 45-60 degrees of external rotation and about 35 degrees of internal rotation. These values allow adequate hip mobility to perform a squat below parallel with a small degree of toe-out (15-30 degrees).
  - › If pulling your knee straight to your chest was very comfortable, and putting your hip into internal rotation at various abduction angles felt very loose and free, you may be an athlete that is more comfortable squatting with toes relatively straight forward.
  - › If pulling your knee straight to your chest was uncomfortable versus out to the side, and you felt you had substantially more hip external rotation than internal rotation, you are probably going to squat with your toes out a bit more. The exact amount is to be determined. This is also not "bad", as many have come to believe—it's simply a matter of anatomy.

Discussion Point: Is hip external rotation really that important in the squat? The answer to this question, of course, depends on context. As a rule of thumb, when your foot is fixed to the ground during a squat, we need enough hip external rotation to keep the knee in line with the feet. There are subtle variations to this from lifter to lifter. With this in mind, think back to the hip external rotation test described above. Most of you probably had roughly 45 degrees of hip external rotation with the hip flexed to 90 degrees. Let's say some of you were limited to 30 degrees, or even 20 degrees. Are our knees ever 20 degrees outside of our feet when we squat? No. They are not. The point here is that hip external rotation as a stand-alone does not make or break squatting position. It must be viewed in context with the relative amount of hip flexion and abduction needed to maintain the foot-over-knee position regardless of stance width, which we will look at later in the section.

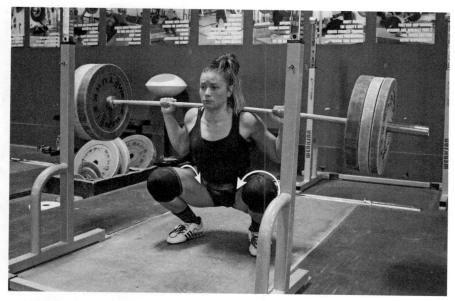

Figure 5.25 A certain degree of hip internal rotation allows an athlete to sit comfortably in between the hips. Note that internal hip rotation does not equal valgus knee collapse. One can express internal hip rotation mobility at the bottom of the squat and still stack the knee over the foot.

Supine Wall Hip Internal Rotation Test

With the above said, in regard to the importance of hip external rotation (or lack thereof) in the squat, accessory hip *internal* rotation has just as much importance in order to comfortably maintain normal hip, knee and ankle tracking throughout the entirety of the movement. It seems counterintuitive to think that hip internal rotation is important for a squat, since it is common to associate such a movement with "faulty" knee position (valgus or "knocked" knees). However, hip internal rotation aids in the ability to sit comfortably between our hips once we hit a very deep squat position—that's the arthrokinematic roll and glide that we discussed in Chapter 2 (Figure 5.25).

Below is a bonus assessment. It is not imperative to perform in regards to finding your optimal individual bottom position, but it is an easy way to determine your hips' capacity for internal rotation, which can guide you to know what type of squatter you will be; and for some, may clue them into the fact that they possess adequate levels of hip IR and need not go cranking away as an intervention.

Starting Position

- Lie on your back with your feet flat against a wall.
- Hold a foam roller between your knees with your feet oriented straight forward.
- Bend the hips to just above a parallel squat position with the knees bent 90 degrees.

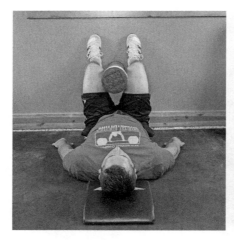
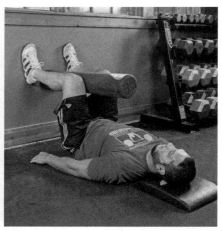

Figure 5.26 Starting position for the Supine Wall Hip Internal Rotation test

- Lay your arms at your sides or on your chest.
- Allow your upper back, lower back and tailbone to rest comfortably on the floor. (Figure 5.26)

Execution

- Exhale through your mouth to get the front/bottom ribs down; you may feel your low back flatten toward the floor slightly, but it should not be pressed completely flat. For the purposes of this test, we want the spinal curves to mimic a neutral spine in a squat—the lower back should remain *slightly* lordotic.
- While gently squeezing the foam roller between your knees, walk your feet straight out to the sides about 30 degrees, putting the hips into internal rotation.
  > Note any feelings of side-to-side differences or limitations.
  > Bring your feet back to the center and move your hips 1-2 inches closer to the wall.
  > In this new position, walk your feet straight out to the sides while keeping roller between your knees, making note of what you feel.
  > Bring your feet back to the center and inch your hips closer to the wall. Repeat the internal rotation test by walking the feet back out to the sides.
  > Continue this process until you have moved your hips past 90 degrees of flexion, and/or you begin to feel significant limitations in your hip range of motion. (Figure 5.27)

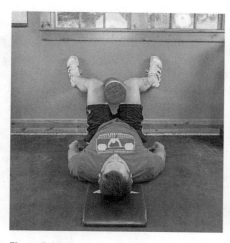
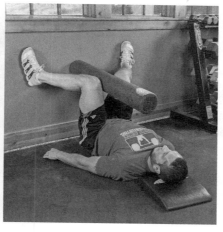

Figure 5.27 For the Supine Wall Hip Internal Rotation test, continue to inch your way toward the wall, walking your feet out to the sides roughly 30 degrees every time you renew a position.

Key Points

- Did you feel a limitation in one or both hips to internally rotate as you approached the wall?
  - › If yes, this may be an area of mobility that should be addressed, especially if that feeling of restriction was also experienced with previous tests and during training.
    - Refer to the Snatch, Clean and Jerk chapters for hip mobility corrections.
- Did the athlete feel no apparent asymmetry or limitation, or did a bilateral limitation occur only when the hips were well past 90 degrees?
  - › If so, then hip internal rotation will probably not be a primary focus for his or her mobility strategies.
  - › **Important** Hip structure/anatomy may dictate the hip's capacity to rotate to a large degree. We have seen individuals who W-sit without difficulty but cannot sit cross-legged and vise versa. This has much more to do with the bony anatomy that they were born with versus some kind of mobility restriction that we can correct. This point will be reiterated as we go through corrections.

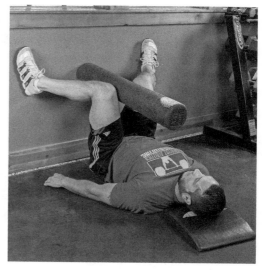

Figure 5.28 This lifter likely does not need to spend any more time mobilizing his hips into internal rotation.

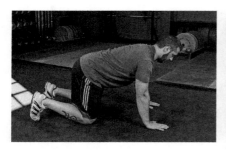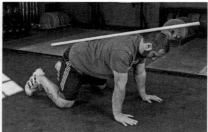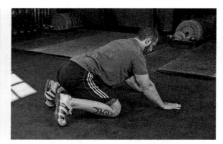

Figure 5.29 The Quadruped Rockback test

Quadruped Rockback with Neutral Spine

The quadruped position is a great tool because it resembles a squat but requires less internal stability from the athlete and provides more external stability from the floor. This allows us to better evaluate without subtle compensations that are hard to pick up.

Starting Position

- Place your hands and knees on the floor with your elbows directly underneath your shoulders and your knees flexed to 90 degrees and outside of your hips at the approximate width they would be in the squat when standing.
- Keep your toes and ankles flexed underneath with your feet approximately the same width as they would be in a standing squat.
- Set a neutral spine for weightlifting posture. A partner or a coach can use a dowel to cue this position.
- This position should mimic a slightly-above-parallel squat. (Figure 5.29)

Execution

- Rock your hips back toward your heels so that the hips flex past 90 degrees without changing spinal position (you may keep the PVC there to cue) (Figure 5.29).
- Make note of how free and mobile the hips feel in this position and return back to start position.
- Now, widen your knees approximately an inch and bring your feet closer together. This will put the hips into relative external rotation. Repeat the rockback test, making note of how free and mobile the hips feel. Return to the start position.
- Return your knees back to the original width that you used for your normal stance and widen your feet so that they are even with your knees. This puts the hips in relative internal rotation. Repeat the rockback test, making note of how free and mobile the hips feel in comparison to the other two positions.
- For a truer representation of a squat, perform the above sequence on your forearms. This will incline the torso forward more like it will be in a squatting pattern.

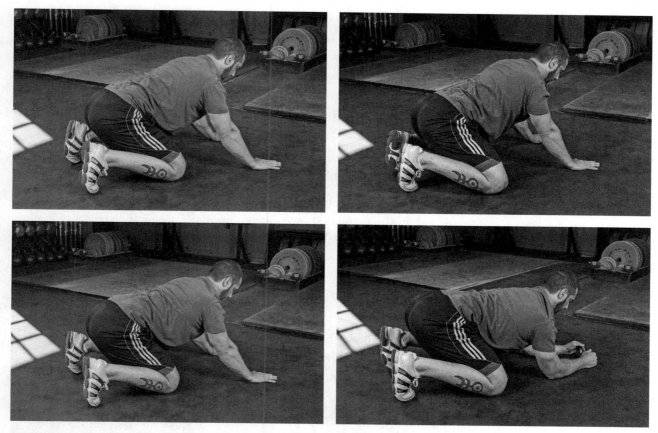

Figure 5.30 Perform the Quadruped rockback test with the knees slightly wider than the feet as a starting point. Gauge how far you are able to rock back with minimal change in lumbar curve. The perform the test with the feet narrower and hips wider, putting the hips into more relative external rotation. Next perform the test with the feet wider and knees narrower, putting the hips into more relative internal rotation. Finally, repeat the sequence on the forearms for a more accurate representation of the hip mobility needed for a deep squat.

- Find a combination of knee and foot width that allows you to rockback into the deepest position while maintaining a neutral spine. This will likely be a close representation of your comfortable squatting stance when you are standing. (Figure 5.30)

Movement Discussion Either you or your athlete may demonstrate much different movement patterns when comparing the previous *standing* squat tests to the quadruped test above. Commonly, novice lifters have difficulty achieving a full squat without compensation, yet the athlete can rock both hips back past 90 degrees of hip flexion without changing his or her spinal curves. If this is the case, and the ankle screen was clear, the lifter is demonstrating adequate mobility in the lower body to perform a squat—at least to the depth where the athlete is able to rockback without any change in back position. If you were to flip the lifter onto his or her feet, it would look like a pretty good squat.

Yet the athlete's standing squat tests did not look like that. So where is the disconnect? His or her hip and ankle structure does not change suddenly when that athlete is standing, does it? What *does* change is the amount of external stability the athlete is given. Theoretically, the athlete has the same joint mobility in a quadruped position that he or she has when standing. However, he or she does not have the ability to demonstrate that mobility when standing because he or she does not possess the internal stability/motor control to maintain the position. In quadruped, with the added external stability from the floor, he or she is able to demonstrate full mobility.

Counterbalance Squat with Varied Stances

We return to the counterbalance squat as an experimental tool to find a lifter's optimal squat stance. The counterbalance of the weight will allow the athlete to comfortably try several different stance widths and foot position combinations. While moving through various options, keep in mind what the previous tests have revealed about your hip structure.

Execution

- Hold a weight 6-12 inches away from the chest (whatever is most comfortable) just as you did previously. Assume your previously normal squat stance (in terms of both width and

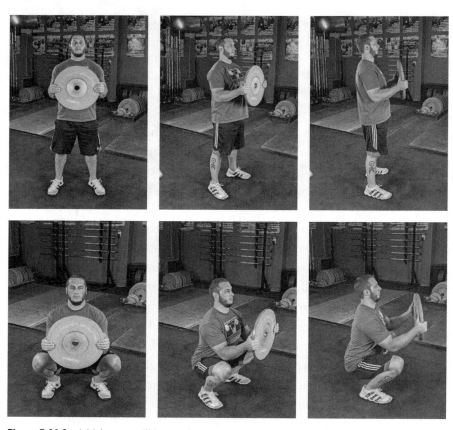

Figure 5.31 Our initial stance will be with feet roughly shoulder width apart and toes turned out slightly. This will be the baseline that we compare other positions to.

amount of toe-out), or place your feet roughly shoulder width apart with the feet pointed out about 15-20 degrees.

- Perform 5 counterbalance squats, focusing on sitting straight down between your feet. Make note of how free and mobile your hips feel here, and the ease with which you are able to squat down. (Figure 5.31)

- Now perform the test with the same stance width, but point your feet completely straight. 5 squats. Make note of how this feels in comparison to the previous position in regard to ease and comfort of the movement.

- Now perform the test with the same stance width, but point your feet out more than in the first squat. Try to maintain each knee directly over the middle of the corresponding foot. 5 squats. Compare the feel of this position to the previous two.

- You will now perform this exact sequence but with a narrower stance and a wider stance than the initial test. Within each stance width, experiment with your normal amount of toe-out, feet completely straight, feet turned out more than normal, and anything in between.

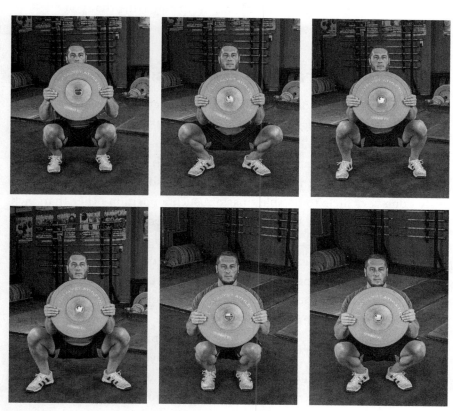

Figure 5.32 Stance variations for the counterbalance squat. Initial stance width with feet straight forward; initial stance width with feet turned out more; wider stance with feet straight forward; wider stance with feet turned out; narrower stance with feet straight forward; narrower stance with feet turned out.

- As long as previous testing was pain free and the lifter has no other existing injuries, this squat series is appropriate to implement for the barbell back squat, front squat and overhead squat in order to find the lifter's optimal stance for those lifts. It is not uncommon for the lifter's stances of those three squat variations to differ from each other slightly as we take into account the subtle variations in torso angle that accompanies them.

Key Points

- You are looking for the stance that allows you to sit into the most comfortable squat position with minimal change in spinal curves while keeping your feet flat and your knees over your feet. Of course, squat depth is a consideration here, but you do not want to sacrifice the abovementioned parameters for the sake of maximizing squat depth. This goes back to our need to balance both mobility and stability. The stance width and foot turnout combination that gives you the deepest squat may not be the one that gives you the best control of your spinal curves or knee and foot positions. These considerations pertain to all variations of squatting that you implement this series with.

Summary of Screening & Assessing The Squat

Do not deem a muscle or joint as tight or restricted just by looking at a squat. What looks like tightness can in fact be weakness and/or instability. Screen and assess—don't guess.

Not everyone is meant to squat narrow with toes forward. It is not some type of badge of honor to be able to do so. Lifters who can have likely done very little to be able to attain such a position other than pick the appropriate parents. We have to respect anatomy and understand that there are simply some things that cannot be changed. Your hip and pelvis structure will dictate your squat stance to a large degree. This is not to say that focused work on specific movement parameters will have no impact on how you squat. Of course it will—that's the point of this book. But we will respect the laws of nature.

Some of you probably identified asymmetries in your ankles or hips, especially during the squat stance series. You may have identified one hip that rotated further externally or internally than the other, one side that felt restricted or "crowded" while you were testing your rockback or squat, etc. Many asymmetries are just a normal part of being a human and will have little bearing on your weightlifting performance. Sometimes they will have more of an effect. Obviously, pinpointing exact mechanisms for individual asymmetry through a book is impossible. This is why we will always work the corrections on both sides initially, and if we find that one side is giving us more trouble than the other (which may correlate to what you found during the screen and assessment), then you will simply spend more time there. Most things will balance out over time with consistent, focused work.

In regard to the Squat Stance series, you can easily reverse the order of the tests. In fact, logistically it makes more sense to reverse them. I chose the order that I did for the purposes of teaching the reader what pure hip motion feels like first. This is much easier to explain in supine, as other variables are taken out of the equation. You may never do it in that order again, and that is totally fine. To summarize this point, the tests were laid out in the following order:

Screen

- Ankle Dorsiflexion
- Overhead Squat
- Front Squat

Assessment

- Overhead or Front Squat with Elevated Heels
- Air Squat without & with Elevated Heels
- Counterbalance Squat without & with Elevated Heels

Squat Stance Series

- Supine Passive Hip Flexion with External & Internal Rotation
- Supine Wall Hip Internal Rotation
- Quadruped Rockback with Neutral Spine
- Counterbalance Squat with Varied Stances

Below is an example of an order than may be more time efficient. You may find that the last 2 or 3 squat series tests are unnecessary to perform if the lifter is able to move through the previous tests without incident.

Screen

- Ankle Dorsiflexion
- Overhead Squat
- Front Squat

Assessment

- Overhead or Front Squat with Elevated Heels
- Air Squat without and with Elevated Heels
- Counterbalance Squat without and with Elevated Heels

Squat Stance Series

- Counterbalance Squat with Varied Stances
- Quadruped Rockback with Neutral Spine
- Supine Wall Hip Internal Rotation Test
- Supine Passive Hip Flexion with External & Internal Rotation

The Squat: Screening & Assessment Example Cases

Here are different examples of what you might see when taking a lifter through these tests. The cases reveal slightly different placement in regards to the Mobility-Stability Continuum, and in turn, slightly different strategies are used to correct.

Example Case 1

Findings

- Screen
  - › Ankle: normal
  - › Overhead squat: unable to achieve full depth
- Assessment
  - › Overhead squat with heel lift: all required squat parameters passed

Correctives Implemented

- Stability and movement corrections in standing, focused on teaching the lifter optimal trunk and pelvic position to attain a full squat.

Example Case 2

Findings

- Screen
  - › Ankles: normal
  - › Overhead squat on flat ground: bar comes forward, poor depth.
  - › Front squat on flat ground: elbows drop, poor depth.
- Assessment
  - › Overhead and front squats with elevated heels: findings unchanged
  - › Restricted internal rotation on right side.
  - › Air squat on flat ground: full depth, upper back rounding.
  - › Counterbalance squat: all parameters passed.

Correctives Implemented

- Ground-based: ribcage positioning, thoracic spine and overhead mobility-stability training.
- Integrate improved overhead mobility into squatting variations with counterbalances, then progress to flat ground.

Example Case 3

Findings

- Screen
  › Left ankle: 2 inches away from wall; right ankle: 2.5 inches away from wall.
  › Overhead squat and front squat on flat ground: feet spin out as lifter descends; poor depth; lumbar flexion at bottom.
- Assessment
  › Overhead and front squat with elevated heels: all parameters passed.

Correctives Implemented

- Ground-based ankle mobility strategies with focus on maintaining a stable foot position. Integrate this into barefoot counterbalance squat variations, with focus on using newly acquired range of motion.

Summary Of Screening & Assessment

As stated previously, the tests in this section are simply tools and recommendations that can help to point you in the right direction. It would be helpful to run through all of them as a coach or athlete to become familiar with the movements and to establish a baseline of movement competency with yourself or your lifters. You may find a certain combination of tests (different than how I presented it here) that you feel generally covers your bases, and that's great. Regardless, I would also suggest retesting certain things frequently throughout a training cycle to gauge improvement or maintenance.

With these tests, we use movement to identify competency. We started broad and narrowed down. If the lifter felt a "sticky" joint during one of the movements, perhaps that's an area to mobilize, but you used focused movement and positions to figure that out, as opposed to blindly trying to stretch or mobilize every body part at once. This is where the 45-minute warm-up can occur. Trust me, I've been there.

For the coach, initially you'll want to limit cueing for the athlete during a screen or assessment, but you will begin to identify common patterns very quickly using this approach. After a short while, you will be able to devise your corrective plan in your head before the tests are finished, and may be able to make improvements in perceived quality of movement almost immediately simply from coaching.

Of course this is not an "anti-mobility work" message; however, if all you have been doing is stretching and mobilizing and your weightlifting positions are not easier to attain or have not improved, then you are probably not paying enough attention to the other side of the mobility-stability continuum. As many of you will see when you go through a few of these tests, having all the mobility in the world means nothing if you cannot stabilize enough to demonstrate it.

You saw that with the "positional hacks" you could become more or less mobile simply by changing your bony position without mobilizing or stretching a thing. Pelvic position influences hip mobility. Ribcage position influences shoulder mobility. Go back to any of the other tests that were difficult and focus on the breathing sequence that we have discussed and stabilizing your "can of stability" to see if you can create more change.

Finally, what exactly are you supposed to do with the information that you gathered in this section? Try the drills that are to follow, keeping in mind what was observed and discovered during testing, and spending the majority of your warm-up and corrective time there. Any corrective drill is meant to be a teaching tool that will be integrated into your barbell training and will aid to optimize MV and facilitate MSA.

Here are all of the screening tests listed in a way that is easy to progress through logistically in case you would rather implement things that way. Then, incorporate the appropriate assessment tools from each section if limitations are identified.

Screenings

- Forward Bending
- Backward Bending
- Hip Hinge
- Upright Row with Snatch Grip
- Apley Scratch
- Overhead Squat
- Front Squat
- Standing or Half Kneeling Back to Wall Shoulder Flexion
- Ankle Dorsiflexion
- Wrist Extension
- Active Straight Leg Raise
- Thomas Test

■ PART III

Building The Weightlifting Movements

This section is a monster and most likely contains the information that you have been waiting for. As we progress through the following chapters, keep in mind what we have continuously reiterated—that motor control and motor skill acquisition is a process. Movement is a skill like any other, which requires consistent and focused practice, including the sport-specific skills of the snatch and clean & jerk. There is a theory of the stages of learning that looks like this:

1. Unconscious Incompetence
2. Conscious Incompetence
3. Conscious Competence
4. Unconscious Competence

Essentially, we go from screwing up a skill without even knowing it, to performing that skill well without having to think about it. It becomes automatic. In the chapters to come, many of you will be moving *back and forth* through these stages of learning, and that is normal. We start with focused and conscious practice on more general movement skills, and eventually integrate our newly acquired skills into our sport practice. This sequence follows the training law of specificity, in which we build a competent foundation of general movement and slowly funnel it to movement skills specific to the sport of weightlifting.

Objectives

1. Learn how to use ground-based/positional drills to not only prepare the body for movement, but to teach the lifter

optimal body positioning for the weightlifting movements before the barbell is used.

2. Provide appropriate strategies for the optimal balance of mobility and stability to improve movement related to the snatch and clean & jerk.
3. Learn to integrate newly acquired mobility and motor control into the barbell lifts and their variations.
4. Provide a feasible, time efficient warm-up and movement preparation template that an athlete can utilize before or during daily training or competition.

CHAPTER 6

Programming Considerations

In this chapter, we will discuss how to implement training preparation and corrective strategies for the weightlifter. By following the guidelines that will be discussed, the lifter or coach should be able to devise a strategy based on the athlete's individual needs, which may have been determined in our screening & assessment chapters. The goal will be to maximize time efficiency while making a perceptible positive change in movement based on your standard. We then integrate that change into the barbell lifts.

We start by outlining guidelines in regard to corrective programming that form the *hows*, *whys* and *whats*.

Objectives

1. Discuss proposed theories and mechanisms of corrective strategies (how they work).
2. Create a framework with which to structure feasible, time-efficient training preparation and corrective programming for the snatch and clean & jerk.
3. Provide appropriate strategies to address mobility-stability needs related to weightlifting within the proposed framework.

Guidelines To Training Prep & Corrective Programming

1. Focus On Making A Change in Perceived Quality, Not Structure

With any mobilization, stretch, activation drill, core exercise, etc., we are making a *short-term* change in the way you move. You may have experienced feeling looser or more stable after a simple intervention, and that is great. We will take advantage of that over and over. However, understand those types of quick changes are neurologically based and often do not last long. They must be integrated with speed and load (more powerful stressors to elicit adaptation) or they will likely not contribute to MSA. This leads into an important discussion:

Mobility Implements: Self-Soft Tissue Work AKA Myofascial Release

"The greatest enemy of knowledge is not ignorance, it is the illusion of knowledge." —Stephen Hawking

Self: Performed without someone else's assistance, typically with various types of implements (e.g. foam roller or lacrosse ball).

Myo: Muscle

Fascia: Soft tissue component of connective tissue that is part of a body-wide force transmission system (we think).

Release: Eh. We'll talk about it.

Self-myofascial release (SMR) is all the rage, and for good reason. It works really well to decrease *perceived* tightness and restrictions in range of motion, which is why we will use it.

Having Said That... It's important to know the mechanism of *how* a technique or corrective strategy works (or maybe more relevant in this case, how it *doesn't* work) in order to implement it most appropriately and effectively. The use of a foam roller is a common form of SMR and has been studied a bit. Here is what the literature says:

- Foam rolling may improve joint range of motion *acutely* with bouts ranging from 30-60 seconds with effects lasting 1-10 minutes afterwards, but the effects may not differ from static stretching.
- There is no change in strength or power output when foam rolling is performed, versus static stretching which *trends* towards *decreasing* these measures of performance.
- There is preliminary evidence that foam rolling *acutely* improves arterial function by increasing nitric oxide (which dilates blood vessels) compared to no treatment.
- Foam rolling may decrease perceived muscle soreness associated with exercise when performed at 0, 24, and 48 hours after a hard training session, compared to no treatment. Similarly, acute levels of muscle soreness associated with exercise

were reduced for 30 minutes after one bout of foam rolling, versus no treatment at all.

To summarize the relevant points:

- SMR can provide *short-term* mobility improvements.
- We do not know what time duration is ideal. 30 seconds may be as beneficial as 60 seconds.
- Short bouts of SMR probably do not significantly reduce power output.
- SMR may reduce the *perception* of muscle soreness and tenderness up to 2 days following the training session.
- SMR may temporarily improve blood flow to the area.

How It *Doesn't* Work (to improve range of motion, decrease soreness, etc.):

- Research seems to indicate that the external forces required to cause true, structural deformation of deep fascial tissues that we would be targeting with a foam roller are well beyond that which we can tolerate. Based on this info, we can infer that the force that a foam roller provides on our tissue is not likely to be high enough and is not applied long enough (the duration needed would be impractical for any athlete) to cause the shear for true structural deformation/change *in that moment*.
- In other words, with the research that we have at this time, it is inaccurate to say that foam rollers, lacrosse balls, bands, (insert favorite mobility toy here), etc. are "breaking up scar tissue", "releasing adhesions", changing the "viscosity" of tissue, etc. And if you think about it, THANK GOODNESS our tissues are not that fragile. We'd all have huge dents in our upper traps from the barbell and our shoulders would disintegrate when we caught a snatch. Tissue adaptation is a *process*, it is not a single event, and we are not made of clay.

How It *Might* Work (to improve range of motion, decrease soreness, etc.):

- **Theory 1** Pressure from the implement redistributes water content in the tissue and rehydrates it.
- **Theory 2** It stimulates sensory receptors in the affected area, which send a message to your brain, which then sends a message back to the corresponding muscle to relaxed its contracted state.
- **Theory 3** (most likely) Inhibits pain signals from the central nervous system, subsequently increasing tolerance to stretch and pressure, and reducing the *perception* of soreness.

Now you may be saying, "Who cares *why* it works, as long as it works?" It matters with respect to *how* you implement these techniques:

- **Intensity** Since you are probably not "breaking up your tissues", you do not need to cause pain or use these implements with intense pressure. In fact, that's likely defeating the purpose, since we are looking for sensory inhibition. Making your eyes pop out with pain will likely just cause you to tighten up more to protect.

- **Duration** since it seems that the mobility benefits from SMR are short-term, it is important to keep the bouts as short as possible, in order to then integrate that new mobility with some type of movement. Think *least investment, maximum return* or *minimum effective dose*. If your low back erectors feel tight, and you foam roll them for 20 seconds and they don't feel tight anymore—Boom! Foam roller did its job. Doesn't have to be more complicated than that, and 5 more minutes in the same spot is not going to provide 10 times the relief. That's the mistake we see athletes making—spending 20-30 minutes rolling around, because the mobility benefits that they gained 15 minutes ago have probably dissipated. Remember: short bouts—make a perceived change and move on. Now, because there are reported benefits of SMR on delayed onset muscle soreness, implementing it for longer bouts after training or on your free time is fair game. If you've got the free time, go for it. Just remember our discussion on intensity—it's supposed to *inhibit* soreness, not create it.

Static Stretching

It is important to have a similar discussion on the topic of static stretching as it relates to mobility and performance, as it is very commonly implemented in lifters' regimens. Here is what the literature says:

- Static stretching has not been shown to prevent injury, and flexibility measurements have not been shown to predict injury.
- ROM improvements from a single stretching bout typically last less than 30 minutes, with dosing extremely varied across studies.
- The increases in muscle extensibility observed after single bouts or short-term stretching programs (3-8 weeks) are due to modifying sensation, or increasing the *tolerance to stretch* rather than structural changes in the musculotendinous unit.

- There is evidence to show that static stretching bouts can decrease top-end power output (vertical jump for example), especially if held for longer than 60 seconds. HOWEVER, when post-stretch dynamic activities were included, the decrease in performance was mitigated.

To summarize the relevant points:

- Flexibility is not a gold standard to prevent injury. To support our bias, we'll *infer* that stability and strength need to be incorporated to that range of motion in order to be protective against injury.
- Stretching can certainly increase range of motion, but similar to mobility implements, the changes seem to be transient and more neurophysiological in nature than structural.
- Static stretching may decrease power output momentarily, but most lifters perform enough empty bar and lighter warm-up sets that these power decreases are likely minimal.

So, we will incorporate static stretching in the same way that we do SMR:

- Interspersed when desired.
- Short bouts—minimum effective dose.
- Intensity—enough to make a perceived change in range of motion, tightness, soreness, etc.
- Coupled with a stability and/or loading strategy.

What *does* cause permanent changes in structure you ask? Repetition, load and time. Moving through a desired range, loading it, and doing that over and over for the course of months. Your tissues will adapt accordingly. It's a process, not a single event.

Developing that range along with the MSA is our priority and short bouts of SMR and/or stretching in combination with a corrective strategy can augment that. It's useful, but probably the least important component of our strategies.

2. Anatomy Will Dictate Some Things

- Not everyone is meant to squat narrow with the toes forward.
- Some internal rotation of the shoulders may actually be a more comfortable, stable position for some lifters.

These are just a couple of examples of things that will be exemplified. Striving to improve certain joint ranges of motion will be a focus of ours in many cases, but at the same time, trying to force your body into positions where your bones are not built to go can be an exercise in futility. Of course, there are plenty of people who can squat beautifully with their feet perfectly straight, and that absolutely works for them; however, it's probably not because of their go-to mobility drill, and has much more to do with the parents that they picked.

Hopefully, you got a sense of your individual structure in our screening and assessment chapters. We must respect anatomy.

3. Position Regressions & Lift Variations

As we know, our ultimate goal is MSA as it relates to the fast and powerful moves of the snatch and clean & jerk. Any training modality that we utilize will have varying levels of specificity and carryover to those two lifts—with the snatch and clean & jerk themselves eliciting the most specific adaptation for weightlifting MSA, and something like foam rolling the quadriceps having very low specificity and eliciting low levels of adaptation in regard to the sport. Ideally, we use the snatch and clean & jerk to develop the positions for the snatch and clean & jerk. This is probably obvious to most.

But many times, utilizing regressed positions and/or lift variations can facilitate the process, by reducing the stress/threat of the activity for motor learning purposes. They are teaching tools. For example:

- For a lifter who struggles with overhead position, a supine overhead exercise in which he or she is much more supported will allow him or her to be able to focus on the specific motor task of controlling overhead range with a neutral trunk (dissociating shoulder movement) without having to deal with other variables. Of course, a supine exercise has much lower correspondence to something like the split jerk, so we will want build back up to standing as soon as possible. From there, perhaps we progress to an overhead variation that allows the athlete to slow the movement down to practice the overhead movement that they rehearsed in supine. A strict press in the split position is an example of that.
- For a novice lifter who struggles attain the squat depth that he or she desires, spending time in the quadruped position rocking the hips back and forth in order to *feel* that triple flexion pattern of a squat can be a useful teaching tool. Then moving that athlete to a standing squat variation with heels elevated, trying to recreate the exact same torso position as in quadruped, is a logical progression.

The point is to provide an environment where MSA can occur with as much specificity to the snatch and clean & jerk as possible. That will vary depending on where the athlete is in the training process. Positions such as supine, sidelying, quadruped, half kneeling and tall kneeling may lack specificity to standing exercises, but they provide the athlete an environment to learn novel tasks or positions. Increasing ground contact compared to standing provides more sensory feedback and facilitates proprioception for the athlete to *feel* certain movements and positions more effectively. This is where conscious, mindful practice can take place in an effort to build confidence and control with a movement or position, so that it can then be used reflexively for performance. Once the weight is on the bar, thinking turns into reacting; but the position should come more fluidly because you ingrained the pattern previously. This can also reduce cueing for the coach, as sometimes a lifter just doesn't understand what position you want them in, no matter what cue you use. Breaking it down to the next most difficult variation or even further (supine, sidelying, quadruped, half kneeling and tall kneeling) now gives you more options to regress and build back up.

This is often where "PT exercises" go wrong. 3x10 mindless, half-assed glute bridges at a random time of the day will do little to nothing to elicit an adaptation for the positions of weightlifting. However, 5 slow, controlled glute bridges, with focused intent on maximizing true hip extension done before your pulls or in between light warm up sets... now you have a useful little tool to augment the MSA process. You felt the hip extension in a low stress environment; now you try to recreate it while layering on speed and load.

4. Using Tension/Threshold Strategies for MV and MSA

As alluded to in Chapter 2, we can utilize different core and breathing tension strategies based on the MV or MSA goal at hand.

Examples

- Cueing an athlete to relax and breath calmly in the bottom of an overhead squat (low tension), when his or her typical strategy is to breath-hold and create global muscle tension, which affects squatting mobility.
- Cueing an athlete to exhale forcefully and create core tension and stiffness in the bottom of an overhead squat (high tension), when he or she has hypermobile tendencies that sometimes create an unstable bottom position.
- "Stretching" the hip flexors in a half kneeling position while creating tension through the core and other three limbs (high tension) in an effort to elicit a perceived range of motion change in hip extension. Adding internal tension in a position of stretch (either at the muscle or through the core) is

one way for us to add a bit of "load" to the technique for a more powerful response.

■ Not only can we utilize internal tension strategies during static stretching, but we can also utilize external load and take advantage of the benefits of eccentric loading. Think of this as *loaded mobility*. There is evidence that eccentric muscle training improves range of motion more effectively than an unloaded static stretch or control group.

■ Having an athlete pause in the front rack with heavy load, relax his or her face, hands, neck and breath, while maintaining a position used for the dip and drive—here we are teaching an athlete to utilize a low(er) tension strategy, in a generally high-load, high-stress situation, in order to facilitate fluid movement even under heavy load.

■ Taking the slower, more static control of an overhead squat, and following it up with a more dynamic higher tension snatch balance, but trying to receive the snatch balance in the same position that you were in locking in your overhead squat: dynamic correspondence.

Combining this concept with Guideline 3 can be a very effective strategy for lifters to induce some quick changes in movement and mobility that can be integrated in the barbell lifts with increasing specificity. When in doubt, find a way to load a position in one way or another, because don't forget, that's how we change tissue.

Components & Goals of Training Prep & Corrective Programming

The following are physiological objectives that we are trying to accomplish when prepping for training. They work in a continuous flow and are not mutually exclusive, and do not follow an order of operations. They facilitate each other.

Circulation & Lubrication

It's called a *warm-up* for a reason: it should literally make you warm, whether that's enough empty bar and warm-up sets that you feel sufficiently loose, or it's performing a "cluster" of corrective strategies. The tempo and focus should be such that it naturally begins ramping up your temperature regardless of what you're doing. We know that increased core temperature improves neuromuscular signaling by increasing the speed of nerve impulses and improving the rate of muscle contraction and reaction time, drives a psychological state conducive to hard training, etc. You are literally a better, faster-reacting athlete if you are warm compared to not.

A common mistake we see is an athlete who wanders into the gym, and in the course of 30 minutes, performs 3 half-assed stretches and foams rolls for 10 minutes while texting on the phone. Nothing productive has been done to prepare that person for training, and he or she will likely jump into relatively heavy weights without optimally priming mobility and movement patterns, because they ran out of time dicking around. Focused intent. Tempo. We are priming and ramping up the nervous system for a heightened couple of hours—warm up that way. This could easily be Guideline 6.

The lubrication aspect of this component refers to the fluid in our joints. Cycling through full ranges of motion lubricates the joints and prepares them to absorb the load that will soon be upon them. You'll often see weightlifters performing "joint circles" starting at their ankles and working all the way up.

It should be noted that things like arm swings, leg swings, jumping on the bike or rower, and various generic dynamic warm-up drills are all fair game for C&L and for your general warm-up.

Inhibition

This is all about perception. Whatever range of motion, position or movement we are trying to acquire or perform, we are looking to decrease the restriction, soreness, tightness, etc. that is perceived to be inhibiting it. This could be through the use of SMR, the lower level breathing drills outlined in Chapter 2, corrective drills, a more extensive barbell warm-up, etc.

For example, if we are looking to achieve full hip lockout at the finish of the pull, we'll work to inhibit any perceived tension in the anterior hip. If we are looking to achieve ankle mobility, we'll look to inhibit any perceived limitation in that calf musculature or front of the joint. Your regular warm up routine, performed with tempo and intent, may do the job of the inhibition we speak of. It's not any one drill or trick, and it doesn't mean that certain muscles literally "turn off"—it's a perception. A perceived reset. What was once tight or sore is no longer so.

Facilitation

As much as we want to inhibit feelings of restriction or tightness, we want to facilitate areas that will aide in achieving our desired range of motion, positions and movement. While we are working to inhibit any anterior hip tightness in our hip lockout example above, we are also working to facilitate active hip extension—sending drive to the glutes, hamstrings, abs, etc. in a purposeful, tension/loading strategy as mentioned in Guideline 4. For our ankle mobility example, perhaps we are pulling forward with the anterior shin muscle into active dorsiflexion, and holding at end range maximally at the bottom of a squat, utilizing tensioned breathing strategies.

For overhead movement, perhaps we are warming up with the empty bar by reaching up on it, making our arms as long as possible, and alternating that with perceived inhibition to the lat with SMR or the standing wall press drill from Chapter 2. All the while, our C&L tempo is facilitating and increasing perceived nervous system drive, ramping us up for training.

For the snatch pattern, maybe this means going from an overhead squat with the empty bar or light weight into a snatch balance, with deliberate snappiness and focus on something like a strong elbow lockout. Even though it's light weight, you're grooving the pattern and priming the nervous system.

We take these three continuous components and implement them into the phases below.

Phases of Training Prep & Corrective Programming

The proposed terms to describe the preparatory phase of training are below. They work on a continuum, and are also not mutually exclusive. The order is leading to specificity of the snatch and clean & jerk, but any one strategy may be satisfying criteria for multiple phases.

1. Mobilization

In this phase we are implementing strategies to increase a desired joint range of motion. We can use some type of test before and after to gauge change. For example, in regard to the ankle:

- Pre-test: Half kneeling dorsiflexion test.
- Intervention: Half kneeling ankle rocking with anchored foot alternated with SMR of the calf soft tissue for 3 rounds.
- Post-test: Half kneeling dorsiflexion test.

We are interested in increasing movement potential in a specific area utilizing a combination of active and passive techniques for focused tempo and a specific goal in mind to make a temporary but perceivable change. Open a mobility window of opportunity.

2. Stabilization

In this phase, we utilize the range of motion gained in the mobilization phase actively in some way in an effort to layer on control in that new range. The activities here may still involve conscious focus on movement and position, but we are looking to solidify mobility with increased load and increasing specificity to the snatch and clean & jerk. Continuing our ankle example:

- Pre-Test: Barefoot air squat—athlete gauges ease of movement and any feelings of restrictions in the ankle.
- Intervention: Compact split squat holding 10kg plate, with emphasis on maximal forward shin angle and active assisted dorsiflexion with anterior shin muscles.
- Post-Test: Barefoot air squat—athlete gauges ease of movement and any feelings of restrictions in the ankle.

Remember you are not going to make long-term structural changes in any one session, but you can make short-term changes in mobility, and over time, *using* that mobility through the desired range of motion will create long-term tissue adaptation. In this phase, you're really trying to create awareness of how your body moves.

3. Integration

This is barbell skill work, as the athlete will have a bar in his or her hands during this phase of prep. This includes any lift variation or modification up to the full snatch and clean & jerk. The goal is to take the solidified movement pattern primed and practiced in both the Mobilization and Stabilization phases and incorporate it into the barbell lifts in some capacity—specificity. Continuing with our ankle example:

- Pre-Test: Front Squat with weightlifting shoes on—athlete gauges ease of movement and any feelings of restrictions in the ankle.
- Intervention: (1) Muscle clean + front squat with conscious focus on allowing the shins to translate forward, just like in the split squat of the Stabilization Phase; (2) Power clean + front squat with same focus; (3) Full clean committing to same receiving position as practiced previously, but implementing increasing speed.

It's important to reiterate that these phases are not mutually exclusive. In the above example, the lifter could perform the split squat from the Stabilization phase in between sets of lighter percentage clean variations. The lifter could also alternate between sets of split squats with dorsiflexion focus and half kneeling ankle rockers. He or she could perform half kneeling ankle rockers in between muscle clean + front squat. The point is that the work is done with focused intent and the goal of creating a perceivable change in the range of motion, fluidity, control, etc. of the desired weightlifting related position or movement. It is also done with the previously discussed guidelines and components in mind.

Just keep in mind that the regressed positions and increased ground contact are for slow learning environments, but then you must progress the specificity of position and layer on increased rate of force while minimizing conscience cueing/thinking. The speed at which the snatch and clean & jerk are performed preclude reliance on conscious body sense. At that point, it's time to just "react" and trust that you will attain the body positions needed automatically based on the work that you put in previously.

Training Prep & Corrective Programming Implementation

Clusters

We've alluded to this already—alternating between and combining strategies for mobilization, stabilization and integration purposes with a specific weightlifting-related position or movement in mind. This could be SMR/stretch + regressed position exercise + barbell variation. It could be a barbell variation + specific joint mobilization. We'll refer to these combinations of corrective strategies as *clusters*. Movement clusters that circulate and lubricate, inhibit and facilitate.

Before Training

Clusters can be performed before touching the barbell or putting on your shoes, typically with a focus on inhibiting and facilitating with regressed positions, concentrating on the mobilization and stabilization phases. This can be as general body prep or specific to a pattern.

Example: For an athlete who typically feels restriction in the hip joints when squatting below parallel, it's a great idea to inhibit those feelings of tightness with some positional practice before putting on weightlifting shoes. If you can open a short term mobility window and acquire a barefoot air squat without weightlifting shoes that's without your usual feelings of hip tightness, then you will feel like superman when you put your weightlifting shoes on. You will have given yourself a buffer zone, i.e. increased your MV, which will make it much easier for your body to acquire new motor skills.

There is no set time limit or perfect duration for pre-training prep. Based on experience, however, quality and focus start to go downhill after about 15 minutes. This is why tempo and focus is so important, and don't forget that our mobility windows of opportunity don't stay open forever. Choose 1-2 movements/positions to focus on based on your screening and assessment.

During Training

This is an underutilized but valuable period of time to add in some extra work for movement clusters. The recommendation is to implement clusters specific to your goal in between empty bar sets or lighter warm up sets, *only* if you feel it provides you better positioning that simply working the lift doesn't seem to attain. The advantage of performing something like a regressed position drill in between barbell sets is that you get to immediately integrate that practiced motor pattern in the lift. It's immediate feedback. Just remember, at some point, it's time to shut off the thinking and "corrective mode" and just react. Once you're hitting 60%+, it's a good time to shut down any cluster work, rest like normal between sets, and focus on weightlifting.

Another good time to throw in some focused movement cluster work is in between components of training—specifically lifts that use different movement patterns in order to prepare for that next exercise. For example: going from muscle snatches to split jerk. You prepped the rotational capacity of the muscle snatches well and felt great. However, now in your next training exercise, you have a movement pattern that involves a narrower overhead grip and a split hip position. Perhaps you hit a couple rounds of a front foot elevated half kneeling plate press with high tension active hip extension on the down leg + SMR to the lat for a couple of rounds before hitting the jerk blocks. Or as a barbell skill complex to prepare for the full split jerks, you perform split strict press behind the neck + jerk balance + overhead split squat. Then you do the same complex starting in the front rack. This will develop balance through the feet and teach the lifter how to stack the torso and hips in order to support to load most optimally.

As you can probably tell, the options for corrective strategy combination can be endless. It's not about the perfect stretch or drill, because everyone responds differently to things. It's about concepts and guidelines. Follow those, and the corrections in the rest of the book will flow naturally.

■ The Snatch

The snatch seems to get the most attention out of the three lifts. Maybe that's because it's first in competition. Maybe it's because when performed by experienced lifters, it looks very powerful and athletic. The combination of speed, technical prowess and movement competency required to perform the lift and attain the receiving position make for something that seems to be a never-ending work in progress.

We will break the snatch down into each of its components, giving you various options for corrective programming based on what you wish to work on. We are starting from the setup and building up to each phase. It's done this way for logical flow, but the true starting point will be individual to the lifter. Also, understand that you will not need every drill, variation, mobilization, etc. in this chapter, and most certainly cannot implement everything in any one period of time. Pick 1-2 things you wish to emphasize, and address them with focus and intent.

Lastly, the suggested drills are sequenced for each phase as follows: mobilization, stabilization and integration. We will consider this a "bottom-up" approach, as it takes us from less stressful and specific to the snatch, to more stressful and specific. Again, it is ordered this way for logistical purposes. For experienced lifters, consider implementing a "top-down" approach, where you begin with specific barbell variations for the lifts and regress to lower level loading strategies and/or mobilizations if needed.

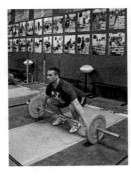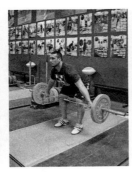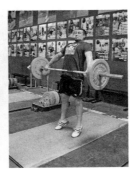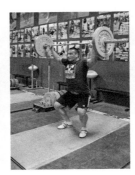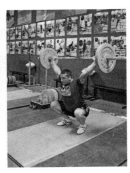

The snatch

CHAPTER 7

Snatch Starting Position

Because the successful completion of a snatch depends so heavily on technique, attaining a consistent starting position is critical for proper execution of the lift. Due to the wider grip, the snatch setup poses more of a challenge for lifters to find a comfortable yet stable position to begin the pull from.

Finding *Your* Stance

As was the case with individual squatting stances (as discussed in Chapter 5), the optimal starting position will be specific to the lifter's preference and proportions. Some very common coaching cues for teaching the starting position are:

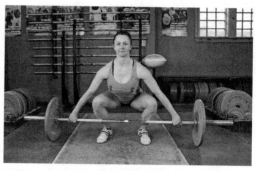

- Feet hip-width apart.
- Barbell over the balls of the feet (where the toes connect to the foot).
- Shins touching the bar or as close as possible.
- Hips at or slightly higher than knee level (when the bar actually breaks from the floor).
- Shoulders directly over or slightly in front of the bar.

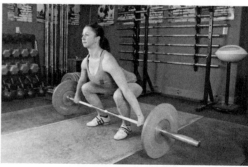

Again, these points may differ from coach to coach based on pulling style, and may need to be adapted from lifter to lifter based on body proportions. What is universally agreed upon is the curvature of the spine—where the spinal curves start, they should generally stay throughout the duration of the pull. This will aid in transferring maximum force through the core and into the bar. Some lifters may increase the relative amount of extension of the spine as they begin to pull the hips through to meet the bar for the final extension. However, a noticeable increase in *flexion* of the spine during

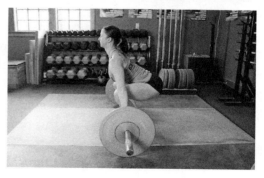

Figure 7.01 Starting position of the snatch

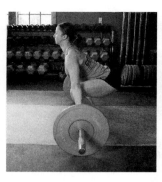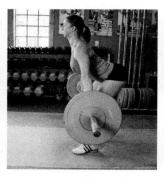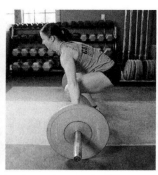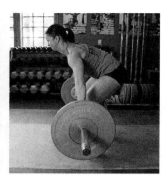

Figure 7.02 In the first sequence, you see the lifter maintaining a consistent spinal curve off the floor to the knee. In the second sequence, you see a position in which the lifter has not set a sustainable spinal position off the floor, which commonly results in a greater loss of posture as the lift progresses.

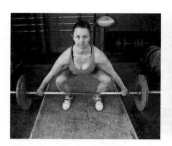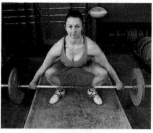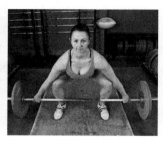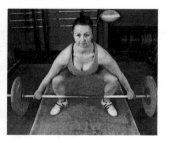

Figure 7.03 As you did with the squat, experiment with various levels of foot width and rotation that allow you to achieve a starting position in which you can maintain a set spinal position.

the pull will likely result in a leakage of power, making it difficult to impart maximal force into the barbell at the top of the second pull. (Figure 7.02)

Lifters need to find a stance that allows them to set up with a spinal position that they can maintain through the pull to final extension. It starts with the feet and ankles.

Stand with the barbell over the balls of the feet and with feet hip-width apart. From this position, squat straight down to the barbell, attempting to maintain the neutral curvatures of the spine (more concerned with maintaining a relative amount of lumbar lordosis at this point). Repeat this procedure just as you did with squatting stance—experiment with various foot widths and *within* different widths, experiment with pointing the toes out to varying degrees. (Figure 7.03)

The goal is to find the position that allows you to set a sustainable, consistent spinal position that you can maintain throughout the lift. You can also repeat this sequence by allowing your lower back to round at the bottom, then use leverage from the barbell to pull your spine back into a more extended position. The goal and sequence of squat width and toe-out remain the same. A coach, lifting partner, video or mirror is useful during this time to provide the lifter immediate feedback regarding position.

Important Points From a biomechanics standpoint, the ideal stance would put the feet directly underneath the hips (when standing) to maximize the upward drive of the legs during final extension. Do not sacrifice the integrity of your spinal position to attain such a stance if it does not allow you to set up comfortably and maintain your spinal curves. It is also common for a lifter's starting position to evolve subtly over the course of his or her career as strength levels, movement patterns, tissue leverages, etc. change.

Ankles

Although the ankles may play a larger role in a full squatting pattern, the nature of the snatch start position (hips generally lower than in the start of the clean) is such that ankle dorsiflexion is utilized to attain a comfortable position. A shin that is unable to translate forward (and instead stays closer to vertical) in the start position may cause the lifter to be shifted back on his or her heels excessively during the first phases of the pull. This can result in an unnecessary jump back or kicking the hips forward into the bar at the top of the pull, causing the bar to sail away from the body. Going back to the ankle-screening test in Chapter 5, for those with restricted ankle dorsiflexion, a wider stance may be what you need to be able to sit your hips down adequately.

To improve function of the ankle, we will move through a series of positional options for the lifter to experiment with.

Mobilization: Half Kneeling

The test position now becomes the corrective position.

- Half kneeling with the down knee directly under your hips and shoulders.
- Remind yourself how to create a stable midfoot by lifting your toes while keeping the balls of the foot down. Spread your toes and place them back down flat (not scrunched), while attempting to maintain that midfoot position. It's kind of like a little foot push-up, balancing your foot between three points of contact—your big toe, little toe and heel. (Figure 7.04)
  > Rock your shin forward toward the wall and back to the start position while lightly but actively pressing the toes into the floor (especially the big toe) to maintain a stable foot. This will ensure that the movement is coming from the ankle. Perform 10 reps, then scoot the foot back half an inch or so and repeat. Be mindful that you are not rolling to the outside edge of your foot, and the foot remains broad and stable from side to side. (Figure 7.05)

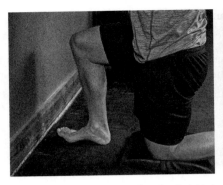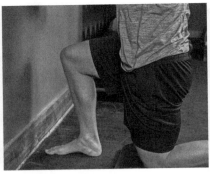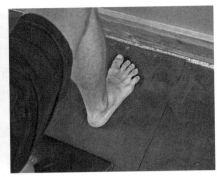

Figure 7.04 We want the foot broad and stable to ensure we are isolating motion at the ankle joint.

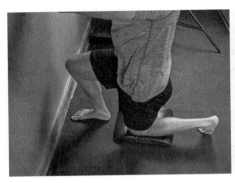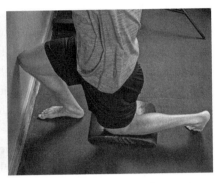

Figure 7.05 In the Half-Kneeling Ankle mobilization, rock the shin forward, mobilizing the ankle into dorsiflexion, without altering foot position or allowing the midfoot arch to collapse.

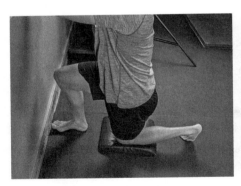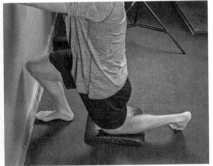

Figure 7.06 Keeping the toes pulled up in the Half-Kneeling Ankle mobilization will add a mobilization component to tendons of the foot.

Toes-Up Variation To maximally stabilize the midfoot and ensure we are isolating the ankle, perform the rocking mobilization with the toes actively pulled up throughout the entire set (Figure 7.06). This may limit total excursion because we have now put intrinsic foot tendons on stretched, which is a nice way for them to get some active length.

It's recommended that you always follow this option up with at least one set in which your toes are back down on the ground, since this will mimic performance and we are always trying to "grease the groove," so to speak, in regard to movement patterns.

Active Dorsiflexion Variation Another way to facilitate as much ankle dorsiflexion as possible during this drill is for the athlete to actively pull forward with his or her anterior shin muscle (anterior tibialis) when rocking toward the wall (Figure 7.07). Holding at end range for 3-5 seconds can enhance the mobilization.

This can be done both with the toes up and toes down. When performing this option with the toes down, be mindful that the toes are not scrunching together as you are actively rocking forward. We do not want make the area of our foot smaller. It is our base, so we want it broad.

Weighted Variation All of the above options can be performed with an external load being applied on top of the knee (Figure 7.08). *Do not sacrifice foot position* for the sake of adding more weight or gaining more range of motion. Blowing through your midfoot is not what we are after, so be disciplined and maintain your "foot push-up" while applying the weight gently to increase ankle dorsiflexion range of motion.

Mobilization: Foot on Box

- The foot can be placed on a box to improve the leverage that you can push forward with (Figure 7.09). All of the same cues above apply to this variation.

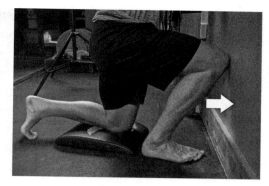

Figure 7.07 Actively pull the shin forward with the anterior shin muscle to assist in the Half-Kneeling Ankle mobilization.

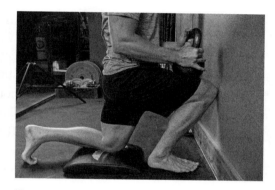

Figure 7.08 Adding a load to the mobilization can increase the range of motion. Utilize this with any aforementioned variation—toes down, toes up or adding active dorsiflexion with the anterior shin muscle.

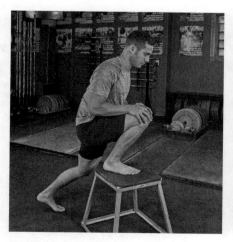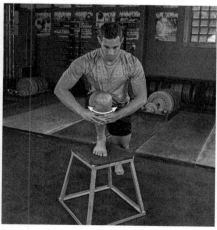

Figure 7.09 Put the foot on a box if you feel it increases your leverage to rock the shin forward for ankle mobilization. Utilize this with any aforementioned variation—toes down, toes up, adding active dorsiflexion with the anterior shin muscle, or adding load. Implementing a tibial rotation component may aide in minimizing any pinching sensation in the front of the ankle.

- One can also add a manual tibial (shin bone) rotation component, either internally (makes more sense based on tibia mechanics with knee flexion) or externally, as the shin rocks forward. Tibial rotation naturally occurs during knee flexion and extension. During the squat (knee flexion), the tibia internally rotates slightly. This is not a conscious motion, and the degree is extremely small; however, anecdotally, some athletes report slightly better increases in forward tibia angle when a manual tibial rotational component is added to this mobilization. Whichever direction you choose should limit any pinching sensation in the front of the joint and shouldn't alter foot position.

Mobilization: Standing

- Perform the same forward rocking of the shin while in a standing position (Figure 7.10). All of the previous cues apply here as well. You can put your hands on the wall for balance.
- Experiment with toes up, toes down and active shin muscles.
- This is obviously a convenient option if there is no box available, if the athlete is sensitive to kneeling, or kneeling is just not feasible. A potential benefit to standing is that the athlete can really use bodyweight to leverage forward.
- Potential drawbacks are that you cannot really add external load, and it is also easy to get lazy with foot position—maintain a stable foot.

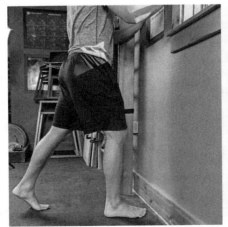 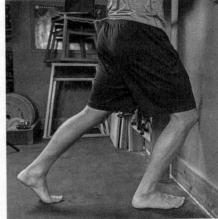

Figure 7.10 One can perform the ankle mobilization in a standing position utilizing any aforementioned variation—toes down, toes up, adding active dorsiflexion with the anterior shin muscle, or adding load. Implementing a tibial rotation component may aide in minimizing any pinching sensation in the front of the ankle.

Every student who goes through Physical Therapy school learns the test/retest principle. It's PT 101. It should also be movement 101. With the above mobilizations, the goal is to make a change in your half kneeling dorsiflexion screening. So make sure you are doing that by re-checking your range of motion afterward to gauge improvement. Any range of motion increase is a victory.

Movement Cluster Options

- Alternate any of the above ankle mobility drills with SMR of the back of the lower leg (calf area) if that is where you feel the restriction during the half kneeling dorsiflexion test. If it is the front of the ankle where you feel the restriction, you will want to reposition the foot as mentioned above, but SMR to the front of the shin may inhibit this feelings. Perform approximately 20 seconds of SMR + ankle mobilization of choice for 2-3 rounds or until a perceptible change in range of motion is made.

Stabilization: Split Squat

Now we work to control our newfound range of motion.

- In the half kneeling position, lift the toes of the down foot and rock your ankle forward until it hits it end range. Then, spread the toes and place them back down flat and apart. You should maintain the arch of your foot while doing this. (Figure 7.11)
- A dowel can be used for balance here.

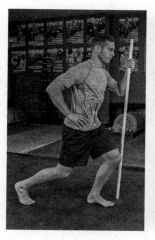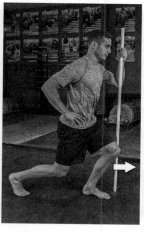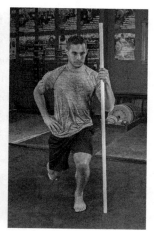

Figure 7.11 The start of our Split Squat Ankle stabilization drill

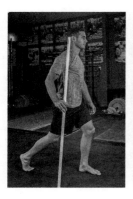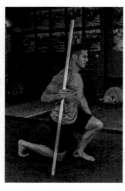

Figure 7.12 Intentionally emphasizing dorsiflexion during a squatting movement can help the mobilization "stick." Maintain a broad, stable foot and try to avoid rolling to the outside edge.

- Now use the muscles of the front of the shin to help pull your ankle into even more dorsiflexion. You can rock back and forth here for 1-2 sets of 4-5 reps before performing the split squats if you did not start with a prior mobilization.
- Now perform half kneeling split squats with your ankle in end range dorsiflexion, but while maintaining that stable midfoot (Figure 7.12). *This does not mean rolling to the outside edge of your foot.* The shin will undoubtedly come to vertical at the top of the movement, but you are looking to return to full dorsiflexion as soon as possible on the way down. The goal here is that you are moving through and maintaining end range dorsiflexion through as much as the split squat as possible.
- Really FEEL what it is like to have an angled tibia in a squat. Own your dorsiflexion. For many, it may be a foreign feeling to be controlling a squat utilizing such a position.
  - › Some may be concerned with stresses at the front of the knee here. If this hurts the front of your knee, you should discontinue or get checked out. However, it is the clinical experience of this author that if the athlete has stabilized the foot through the entire range, keeping the big toe actively pressed into the ground, knee issues are not present, as the forces are distributed appropriately through the hip, knee and ankle.
    - We are not concerned for the knee for several reasons:
      - › It is completely normal and necessary for the shin to travel forward over the toe in human activities such as running, jumping, squatting and going up and down stairs. With the foot flat, forces are distributed across the hip, knee and ankle.
      - › You are allowed to use a dowel, rack or bench for support.
      - › We are emphasizing position and control.
- Perform 1-3 sets of 5 split squats on each side.

Movement Cluster Options

- Alternate the split squat with around 20 seconds of SMR to the calf area.

Integration: Barbell Mobilization & Setup

An ageless classic. Many would consider this a mobility rather than stability exercise (remember we are usually training both to some extent, so semantics play a part). However, the lifter is on his or her feet, most likely with weightlifting shoes on, so this is a drill that we can really integrate into finding our comfortable starting position, and then take us right into a pull.

- Place the barbell over the tops of your knees in the bottom of a squat.
- As you did to test for optimal starting position, perform this drill with varying foot widths and degrees of toe-out. This is to teach yourself how to utilize true ankle dorsiflexion in several planes.
- Lifting and spreading your toes becomes futile in weightlifting shoes, but apply the concepts of actively pressing your big toe down and using your anterior shin muscle to assist in pulling your shin forward.
- Spend around 20-30 seconds oscillating back and forth or holding a prolonged stretch, but then take this right into your start position and practice the pull. Utilize this new

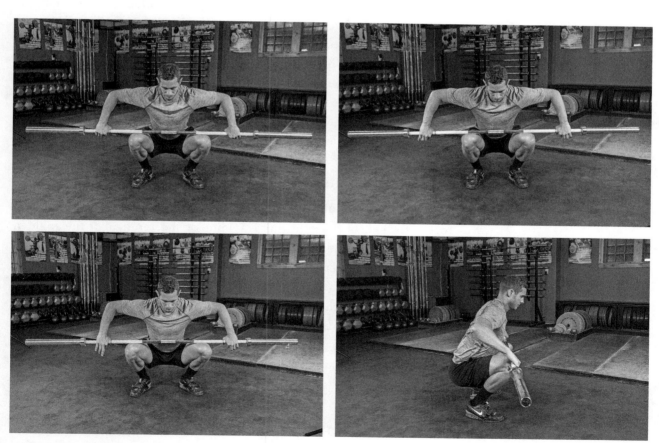

Figure 7.13 Use the bar to push your ankles into dorsiflexion while experimenting with varied stances.

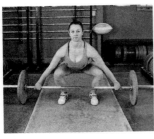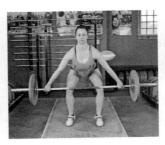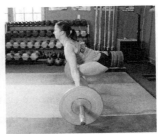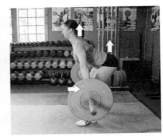

Figure 7.14 Drill components of the pull to integrate the short-term improvements in ankle dorsiflexion that you made with the mobilizations. Find a balance point in the starting position where you can push with the legs to reach the knee with vertical shins, then return back to the ground with deliberate utilization of ankle dorsiflexion.

window of opportunity that you have with increased range of motion, and put it to use right away. This will allow it to "stick." However much dorsiflexion you utilize in your start position (dependent on the lifter), it should feel as stable as when you were performing your split squats.

- Perform 1-3 rounds alternating the bar ankle mobilization with light pulls or lift variations, with a focus on "owning" ankle dorsiflexion. Going back and forth from pulling from the floor to pauses at the knee is a great way to integrate ankle dorsiflexion and help you figure out which pull position works best for you. At the knee, the shins are vertical and the shoulders and hips should rise as one unit with the feet staying flat and balanced. When returning from the knee back to the floor, the ankles will dorsiflex, and the shoulders and hips lower as one unit. The bar placement in the starting position and whatever amount of ankle dosiflexion you use should allow for these smooth transitions.

Discussion Points & Summary Of The Ankle

Impingement Is Not a Stretch You should not feel pain or sharp discomfort in the side of the joint that is folding or shortening. For the ankle in dorsiflexion, this means the front of the joint where the "crease" is. The tissue is slacking here, so in theory, there should be no restriction. You should feel a stretch on the side that is lengthening (your lower calf and Achilles tendon in this case), but not much of anything, other than some general pressure, in the side that is shortening (front of the ankle).

However, if you do feel an uncomfortable pressure or pinching in the front crease of the ankle, this is commonly referred to as *impingement*—not tightness—and may indicate faulty mechanics of that joint. Do not jam into this feeling in an attempt to "release" it, because impingement is a positional problem, not a tightness problem. To correct it, we will alter position/mechanics. Do this by:

- Focusing more on maintaining an active "foot push-up" through our midfoot by actively pressing the big toe down with more force as the shin rocks forward.
- Spending more time with the Toes-Up variation in order to work just short of end-range joint motion.

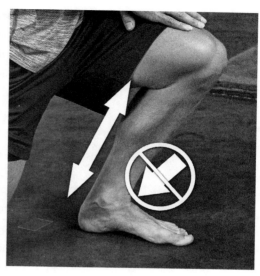

Figure 7.15 A stretching sensation in the back of the ankle is what we would expect when mobilizing the ankle into dorsiflexion since those tissues are lengthening. If a pinch or block is felt in the front of the joint, then we will alter the position in an attempt to change this.

The Foot Is Our Base The foot is important because it is our only relationship with the ground when snatching and clean & jerking. It is our stable (or unstable) platform. We want our base to be as broad and steady as possible. When we push through the floor with a stable, balanced foot during the pull or squat, this provides the body's joint systems with the compression they need to send the brain proprioceptive and kinesthetic signals. These signals tell the brain where your body is in space without having to consciously think about it. In turn, your joint systems react reflexively, with the right muscles doing the right thing at the right time. Weightlifting is about *reflexive* reactions. When you start consciously thinking about where your body is in space with a heavy weight, the barbell usually wins.

Lifting your toes or losing your three points of contact as you pull a weight off the floor or squat may result in several issues: (1) It decreases the area of your foot, meaning your base of support is smaller and you are more likely to be off-balance up the chain; (2) Without your entire foot on the ground, you are decreasing the signals being sent to the brain about your body position. Clinically, we find that lifters who move their feet during the pull or when squatting are much more inconsistent in their dynamic motor patterns, theoretically because they subconsciously are less aware of where they are in space. And as the weight gets heavier, the movement becomes less consistent; (3) With an unstable, unbalanced foot, you have less to push with in order to get the strong finish that we desire during the top of the lifts or when coming out of the hole of a squat.

We cue three points of contact because it puts your center of balance right in front of the ankle. Getting rocked *too* far back on your heels makes it difficult to put an upward trajectory on the bar during the pull, and makes it more difficult to drive straight up out of a squat. We have all had that moment when a clean rocks us backwards, and we have to shift forward in the hole in order to balance over the center of the foot and stand up. On the other side of the coin, getting pulled too far forward toward our toes during the pull or squat also has obvious consequences of instability.

When barefoot, we cue to lift the toes first, and then spread and plant them down because: (1) Lifting the toes (especially the big toe) creates a natural arch in the midfoot via the windlass mechanism (stretching of the plantar fascia that stabilizes the midfoot); (2) Spreading the toes creates a broad platform; (3) Planting them down flat reinforces the stable, balanced position. Planting or pressing down does *not* mean scrunching, as that would make your foot shorter and unbalanced. Obviously, in weightlifting shoes, it is difficult to spread your toes. You can, however, make sure you are actively pressing them down during a movement in which your feet are planted—especially that big toe.

Lastly, I want to address the medial side of the arch/foot. It has become popular among athletes these days to avoid letting the inside/middle of their foot come in contact with the ground. As a result, they roll to the outside of the foot, totally losing a large portion of input, push, balance, etc. I'm here to tell you that it is A-Okay for you to feel the middle to inside edge of your foot when you pull or squat. This will differ among individuals as far as comfort, but collapsing or pronating the foot is much different than relatively slight degree of ankle eversion allowing us to simply "feel" our arch. If you are following the rules of a stable foot and allowing your knee to naturally hinge and track over your second toe, it will likely naturally happen anyway. (Figure 7.16)

It is true that there are many elite level lifters will pull from the floor by shoving their knees way out and seemingly rolling to the outside edges of their feet. I would argue that this is for a straighter bar path (technical nuance vs. basic human movement), rather than to create more power. It's a tradeoff that the experienced lifter can benefit from. For those lifters not so established, focus on maintaining a balanced foot through the pull.

This is where allowing for some toe-out in the snatch start position can aid in maintaining proper balance through the foot for many lifters. It is simply more difficult to move the knees back and out of the way of the bar if the feet are narrow and straight (easier to do on the clean). It

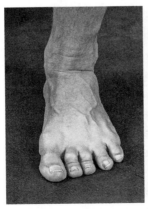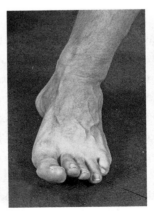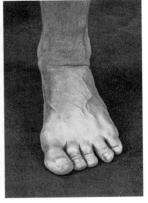

Figure 7.16 The first picture demonstrates a stable, balanced foot position, with which the athlete can impart a vertical force into the ground, while the other pictures demonstrate unstable foot positions (rocking outward or collapsing inward).

all comes back to individuality and understanding that there is rarely a one-size-fits-all approach to this sport. Figure out what work best for you with the above tools.

Thoracic Spine

The thoracic spine is another point of emphasis in the snatch starting position, as attaining the relative amount of upper thoracic extension (or at least intense "anti-flexion") that we discussed in Chapter 2 will aid in maintaining a consistent torso position over the bar during the pull. As we address this, please understand that thoracic spine position is not mutually exclusive to the hip, knee and ankle position discussed previously, which is why we focus on alignment from the ground up.

Mobilization: Quadruped

Here we work to attain movement through the thoracic spine in the sagittal plane (flexion and extension). Restoring a natural kyphosis of the upper back will restore congruency of the shoulder blades with the ribcage and will give us more room to train thoracic extension. The lower back shall remain relatively neutral and motionless to mimic the position of the pull and teach the lifter how to dissociate those portions of the spine. The quadruped position gives an ample amount of external support to focus on specific areas.

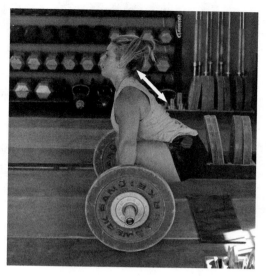

Figure 7.17 Lifter demonstrating a relative amount of upper thoracic extension in the starting position of the snatch

What is great about this drill is that it will show you that extending the upper thoracic spine is not a large movement. On the contrary, the excursion is relatively small, contrary to popular belief. What's more important than the amount of movement is the ability to maintain it. Think about it more as *anti-flexion* than extension. This can be a teaching drill if a lifter has difficulty setting and maintaining a consistent upper back position during the pull.

Starting Position

- Start on hands and knees.

Execution

- Initiate with an inhalation through the nose.
- As you exhale, smoothly reach through the shoulder blades (protract) and flex/round the upper back spinal segments from the base of the neck to the middle/low back without shrugging towards the ears. Focus on moving each individual vertebra.

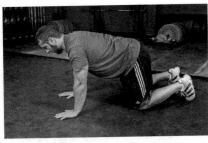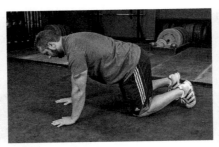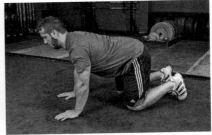

Figure 7.18 Starting position for quadruped thoracic spine mobilization; athlete flexing the thoracic segments; athlete extending the thoracic spine segments. This subtle amount of T-spine extension is typically all we need from a range of motion standpoint to perform the lifts. Notice that the position of the lower back stays constant.

- Maintain this position and inhale again, focusing on placing air into your upper back (expand). Keep the neck relaxed.
- As you exhale through the mouth, smoothly extend the same upper back segments that were just flexed.
  - › *Keep the lower back motionless at this time.* The movement should primarily be coming from the spinal segments between the shoulder blades, not the T/L junction.
  - › The chin should be tucked slightly and the neck in an even, uniform lordosis.
- Inhale in this upper-back-extended posture, then exhale through the mouth and repeat the process.
- Perform 1-2 sets of 8 total reps, moving back and forth between T-spine flexion and extension. (Figure 7.18)
- Again, notice that the thoracic-spine-extended position does not have to be an exaggerated arch. The excursion of motion is not great, but you will likely feel the musculature of mid and upper back activate.

Mobilization: Back to Wall

Now we work to establish the same pattern of a stable T/L junction and upper back extension in standing, with arm action that mimics the start position of a snatch. This is, again, a teaching tool for the lifter to feel the upper back tension utilized in the snatch starting position.

Starting Position
- Stand with feet approximately 12 inches away from the wall with your back supported by the wall (Figure 7.19).
- With the lumbar spine, we have a couple of options:
  - › For the athlete who has difficultly with cueing of spinal position, he or she can start this drill with the low back completely flat against the wall. This will maximize proprioception and teaching of upper back movement.

> For the more stable and kinesthetically-aware athlete, maintaining a slight lumbar lordosis is desirable, as this mimics the low back position during the pull. A slight lordosis is enough to fit fingers between the low back and the wall.

Execution

- Initiate the drill with an inhalation through the nose, "pushing the air down into the lower back."
- Exhale through the mouth and reach the arms forward (protract the shoulder blades) as you did in the quadruped drill above. You will feel your upper back round and may come away from the wall slightly, but maintain the exact position of your mid and low back.
- Inhale through the nose, pushing the air down and filling the entire trunk.

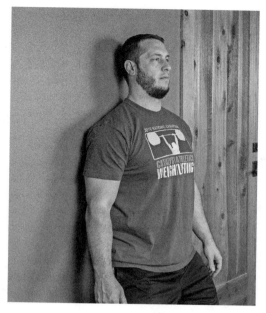

Figure 7.19 Start of Back to Wall thoracic spine mobilization

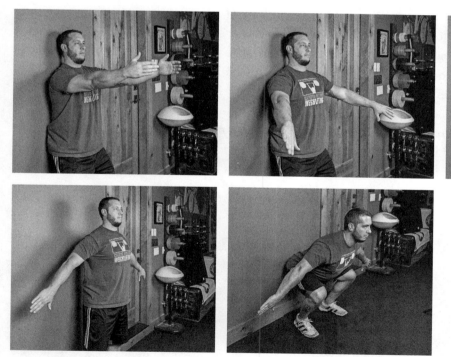

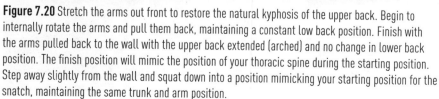

Figure 7.20 Stretch the arms out front to restore the natural kyphosis of the upper back. Begin to internally rotate the arms and pull them back, maintaining a constant low back position. Finish with the arms pulled back to the wall with the upper back extended (arched) and no change in lower back position. The finish position will mimic the position of your thoracic spine during the starting position. Step away slightly from the wall and squat down into a position mimicking your starting position for the snatch, maintaining the same trunk and arm position.

> Toward the end of your inhalation, rotate the arms and hands inward, pulling them back towards the wall at the angle the mimics your snatch grip.
>
> - As you do this, your upper back will naturally being to reverse its flexed posture and move toward extension. You can use the muscles of your upper back to assist in active extension.
> - When the hands are even with your body or against the wall, finish off the repetition with a full exhale without losing position.
> - This entire extension portion of the drill should be done without losing contact or altering position of the mid and lower back.
- Move away from the wall slightly without altering the positions of the spine or arms.
- Squat down slowly into a position that mimics the starting position for the snatch, maintaining the same spine and arm positions.
- Repeat the process for 1-2 sets of 8 total reps (Figure 7.20).

Stabilization: Snatch Pull Setup

Now we simply integrate this into our setup position for the snatch. With the teaching tools outlined above, the athlete should have developed the body awareness to combine the deep hip flexion needed for the snatch setup, with a "tall" spine (upper thoracic extension).

Practice with the steps of the Finding *Your* Stance section of this chapter to find the optimal balance of stance and spinal position for you. In standing, you can literally mimic the actions of the Standing Back to Wall drill to set your upper back position if need be, then squat straight down to the barbell (Figure 7.21).

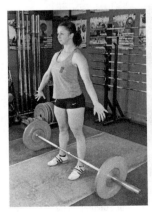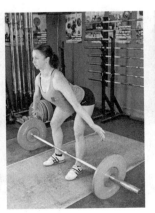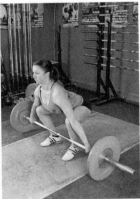

Figure 7.21 Using the position of the Back to Wall T-spine drill to set the starting position of the snatch.

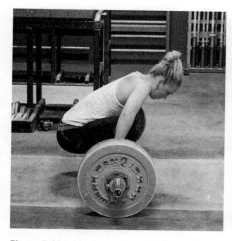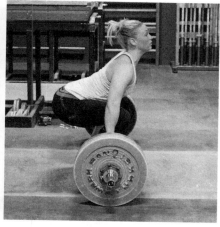

Figure 7.22 Lifter going from slight upper back flexion to extension, just as we did in quadruped T-spine mobilization.

One can also experiment with creating tension off of the bar from a deep squat position, mimicking the upper back extension you created with the quadruped mobilization (Figure 7.22).

Regardless of which practice method you choose, it can also be beneficial to sit in the starting position and take full, deep breaths in through the nose pushing the air down, and exhaling forcefully through the mouth to create core tension. On each exhalation, get "tall" through the upper back, then inhale to reinforce and expand the position 360 degrees. Learning to breathe and brace in the snatch starting position will have carryover to when you're working with weights closer to maximum.

Integration: Pauses

Accessory work that does a fantastic job of reinforcing and developing the static strength required of the upper back to hold position is the utilization of *pauses*, specifically from the floor to the knee, just as we did earlier for the ankle utilizing lighter weights.

1-inch Pause

- Set up in what has been deemed your optimal snatch pulling position.
- As soon as the bar breaks from the floor (approximately 1 inch off the ground), pause for a 3-count, utilizing forceful exhalations for stability, and strong inhalations into the tension to hold position (Figure 7.23).
- Pausing here will not only reinforce position and develop static postural strength, but it will also give you immediate feedback in regard to whether or not the lifter is utilizing an optimal starting position.

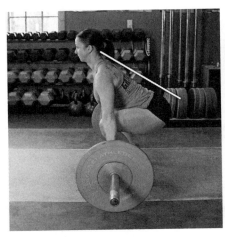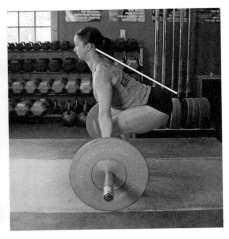

Figure 7.23 1-inch pause off the floor in the snatch pull. Notice that the shoulders and hips rise together, maintaining the same back angle.

› The bar will likely move slightly back as it breaks off of the floor, but other than this, the lifter's shoulder to hip ratio/angle should remain exactly the same from when the bar was resting on the ground, *if* he or she is set up correctly in the first place. It is essentially a "push" with the legs.

› If the lifter's shoulder and hip angle changes as the bar breaks—hips rise, shoulders drop, shoulders pull back, heels come up, etc.—then it is possible that the lifter was not set up optimally and needed to reposition in order to stack his or her joints to break the bar from the floor.

■ This shift could also be caused by general back weakness. To differentiate, incorporate this 1-inch pause with higher and higher percentages of the athlete's 1RM. If positions remain optimal until higher percentages are reached, then it is likely a weakness issue that will be addressed with progressive training. However, if the athlete is altering his or her hip and shoulder angles during the 1-inch pause at percentages much lower than a strength deficit would indicate (60% or less, for example), it is more likely a suboptimal setup based on the lifter's individual structure and/or a learned motor control habit. There will be more discussion on upper back weakness in the subsequent Discussion section.

Pause At Knee

■ Same cues and concepts as the 1-inch pause. The lifter's shoulder to hip angle should remain approximately the same, and the shins should be approximately vertical once the bar reaches the knees. (Figure 7.24)

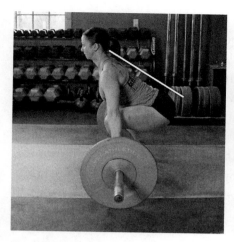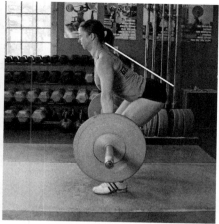

Figure 7.24 Pause at the knee in the snatch pull. Note again that the shoulders and hips rise together to knee level, maintaining the same back angle.

Discussion Points & Summary Of The Thoracic Spine for Snatch Set Up

Understand that the preferred setup sequence of individual lifters will vary and evolve, and will likely not be as deliberate as the standing sequence that was just described. However, from a positional teaching standpoint, this is an effective way to initially learn.

Upper Back "Weakness" When an athlete has difficulty maintaining stability through the upper back during a snatch pull, it is common for the musculature of the upper back to be deemed as weak and supplemental strength work implemented. Such exercises may include rowing variations, back extension variations, etc. These exercises are great and are usually warranted.

However, it must be understood that the spinal erectors of the upper back are smaller and will likely always be weaker than those of the lower back. While the old adage of *we are only as strong as our weakest link* has merit, we must make sure that we have given those inherently weaker muscles the most biomechanically advantageous position to pull from. Supplemental upper back strengthening exercises will have less carryover if the athlete is not utilizing mechanics optimal to his or her individual structure.

Common examples of these errors are:

- Using a foot stance that is too narrow for the athlete to achieve proper hip position
- Bodyweight shifted too far back onto the heels, resulting in compensatory upper back flexion.
- Not utilizing a slight toe-out, if that is optimal for the athlete's hips to achieve the depth needed for setup.

These are examples of faults that can cause athletes to feel "crowded" in their setups, and not allow for adequate hip freedom, and ultimately not allow the athletes to set a stable lumbar (low back) position. If this is the case, then we are relying on the already weaker upper back erectors to keep us upright and stable, which means we are set up for failure.

The positional drills that were outlined in this chapter are designed to teach athletes how to position and *use* the upper back strength that they possess with respect to proper alignment. When combined with supplemental strengthening programmed by a coach and periodic pause work as described above, upper back "weakness" will be addressed adequately in most cases.

Faults With Traditional Upper Back Mobilization Drills It is understood that "mobility" drills will be more passive in nature and do not necessarily need to have exact positional carryover to the weightlifting movements. However, it is important that the drill actually mobilize the body part you are targeting.

Foam rollers and various ball implements (more on these later) are often used for mobilization of the thoracic spine with great success. The common mistake is not isolating the thoracic spinal segments, and attaining much of the extension from the T/L junction and lower back (Figure 7.25). While this can certainly still knock down unwanted tension in that musculature, it is not giving the athlete much of the upper thoracic movement that they desire. It also reinforces a suboptimal overhead position.

These drills are better implemented with knees bent and feet flat on the floor. In this position, utilize an exhalation through the mouth to set the lower ribs down (neutral). Maintain this lumbar and T/L junction position as you are mobilizing your thoracic spine with whatever implement you choose. Exhaling as you extend the arms up and back will aid in

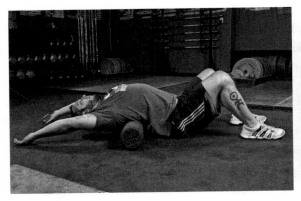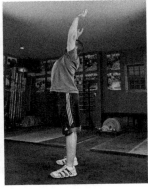

Figure 7.25 How we commonly see athletes mobilizing the T-spine. This is little movement actually coming from the upper back, as most of it is occurring at the T/L junction. It's essentially just a tilting backwards of the entire ribcage, as is more obvious in the standing position pictured here. This position wouldn't translate to a very stable or comfortable overhead position.

keeping your lower half stable. The mobility implement and arms should work as a fulcrum at each upper thoracic segment. And remember, drills like these are only mentioned because of their popularity, but are low on the priority list of movement strategies; but if they are to be done, we'll at least try to maximize the benefit.

■ CHAPTER 8

Snatch First Pull

Once we have established a starting position for the snatch that provides us a nice balance of tension and position, it's time to pull.

Hip Hinging

The initial pull from the ground to somewhere around mid-thigh is generally thought of as a "push" by the legs, with the end of the first pull phase putting the athlete's shoulders over the bar with a slight bend of the knees.

This position resembles a movement that's commonly referred to as a Romanian Deadlift (RDL), where an athlete bends the torso forward, only moving from the hips relative to the knees or ankles. For both the RDL and first pull, this ability to move through the hips is what we will refer to as a *hip hinge* and is an important movement component of pulling or deadlift variations.

Let's go back to our Active Straight Leg Raise test from Chapter 3. There we discussed how that test was looking at the ability for the athlete to hinge at each hip in a relatively stable environment (supine). We will return to that position to teach the pattern initially for those who were limited during the screen.

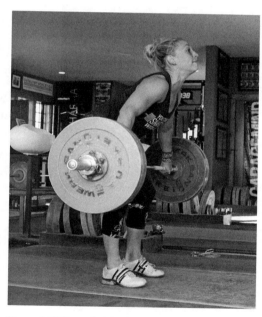

Figure 8.01 The end of the first pull of the snatch

Mobilization: Supine Hip Hinging with Arm, Band or Plate Press

This is categorized as a mobilization because we are getting some separation of the hips (one goes into extension while the other is flexed), and relative length through the posterior chain of the up leg. However, we are doing so with a stable trunk in mind, so this is far from a passive stretch.

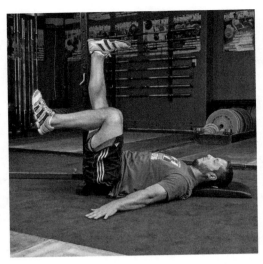

Figure 8.02 Starting position of the Supine Hip Hinging mobilization. The top knee may be bent to mimic the end of the first pull and to allow for individual mobility capacities. The arms are pressed into the floor at the angle of the snatch grip.

Starting Position

- One leg propped to 90 degrees against a doorway or rack. You may bend the knee of the leg that is on the wall to mimic that of the end of the first pull.
- Opposite hip is flexed with the knee bent to 90 degrees and foot in the air.
- Have some head support if possible.
- Toes flexed toward you (dorsiflexion), with feet and kneecaps facing relatively straight.
- Arms outstretched to about 35-45 degrees of shoulder abduction, with palms down. This will maximize ground contact and proprioception, and mimic the arm position during the snatch pull.
- The lower back will be relatively flat against the ground in this position (very slight lordosis). Wherever it starts, it stays through the movement.

Execution

- Initiate the drill with an inhalation through the nose, pushing the air down "into the lower back."
- Exhale through the mouth slowly and forcefully as you slowly lower the heel of the up leg to the floor without allowing the lower back to arch up off the ground.
- Slide the heel out, which will extend the bottom hip, while maintaining all other positions (Figure 8.03).
  - ❯ Exhale through the ENTIRE lowering and heel slide process, even if you run out of air. This will keep you acquainted with your abs. Your lower ribs should remain flush with your abdomen. Reach LONG with the heel of the leg that is sliding to facilitate hip extension.
  - ❯ As this is happening, firmly press your hands and arms into the floor, reflexively engaging your lats and core. This mimics the pressure you need to keep on the bar at the end of the first pull. It will also facilitate upper thoracic extension while you work to keep your low back neutral (integrating concepts here). This is a similar position as the Back to Wall T-spine mobilization in Chapter 7.
  - ❯ Inhale through the nose as you return the leg to the starting position for the completion of the rep.
- The goal is to slide the heel as far as you can until the bottom hip is fully extended, until you cannot hold the position of

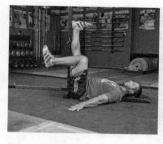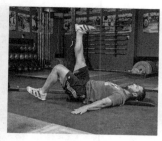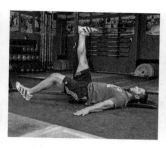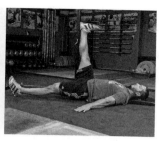

Figure 8.03 Supine hip hinge drill

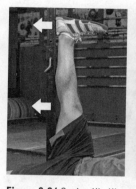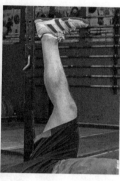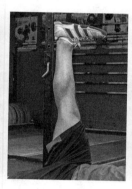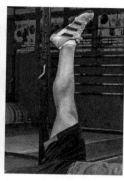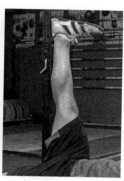

Figure 8.04 Supine Hip Hinge. Actively pushing the up leg into the wall using the hamstrings is a form of PNF that can help to relieve any perceived tightness upon release. Start with a knee that is more bent and slowly straighten the knee with each rep to increase the mobilization. If needed, start with ankle plantarflexion and slowly dorsiflex the top ankle after each rep.

your low back or ribcage, or until the stretching sensation in the posterior side of the up leg limits you.

- Perform 1-2 sets of 5 on each leg.
- For proprioceptive neuromuscular facilitation (PNF) activity, press the up leg into the door frame or rack as you inhale and the opposite leg back to the start position, hold for 3-5 seconds, relax and slide the heel again (Figure 8.04). Repeat that sequence for 1-2 sets of 5 reps on each side.
- Remember, you can manipulate the intensity of the mobilization by bending (reduces intensity) and straightening (increases intensity) the knee; also by dorsiflexing (increases intensity) and plantarflexing (reduces intensity) of the ankle (Figure 8.04).
- The point is to make the position of the end of the first pull more comfortable and attainable, so be sure to retest that hip hinge position in a standing position to gauge any perceived change.

Band Press Variation This drill can also be done with what is commonly referred to as a band press or band pullover. This technique further cues

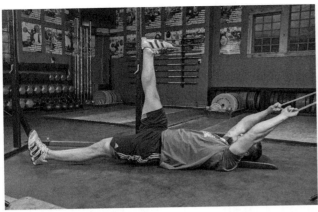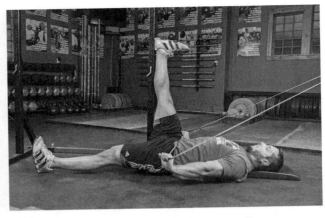

Figure 8.05 Using a band pullover can add some abdominal leverage and further increase control of the movement in the Supine Hip Hinge.

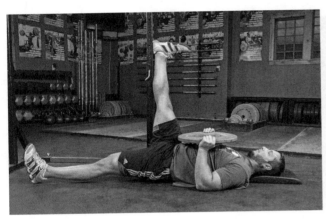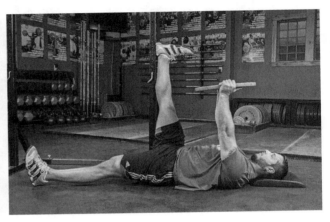

Figure 8.06 The Plate press variation adds more active control to the Supine Hip Hinge mobilization.

and facilitates the abdominal and lat tension we are looking for, and is a great option if resources allow.

Pull the band past shoulder level to begin. During the exhalation and heel slide, put pressure into the band with the lats to facilitate a stable trunk. The arm action should mimic that of the Back To Wall T-spine Extension drill that we performed previously. (Figure 8.05)

Plate Press Variation The athlete can also press a plate up to the ceiling while performing the drill. Exhale, reach the plate to the ceiling, and perform the heel slide. Again, we are looking to add some abdominal leverage and create some higher tension stability to begin ramping the system up for training. (Figure 8.06)

Movement Cluster Options

- Alternate any variation of the previous drill with approximately 20-second bouts of SMR to the glutes, hamstrings or hip flexors.

Stabilization: Standing Single Leg Hinge Test

Taking the control that the athlete has learned from the previous drill and implementing it on his or her feet is now the focus. It is not uncommon to see subtle side-to-side shifting of a lifter when pulling from the floor, as many possess asymmetries from left to right. The body may favor the leg it feels "safer" on (or favor one for other reasons), resulting in a lateral shift. This technical quirk may or may not be a problem for an advanced lifter who is very patterned, but for most, we want to promote symmetry. The following test and drill will identify subtle asymmetries in hip hinge stability from side to side, and teach the lifter how to stabilize on either leg, which, in turn, will help to balance out asymmetries during the bilateral pull.

Starting Position

- Stand with the feet underneath the hips (even if your pulling stance is wider, use this stance to avoid unnecessary loss of balance). The hands can be on the lower ribs, hips, or hanging down. Maintain a slight or "soft" bend in the knees.
- Set the feet with three points of contact—big toe, little toe and heel. Even if you are in shoes, maintain a balanced foot.

Execution

- Initiate with an inhalation through the nose, pushing the air down into the trunk. Exhale and hinge at the hips, allowing the trunk to move forward while keeping the spinal curves constant. The exhalation will aid in setting a neutral position.
- Hinge forward to the point where you feel hamstring tension on both sides, and inhale to reinforce this position (Figure 8.07).
- In a very slow and controlled manner, begin to shift your bodyweight laterally over the top of one leg. As you do this, nothing should change as far as the angle of your torso or the bend in your knees. Your pelvis should remain square and facing forward. Literally nothing changes other than a side-to-side shift.
- When you feel that your weight is centered and balanced over the top of one leg, lift the opposite leg 1-3 inches off of the ground in a slow and controlled manner (Figure 8.08). Hold this position for 3 breaths.
- Shift to center, stand, and repeat the sequence for the opposite leg.

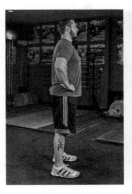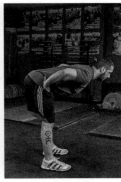

Figure 8.07 Standing bilateral hip hinge. Notice that the spinal curves do not change. Hinge to a depth in which you feel some hamstring tension.

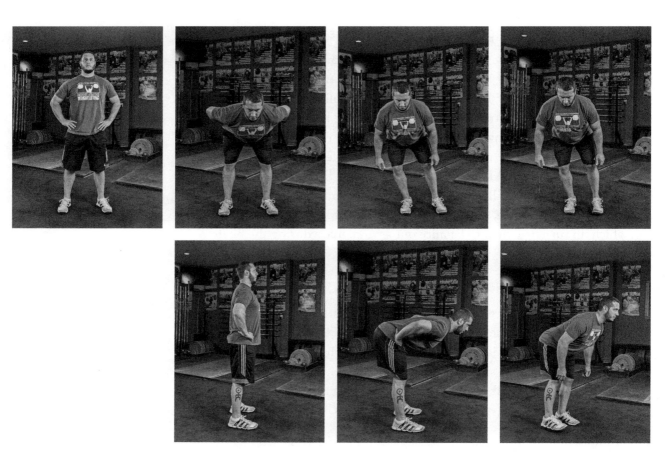

Figure 8.08 Single Leg Hip Hinge test. Notice how the pelvis stays flat and square and spinal curves remain constant.

- You may have felt a difference in stability, difficulty, muscle recruitment, etc. from side to side. If you identify this, it is not a bad idea to spend a little more time on the less stable or "weaker" leg each training day until the imbalance is corrected.

Stabilization: Standing Single Leg Hinge Static Holds & Reps

The test now turns into the correction. This is consistent with our Corrective Programming Guideline 5: Unilateral loading strategies to address asymmetries.

Execution

- Perform the exact same sequence of movements as the test above, and hold for 1-3 sets of 3-5 FULL breath cycles on each side. You can hold a weight in front of you for added challenge and recruitment of the core and hip musculature needed to stabilize the single leg stance (Figure 8.09).

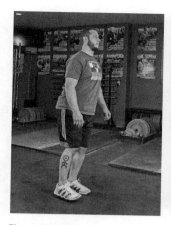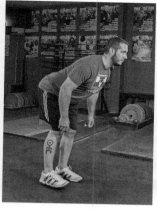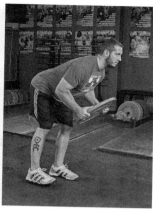

Figure 8.09 Holding a weight can increase the stability demands in the Single Leg Hip Hinge.

- Repetitions can be performed here as well. From the static hold position, perform slow, controlled hip hinge repetitions, trying to recreate the same position on each rep.
  - › 1-3 sets of 5-6 reps on each side
  - › You can add load here as well, but just remember, this drill is not meant to build top-end strength. Pick a weight that is challenging, but does not cause you to compromise position. We are trying to "own" single leg stance on each side.
- It may be beneficial for the lifter to perform these exercises barefoot to really feel and understand the importance of foot balance with the ground. Regardless, maintain big toe pressure down into the shoe or the ground.
- Maintaining a level pelvis actually aides in providing a mobilization to the hips into relative internal rotation, but it is

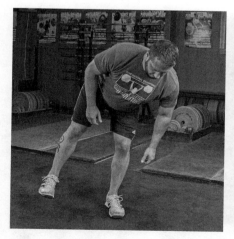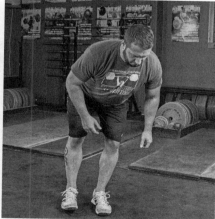

Figure 8.10 In the Single Leg Hip Hinge, do not be in a rush to lift the foot off of the ground if the pelvis tends to rotate without control as shown in the first picture. Keep the foot on the ground until you feel confident you have stabilized and centered yourself as shown in the second picture.

the pelvis moving on the femur instead of the femur moving on the pelvis as is what usually comes to mind. Think of it as being able to "sit into your hip" on both sides. Allowing the pelvis to rotate and open up is not "bad," but may indicate an inability to control single leg stance on that side, and we desire control of both sides for a symmetrical pull. (Figure 8.10)

Movement Cluster Options

- Alternate standing single leg hinge with supine hinge for desired number of rounds.

Stabilization: Standing Double Leg Plate Hinge

This is a good way to immediately utilize the control developed in the single leg hinge into a bilateral stance. It also adds the benefit of eccentric loading to facilitate greater range of motion improvements, but under load, to simultaneously stabilize the position: Loaded mobility work.

Starting Position

- Stand with feet hip-width apart in the same way you did with the single leg version before you lifted the foot.
- Hold a plate 6-12 inches in front of the chest.

Execution

- Exhale forcefully and hinge forward to the limit of your comfortable range, maintaining balance through the foot (Figure 8.11).
- Pause, inhale into your braced position, and perform another exhalation, allowing the weight to help you sink further down into the hinge.

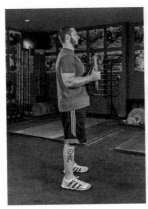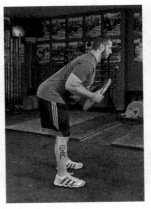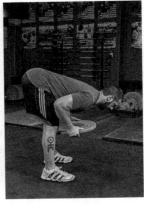

Figure 8.11 Double leg plate hinge, allowing the weight to provide mobility while still maintaining trunk stability.

- Try to resist the urge to deliberately push the hips back as you hinge forward. This creates a counterbalance that not only takes the onus off of the hamstrings, but also does not mimic where the pelvis will be in relation to the feet during the pull. "Own" your hamstrings.
- Perform 2-3 sets of 3-5 reps.

Movement Cluster Options

- Alternate with supine hip hinging or standing single leg hinging for the desired number of sets.

Integration: Snatch Grip Romanian Deadlift (RDL)

Many of you probably already perform this exercise in some form. We are including it because we can implement all of the concepts discussed thus far regarding the snatch pull, and it makes for a great part of an athlete's barbell warm-up or accessory routine. A coach may program these as supplemental strength exercises as appropriate.

Starting Position

- Assume your established pulling stance.
- If the bar is on the ground, with or without weight, set up as you typically would for a snatch and deadlift the bar to the hip in a manner that mimics the snatch pull.

Execution

- In standing, at the top of the deadlift, perform a brief, forceful exhalation through the mouth (not fully this time, since we are holding weight) to reset a stable trunk. As you inhale, pushing the air down, establish the lat and upper back

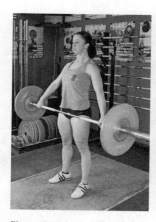 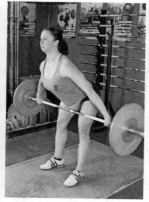 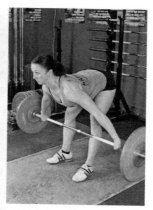

Figure 8.12 Snatch Grip RDLs to reinforce the T-spine position and hip hinge capacity that have been worked on.

tension that you found with the Back To Wall T-spine drill and the two supine hip hinging drills. This will keep the bar close to your mass as you hinge.
- Maintain this upper back position and lat tension as you unlock your knees and begin to perform a snatch grip RDL (hip hinge), just as we did in the standing hip hinges above (Figure 8.12).
- Allow an exhalation through pursed lips as needed to relieve pressure and maintain stability.
- Return to start position and repeat for sets of 5 to 8 reps with the empty barbell or lighter warm up sets.

Integration: Halting Snatch Deadlift

This is a continuation of the pause pulls that we performed previously, and puts more emphasis on static hip hinge and posterior chain strength.

Disclaimer: This drill emphasizes and, in some cases exaggerates, a position which the athlete may not truly achieve during the actual lifts. There are coaches who prefer not to use this drill for these reasons. It is included here because it does a very good job of reinforcing strength in the positions that we have been drilling up to this point. As with the RDL, a coach may program these as a supplemental strength exercise as appropriate.

Starting Position
- Assume your established snatch starting position.

Execution
- Pull the bar from the floor, continuing your leg drive until the bar has reached the upper third of the thigh or the hip, and pause there for a 3-count (Figure 8.13).
  - › The knees never rebend during the pull, and remain in a slightly unlocked position at the top (just like our RDL and hinge drills).
  - › The shoulders should be over the bar or slightly in front of the bar, and tension is created in the upper thoracic spine and lats to keep the barbell close to the lifter's body.
    - This is a GREAT time to practice extending through the upper thoracic spine while maintaining a stable lumbar spine position.
- During the pause, utilizing forceful exhalations through pursed lips and strong inhalations in which the air is pushed down will aid in maintaining stability; the intensity of the breath will be dependent on the weight on the bar.

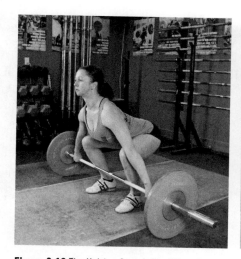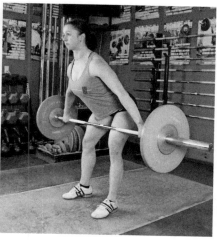

Figure 8.13 The Halting Snatch Deadlift will teach the athlete to push with the legs and maintain the positions we have been practicing.

> This is also a GREAT time to practice maintaining a balanced foot, even amidst the pause. While the bodyweight of the lifter may be shifted more toward the heels at the top of this movement, the foot should still remain flat and in full contact with the ground. The tendency of the lifter will be to lift the toes counterbalance too far back on the heels. DO NOT DO THIS, as it will a very bad habit when it comes time to extend up for the finish. Own the tension. Embrace it.

■ CHAPTER 9

Snatch Finish/Extension

This is the phase of the lift that generates the most power to send the bar upward. Therefore, it is of vital importance that we address the systems and positions needed for optimal execution.

Hip Extension

This is likely the most important joint action during the finish with regard to muscular power generation simply because it involves a larger of amount of muscle—the hamstrings and glutes.

The drills below will teach the lifter how to access adequate hip extension range of motion by coordinating the hamstrings and glutes, as well as the abdominals. Adequate muscle length will be promoted as well based on positioning. Some of these things may be familiar for many athletes—it is *how* we execute them that's important.

Refer back to your Thomas Test from Chapter 3. For those of you who had a limitation in hip extension range of motion, spending time with these drills, along with the hip extension drills associated with the split jerk in Chapter 18, should provide you with an improvement in that plane of motion.

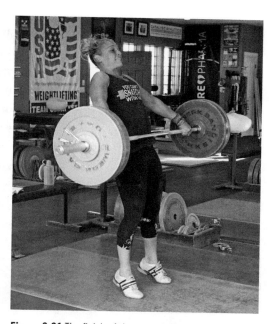

Figure 9.01 The finish of the second pull of the snatch

Even for those who did not demonstrate a restricted Thomas Test, these drills can be useful for you to learn how to utilize the full hip extension range of motion that you possess.

Mobilization: Supine Knee Hug with Heel Push

This drill has both a passive and active component to balance the mobility and stability required to achieve full hip range of motion. It also involves both a hip flexion and hip extension component, which mimics what we need to be able to do during the pull phases of the snatch—hip flexed to hip extended to hip flexed again.

Starting Position

- Supine with both legs extended straight, with heels pressing against a wall, rack or the edge of a platform.
- Ankles flexed to point the toes up.
- Head supported in a neutral position.

Execution

- Inhale through your nose and exhale through your mouth, engaging your abs and pulling your ribs down.
- Inhale into that position as you smoothly flex one hip toward the chest.
- As you are flexing that hip toward your chest, actively reach long through the opposite heel, pushing it into the wall. This should engage the glute and hamstring on the down leg, and aid in actively extending that hip (and knee with help of the quad).
- When you reach maximum active hip flexion of the up leg, exhale fully and use your hands to passively move the hip into more flexion (as is comfortable), continuing to reach long through the opposite heel. The breathing pattern here is key, as stabilizing the pelvis will aid in unlocking hip joint range of motion. Utilize higher tension strategies for more core engagement, and possible increased inhibition of feelings of tightness in the front of the hip.
- Explore internal and external rotation of the flexed hip, as well as adduction and abduction. Stay away from the

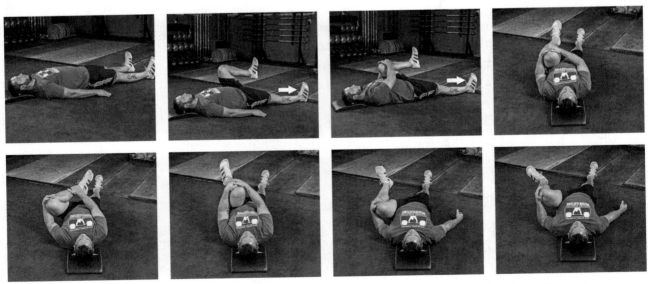

Figure 9.02 An active component of our hip assessment, in the Supine Knee Hug with Heel Push we use leverage from the wall (or substitute—the edge of a lifting platform is being used in these photos) for active hip extension mobility, along with exploring various hip flexion planes of motion.

impinging feeling in the crease/front of the hip. We are look-
ing for pain-free hip range of motion here.
- Think about creating distance/separation from knee cap to
knee cap.
- Perform 2-3 breath cycles for 1-2 sets of 3-5 on each leg
(Figure 9.02).

Movement Cluster

- Alternate with approximately 20-second bouts of SMR to the
hip flexor areas.

Stabilization: Double Leg Glute Bridge Variations with or without Band Pullover or Plate Press

I know what you are thinking—*Really dude? Glute bridges?* Here's the
deal... They can be useful, but people jack them up. They half-ass their way
through 3 sets of 10 super fast, pointless reps. When performed in this
manner, I fully agree that it's a useless exercise.

However, when *we* perform them with specific intent, they are valuable teaching tools to learn how to actively extend the hips, and will light
up the abdominal and hip musculature in a way that grooves a movement
pattern for the finish of the snatch.

Starting Position

- Knees bent to place the feet flat on the floor with 3 points of
contact (big toe, little toe and heel).

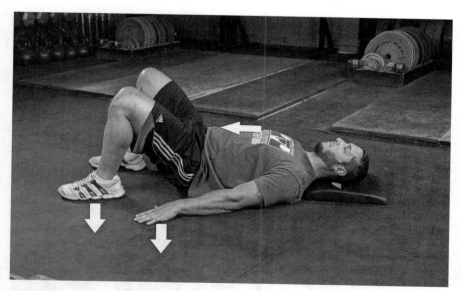

Figure 9.03 We utilize the glute bridge to teach the athlete how to extend the hips while anchoring
other parts of the body to provide stability. Pull the lower ribs down for a stable "can of stability," and
press the arms and feet into the floor.

- Hands flat on the ground with the arms outstretched mimicking a snatch grip.
- Inhale through the nose, pushing the air into the lower back.
- Exhale through the mouth, pulling the lower ribs down with the abs and pushing firmly into the ground with the hands, reflexively engaging your lats and core. (Figure 9.03)
  › This mimics the pressure utilized on the bar at the finish. If will also facilitate upper thoracic extension, while you work to keep your low back neutral (integrating concepts again).

Execution

- As you exhale, push through the *entire* foot and bridge the hips up. Continue forcefully exhaling *the entire way up*, even if you think you are running out of air.
- Hold this position, with the arms pressed into the floor, and inhale through your nose, pushing the air down into your brace and reinforcing your position.
- Exhale forcefully once more as you lower down. Maintain a ribs-down position as you lower the hips. The tendency will be to lower the hips to the floor, but allowing the ribcage to remain flared. Place your hands on your lower ribs to monitor, if necessary. (Figure 9.04)
- Quality over quantity. You can hold the bridge position for longer than 1 breath as well (3 is adequate), to reinforce control, using higher tension breath cycles to begin to ramp up the system for training.
- Perform 1-3 sets of 5-6 reps.

Heels on Bench Variation This variation is performed the same way described above but the athlete will have the heels on a bench (Figure 9.05).

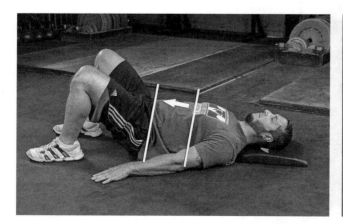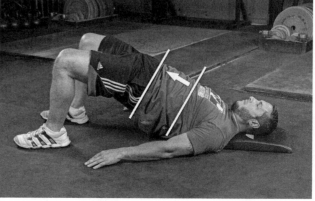

Figure 9.04 The basic glute bridge with pelvis and ribcage moving as a unit. Use the breath to create tension in this position and "own" hip extension.

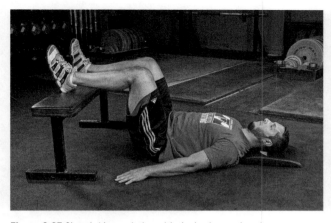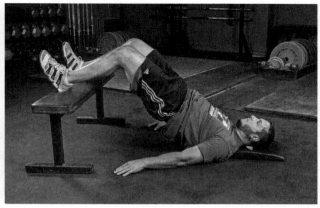

Figure 9.05 Glute bridge variation with the heels on a bench

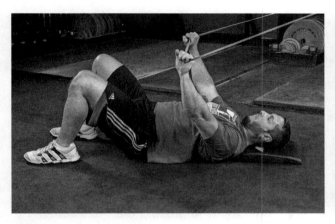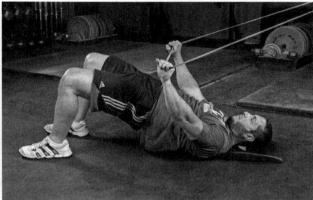

Figure 9.06 Utilize a band pullover for added lat and core leverage in the glute bridge.

This variation is great for those with more significant limitation during the Thomas Test, as it allows more room for range of motion without forcing the issue.

Lat Press/Pullover Variation For added core facilitation, add a banded lat press (pullover) to the same glute bridge movement (Figure 9.06). This will teach the lifter to maintain lat tension while he or she is extending the hips, just as they need to do in the finish of the pull.

Plate Press Variation Another option for adding increased core leverage to the glute bridge is a plate press (Figure 9.07). Exhale, reach the plate to the ceiling, and perform the bridge. Again, we are looking to add some abdominal leverage and create some higher tension stability to begin ramping the system up for training.

Sometimes lifters will experience hamstring cramping or low back tension during these bridge variations. In many cases, this can be remedied by adding more abdominal recruitment to balance the pelvis, or not

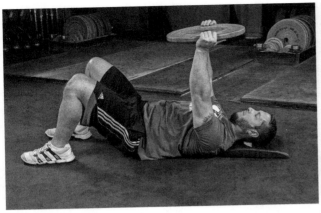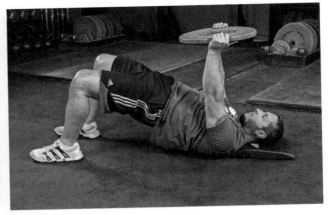

Figure 9.07 Utilize a plate press for another option to add core leverage to the glute bridge.

attempting to push into hip extension range of motion that he or she does not actually possess.

Make sure the starting position is on point—big toes planted into the ground, use a strong exhalation that sets a stable torso, and slightly squeeze the glutes before the hips actually lift off of the ground.

For low back tension, only raise the hips as high as they will go without altering your pelvic or low back position at all. This may stop you short of attaining full hip extension, and for those with a restricted Thomas Test, that's OK and to be expected. Range of motion will come as you gain more control in that position.

And remember, we don't care about improving our glute bridge for the sake of itself. We care about using it as a lower level tool to groove the finish of the pull.

Movement Cluster Options

- Alternate glute bridges with the Supine Heel Push for the desired number of sets and reps.

Stabilization: Tall Kneeling Holds with Lat Press with PVC

Tall kneeling is a great tool to teach an athlete bilateral hip extension, as it lowers the center of gravity and better isolates movement at the hips, but is a progression from the supine hip bridge variations. It is also a useful position to create adequate length through the front of the hips. With the knees bent, a muscle called the rectus femoris is put on stretch at both the hip and the knee. This means that attaining full hip extension range of motion in tall kneeling will be more difficult than in standing, from a muscular standpoint. If you can increase your hip extension range of motion in tall kneeling, then you have given yourself a movement buffer zone for standing.

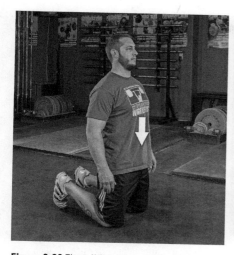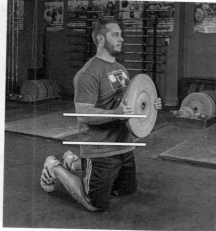

Figure 9.08 The tall kneeling position is used to mobilize and stabilize the hips into extension. Maintain a "tall" spine with neutral torso alignment.

Starting Position

- Tall kneeling position with the toes tucked under the feet and on the floor.
- Place the hands on the lower ribs or hold a weight 6-12 inches in front of the chest. (Figure 9.08)

Tall Kneeling Hold Execution

- Perform a slight tailbone tuck, and perform strong inhalations through the nose in which the air is pushed down into the lower torso, and full, forceful exhalations through the mouth to reset the abs (Figure 9.08).
  - ❯ Performing static holds with focused, forceful breaths will aid to increase neural drive to this movement pattern.
- 1-2 sets of 3-5 breaths

Tall Kneeling Extension Execution

- We can then perform repetitions of hip extension in tall kneeling to reinforce the pattern of flexing and extending.
- Allow the hips to rock back toward the heels (stay within comfort levels) and then extend the hips back to full tall kneeling (Figure 9.09).
- The feet can be flexed underneath or toes flexed up—whichever is more comfortable.
- Maintain the pelvis and ribcage relationship.
  - ❯ The tendency will be to leave the pelvis behind and flare the ribs forward, resulting in lumbar extension rather than hip extension. Exhale as you extend forward to maintain proper trunk alignment. An active posterior

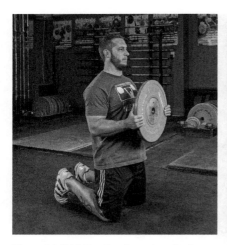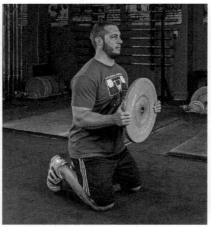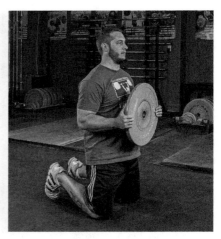

Figure 9.09 Tall Kneeling Extensions. Performing small reps of flexing and extending the hips can further develop control of hip extension. Holding a plate increases the facilitation of the acting muscles while maintaining trunk and hip position during the Tall Kneeling Extension.

pelvic tilt will likely still leave your pelvis and low back in a neutral slightly lordotic position.

- This can be done without weight or while holding a plate in front of the chest.
  - › Holding a weight increases engagement of the abdominal and posterior chain musculature. The hamstrings and glutes have to work hard to maintain hip extension while countering the front load.
- Perform 1-2 sets of 6-8 reps.

Movement Cluster Options

- Alternate tall kneeling drills with glute bridges and/or approximately 20-second bouts of SMR to the hip flexors or low back erectors.

Integration: Snatch Pulls

Most weightlifting programs have some form of pulling variations in which the lifter does not pull under the bar, but performs the movement through the finish (Figure 9.10). This is where integration of the concepts discussed above can be implemented. We've worked to make a transient improvement in hip extension range of motion; now let's integrate that mobility into a powerful finish.

During the lifts, especially at high intensities, the athlete should not have to consciously think about contracting the glutes or hamstrings to attain full hip extension in the finish. This is why practice is key, and along with the outlined drills, pulls can be part of this practice. During empty bar work, light warm-up pulls, and even your heavier working sets, try to feel that full hips-extended position that you created in your movement

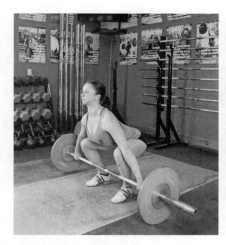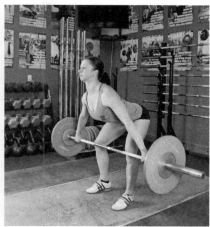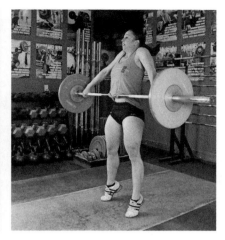

Figure 9.10 Putting all of our previous concepts together into a snatch pull. At this point, less thinking is involved, and more reacting.

drills during your reps. Using a forceful exhalation at the top of your pull may aid in maximizing this drive.

At lighter weights, the lifter can practice pausing at the very top of the pull, balancing on the balls of the feet to indicate that they are controlling what will be an upward trajectory of the bar.

Discussion Points & Summary of the Finish

There are different schools of thought in regard to the finish position and whether or not a lifter should be completely vertical, leaning back, knees locked straight, knees unlocked, feet flat, feet plantarflexed, etc. Much of this can be case-dependent. What is typically universal is that we want to attain as much hip extension as possible for a powerful finish.

We will outline another set of drills associated with the split jerk in a subsequent chapter, which may also aid you in the snatch and clean pull. As was mentioned earlier, there is much overlap between the lifts.

Remember to revisit the Thomas Test from time to time, as well to assess with drills or cues your body responds best to.

■ CHAPTER 10

Snatch Third Pull

This is the phase of the snatch in which the lifter pulls him or herself under the barbell, but has not yet achieved the final receiving position. This phase can be taken for granted as a formality, but is extremely important in the execution of the lift. The positions that we use to pull under the barbell have a direct influence on the trajectory of the bar and subsequent success of the lift. One of the universal weightlifting rules of *keeping the bar close* is dependent on how we execute the third pull.

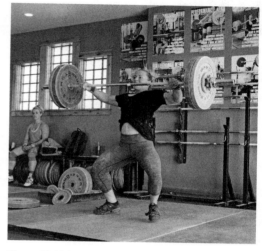

Figure 10.01 The third pull of the snatch

Shoulder Internal Rotation

In the starting position of the snatch (and clean), the shoulders are internally rotated and abducted (10-20 degrees for the clean and 30-45 degrees for the snatch) due to the fact that we use a double overhand grip, and they stay this way for the duration of the second pull. These positions do not pose much risk for impingement in a healthy shoulder, as I rarely see a lifter have such a lack of shoulder internal rotation that they cannot achieve a proper starting position. If they do have a limitation of that extent, they are probably on my treatment table, and not on the platform.

Immediately after achieving full hip extension during the second pull, the lifter will use the bar as leverage to pull under. The shoulders will remain in relative internal rotation in order to allow the inertia of the bar to continue traveling up as the lifter's body travels down. What changes from the starting position is that now we add an element of shoulder elevation coupled with the internal rotation. (Figure 10.02)

As we near the end of the third pull and prepare to receive the bar, our shoulders will transition to a slightly more externally rotated position. This all happens in the blink of an eye. It is this rotational transition that we will focus on, as a smooth transition will translate to maintaining a close and comfortable relationship with the bar.

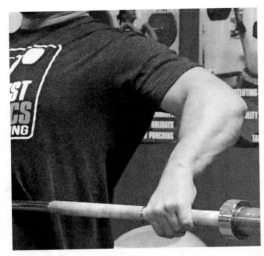

Figure 10.02 Natural internal rotation and elevation of the shoulder during the third pull of the snatch.

Ribcage

Although it is part of the initial screening and assessment, you will notice that we do not include many drills that directly address shoulder internal rotation in regard to specific joint mobilization or stretching in that direction. Although I mentioned it first, shoulder internal rotation as a standalone may not be a barrier to performing the snatch and clean and jerk movements, without consideration of the ribcage and shoulder blade.

As we have mentioned already, shoulder internal rotation is relevant when pulling under the bar in the third pull. Mobility common sense would tell you that if there was a limitation in range of motion to mobilize the joint in the position of restriction, which would involve forcing the shoulder into internal rotation coupled with 80-95 degrees of abduction.

Clinically, I have not seen athletes have great success with such a technique. As a therapist, when I have someone lying on his or her back and test shoulder internal rotation with 90 degrees of abduction, many times what is felt is a block at the end of range—a sudden abrupt halt in movement. Clank. This is commonly where athletes will utilize something like the sleeper stretch (Figure 10.03). However, trying to jam the shoulder through that range just sounds painful. So, we'll take a different approach.

The teaching/positional drills below will show the lifter how to position the ribcage and shoulder in order to move through a smooth transition/turnover, with the goal of carrying over to the bar's path in the snatch.

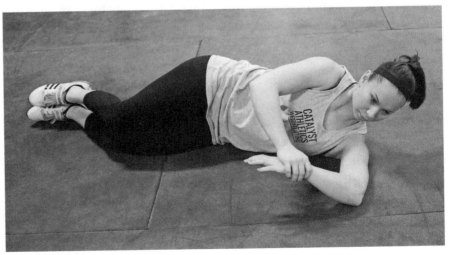

Figure 10.03 The sleeper stretch is a common stretch performed by athletes in an attempt to increase shoulder internal rotation. We will *not* be prescribing such a stretch in this book.

Mobilization: Shoulder Internal Rotation with Ribcage Locked

The following two drills will be used to complement each other to teach the athlete to control the ribcage and shoulder complex. Perform the quadruped variation first, then the standing variation, for 1-2 sets of 5-6 reps each or until you feel improvement with the movement pattern. The "ribcage locked" component simply means that we will be using the floor or wall for leverage and stability in order to isolate motion through the opposite shoulder.

Starting Position

- This is a similar position to our thoracic spine mobilization in Chapter 7.
- Initiate with an inhalation through the nose.
- As you exhale, smoothly reach through the shoulder blades (protract) and slightly flex/round the upper back from the base of the neck to the middle/low back. Think about moving the ribcage backwards. This will restore a natural kyphosis in the upper back and should allow the shoulder blades to sit flush on the ribcage. (Figure 10.04)
- Maintain this position and inhale again, focusing on placing air into your upper back (expand). Keep the neck relaxed.
- The focus here is for the athlete to feel what it's like to move the shoulder blades around the ribcage, as this will be our basis to then teach shoulder internal rotation.
- Hit a set of 5 breaths here, lightly reaching actively through the shoulder blades with each exhalation.

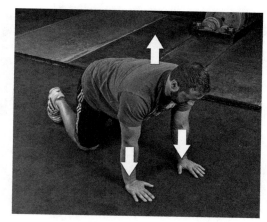

Figure 10.04 Using the quadruped position to teach an athlete to stabilize the thoracic spine with shoulder internal rotation. This is our "neutral" position, which provides a congruent relationship between shoulder blade and ribcage, reducing any scapular winging.

Execution

- While maintaining an active reach against the ground through one arm, slowly lift and internally rotate the opposite arm with the elbow straight to bring it into a position mimicking the pulling position in a snatch.
- Maintaining this internally rotated position, bend the elbow, mimicking a snatch high pull position. The shoulder blade of the moving arm may be retracting slightly to maintain its anchor with the ribcage.
- Turn the shoulder over (external rotation) and lock the elbow out, mimicking the turnover and overhead position of the snatch.
- From here, begin to internally rotate the shoulder, bend the elbow, and return back to the starting position.

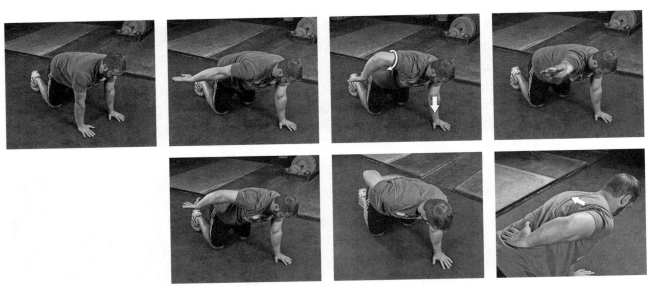

Figure 10.05 Quadruped Shoulder Internal Rotation with Ribcage Locked mobilization. Pushing into the floor with the off hand provides leverage and anchors the ribcage as the athlete performs internal rotation of the opposite shoulder. Further mimicking the shoulder position of the third pull, the athlete works to attain shoulder internal rotation while simultaneously controlling the scapula and torso.

- Alternatively, the athlete may take this into a movement very similar to the Apley Scratch test, in which he or she reaches behind the back while keeping the scapula tilted back and slightly retracted (Pictured). Maintain the reach of the off arm for leverage. Exhale as you pull the arm back. Athletes may find that they have more range here than they had during the Apley Scratch test, which could be an indication that true joint mobility was not the primary limiting factor. (Figure 10.05)
- This is a low-tension drill.

Standing with Wall Press Execution

- This is the same movement with the internally rotated arm but in a standing position. Start with both arms reaching into the wall, pushing the ribcage backward slightly. That will provide leverage and a stable base from which to internally rotate one arm.
- Combine internal rotation and elbow flexion as with previous drills, experimenting with various amounts of scapular retraction and protraction.
- Move back and forth through a snatch high pull position, visualizing maintaining a close bar path (Figure 10.06).
- The off arm is actively leveraged into the wall, and the ribcage is stacked over the pelvis.

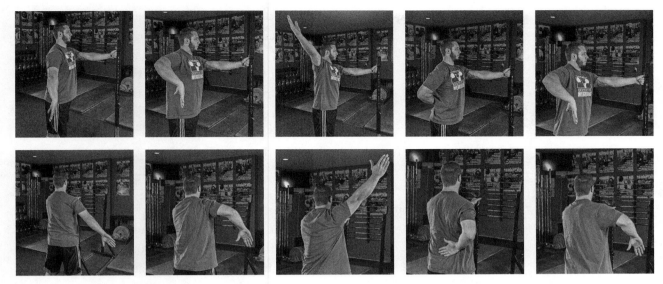

Figure 10.06 Use the wall for leverage to anchor the ribcage and explore shoulder internal rotation mimicking the third pull in the Standing with Wall Press variation of the Internal Shoulder Rotation with Ribcage Locked mobilization.

- The idea with this drill is to teach the athlete how to dissociate movement from the spine, shoulder blade and shoulder joint.

With both of the drills above, you'll likely notice that the shoulder blades on both sides stay anchored to the ribcage, even if this was an athlete that exhibited what would look like scapular winging during the Apley Scratch test. In standing, the athlete can transition to taking the fist off of the wall while maintaining the same trunk position.

Mobilization: Shoulder Internal Rotation Open Chain

Starting Position

- Supine squat position with the feet on a wall and knees bent.
  - With the feet on the wall, pull down with the heels lightly to engage the hamstrings. This will aid in reducing movement through the lower back as we isolate movement at the shoulder.
  - As an alternative to a wall, place the lower legs on a bench.
- Use head support to keep the neck neutral.

Execution

- Lift one arm up toward the ceiling.
  - Initiate the movement with an inhalation through the nose.

> As you exhale, pull the lower ribs down and lightly reach the arm up to the ceiling by moving through the shoulder blade (protraction), just like you did in quadruped. The excursion of movement is not large here. All we are doing is establishing a flush relationship between the ribcage and shoulder blade, and clearing a little bit of space in which to allow the shoulder to move.

- From this reached position, internally rotate the shoulder, simultaneously bending at the elbow and pulling into a 90-90 position at the shoulder. This will mimic the transition phase of the snatch.

  > For some of you, the front of the shoulder will be popped up significantly off the ground. This is not necessarily a problem, but you can attempt to pull the shoulder blade back while maintaining the shoulder 90-90 position.

- Move through this reach to 90-90 transition for smooth sets of 5, or simply remain in 90-90 for 5 full breath cycles on each side (Figure 10.07). Another option is moving through a high-pull type of range of motion. Experiment with packing

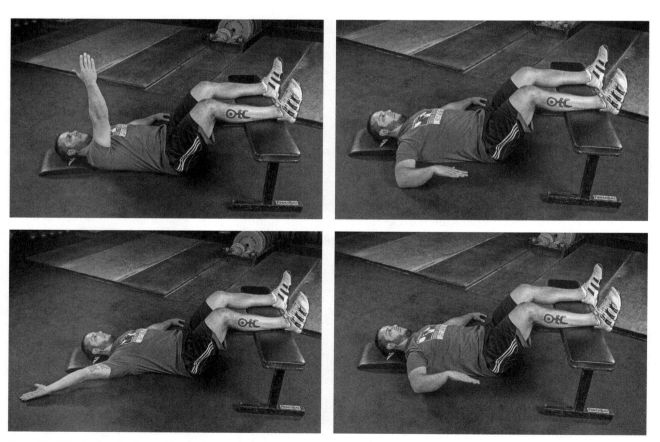

Figure 10.07 In the Shoulder Internal Rotation Open Chain mobilization, we combine slight protraction with shoulder internal rotation and elbow flexion to mimic the third pull.

the shoulder blade down and back versus allowing it to protract forward. Find what affords you the most comfortable range of motion.

> Utilize light exhalations to reset ribcage position periodically.

> Again, this is low tension movement with awareness of position being high.

> One can also load this movement with a *light* training plate. The load should just be enough to increase the muscular effort a bit, but not so much that it changes the path of the shoulder or causes discomfort. For most, keep it *under* 5kg.

Mobilization: Standing Back to Wall Reach with Shoulder Internal Rotation

Now we take what we just did on the floor to a standing position, but with wall support. This is the exact same starting position as the thoracic spine mobilization in Chapter 7.

Starting Position

- Stand with the feet approximately 12 inches away from the wall with the back supported by the wall.
- With the lumbar spine, we have a couple of options:
  > For the athlete who has difficultly with cueing of spinal position, this drill can be started with the low back completely flat against the wall. This will minimize any compensation through the lower back as we isolate movement at the shoulder.
  > For the more stable and kinesthetically-aware athlete, maintaining a slight lumbar lordosis is desirable, as this mimics the low back position during the pull. A slight lordosis is enough to fit fingers between the low back and the wall.

Execution

- Initiate the drill with an inhalation through the nose, "pushing the air down into the lower back."
- Exhale through the mouth and reach the arms forward (protract the shoulder blades) as you did in the quadruped and supine drills above. You may feel your upper back round, but maintain the exact position of your mid and low back.
- At the end of your exhalation and reach OR while beginning your next inhalation, internally rotate the shoulders,

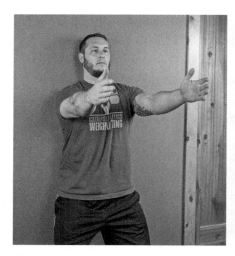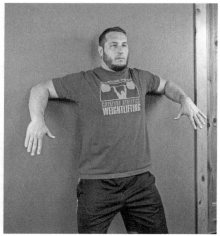

Figure 10.08 The wall provides a cue for spinal position while the lifter works to dissociate shoulder movement, particularly internal rotation, in the Standing Back to Wall Reach with Shoulder Internal Rotation mobilization.

simultaneously bending at the elbows and pulling the arms into a 90-90 position at the shoulder (Figure 10.08).

> This will mimic the transition phase of the snatch, and is exactly what you did in supine previously.

> For some of you, the front of the shoulder will be popped forward significantly off the wall. This is not necessarily a problem, but you can attempt to pull the shoulder blade back while maintaining the shoulder 90-90 position.

> Move through this reach to 90-90 transition for smooth sets of 5, or simply remain in 90-90 for 5 full breaths cycles on each side.

> As you move into the 90-90 position, your upper back may begin to reverse its curve and move into slight extension, but this should be done without losing contact or altering position of the mid and lower back.

> Again, this can be loaded by holding a *light* training plate (under 5kg) as the lifter moves through a range mimicking the third pull.

Dowel Muscle Snatch Variation Repeat the entire process, but while holding a dowel to mimic a bar. When the lifter is comfortable with the 90-90 internally rotated position, begin to experiment with the transition to external rotation overhead. This should be done without having to alter the position of the lower back.

When this is comfortable, the athlete can then transition to eliminating the reaching component of the drill and attempt to achieve the same bilateral 90-90 position and transition by starting at the hip as they would in a pull (Figure 10.09).

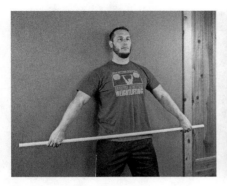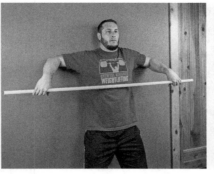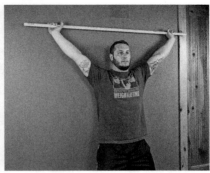

Figure 10.09 With a Dowel Muscle Snatch variation of the Standing Back to Wall mobilization, we can finish the bar path overhead. This is useful for an athlete to learn how to go from a high mobility demand in the shoulder to a high stability demand when locked out overhead.

Utilize an exhalation to set position against the wall, and experiment with various amounts of shoulder blade protraction and retraction to find the most comfortable position to achieve a smooth turnover.

Integration: Muscle Snatch

This is a common accessory lift that will aid in teaching the lifter bar path mechanics. This drill, along with the halting deadlift, is used to varying degrees among coaches. Some do not use this move in fear that it will teach the athlete to "overuse" the arms during the pull. We have included it here as a way to "lock in" the shoulder movement and mobility that we have been ingraining previously.

Starting Position

- Use your established starting position for the snatch.

Execution

- Perform the pull in the same way that you would for a full snatch lift, extending the hips at the top of the finish.
- Instead of pulling your body under the bar, allow the momentum of the bar to continue upward as you stay tall and extended.
- The arms should follow the path that we practiced in the previous drills, transitioning from a 90-90 internally rotated position to external rotation and overhead. (Figure 10.10)
  › Note that this is not a flick of the wrists at the top of the bar's height. It is a deliberate pull to 90-90 then a spin of the elbows under the bar, and a punch up.

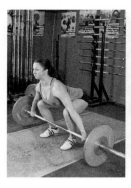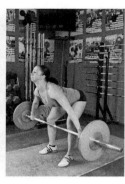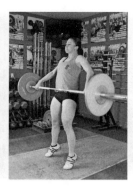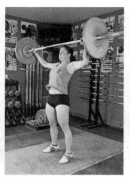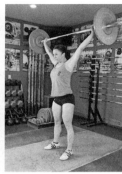

Figure 10.10 The muscle snatch is a way to strengthen the pull of the bar path and add resiliency and strength to the shoulder girdle in this position.

Movement Cluster Options

- Alternate your light muscle snatches with any third pull drill that was previously described for 2-3 rounds before hitting your heavier intensities.

Discussion Points & Summary of the Third Pull

For those looking to improve rotational comfort and capacity in the shoulder, as it relates to the third pull of the snatch, spend some time here exploring and experimenting with various degrees of shoulder rotation and scapular retraction and protraction. Everyone will be different, and the drills can provide feedback regarding what works best for you.

For example, if you move through the transition in supine, quadruped or standing and you feel discomfort in your shoulder, try to alter your position. Reach/protract farther before internally rotating or don't reach/protract as much; retract the shoulder blades more during the transition to external rotation or don't retract as much. Get the idea? If you then find a position that decreases or takes the shoulder discomfort away (and gives you the ability to keep the bar or dowel close to your body), then you have identified the movement pattern/position that you want to practice and ingrain.

And, of course, don't forget to bring it back to where it really matters—the snatch. Perhaps your main focus for that training day is keeping the bar close and pulling underneath with high elbows.

CHAPTER 11

Snatch Receiving Position

Going back to the overhead squat screening, we will break the movement down here to build it piece by piece.

Overhead Position

Pure shoulder mobility may not be *as* significant a limiting factor during an overhead squat, because the abducted position is typically an easier range of motion to attain relative to a narrower jerk grip. It also allows for a faster turnover. However, it can also be inherently less stable, as the joints of the arm are not stacked. When addressing the overhead position of a snatch, it will be about placing the shoulder in a position to support weight with the inherently wider snatch grip.

Mobilization: Supine Squat with Scapular Facilitation

For novice lifters or those who really want to fine-tune their overhead positioning in the snatch, this can be an effective teaching tool. If you identified a perceived shoulder flexion range of motion limitation in the screening, this is a strategy to gain it back actively. This drill requires that the arm move in a plane that mimics the receiving position of a snatch.

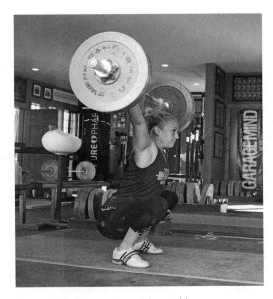

Figure 11.01 The snatch receiving position

The bony structure of your shoulder joint is like a golf ball sitting on a tee. There is very little passive/inherent stability. Due to this, significant amounts of neuromuscular stability is required from the rotator cuff and scapular stabilizers to center the golf ball on the golf tee and provide a firm foundation for the tee to stand on (the scapula on the ribcage). Throughout the following drills, you want to maintain the position of the ball on the tee. This is another example of "stacking" the joints.

Starting Position

- 90-90 position with the feet on a wall or heels on a bench and the head supported in a neutral position.
- Pull the ribs down by fully exhaling.
- Recruit the hamstrings by pulling down with the heels—this will help to limit motion through the lower back and pelvis, as we are looking to isolate movement at the shoulder.

Execution

- Reach one arm up toward the ceiling without shrugging up toward the ear. The reach should come through the shoulder blade, as was the case in the previous drills for the transition.
- If performing on one side only, you can monitor shoulder position with the opposite hand.
- Maintaining a mid-range scapular reach (somewhere between completely down and back and trying to touch the ceiling), move through various angles of shoulder elevation.
- Experiment with various amounts of shoulder blade protraction and retraction, as well as shoulder internal and external rotation, as you move through range of motion that will resemble narrow to wide snatch grips. The goal is to figure out in what position your shoulders feel the most mobile and comfortable overhead. It will vary for everyone, just like squat stance.

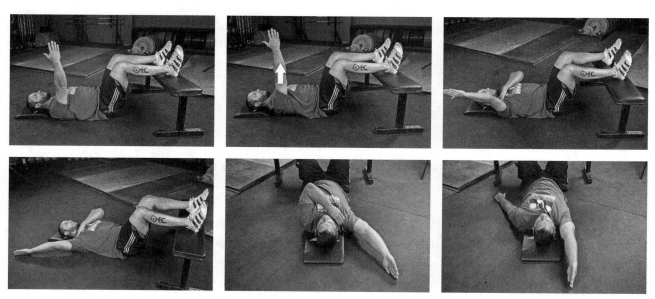

Figure 11.02 Supine Squat with Scapular Facilitation mobilization. Maintaining your scapular reach and monitoring with the opposite hand, move through various angles overhead, keeping your lower ribcage down. Learn to dissociate shoulder movement from the trunk. Find your full, sustainable range of motion.

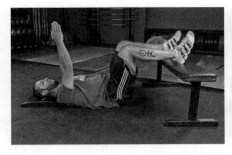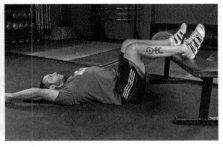

Figure 11.03 In the Supine Squat with Scapular Facilitation mobilization, attempt to dissociate shoulder movement from trunk movement by keeping the ribs down and low back stable as you go overhead. Pictured here the athlete is erroneously arching the lower back and flaring the lower ribs.

- Perform 1-2 sets of 8 reps on each side, or as many as desired (Figure 11.02).
- Experiment with breath control. Exhale as you reach overhead, inhale at the top, or vise versa. Regardless, maintain a consistent ribcage position and low back position in relation to the floor. (Figure 11.03)

Pullover Execution

- Here is another opportunity to add load to our mobility work, taking advantage of eccentric contraction.
- Hold a light plate or dowel rod with a change plate in the air towards the ceiling.
  - > Start with no more than 5kg. I've never prescribed more than 10kg with this exercise.
- Slowly move into shoulder flexion, allowing the weight to pull you into full range of motion, but still under active control. Only move into range in which you feel comfortable and confident.
- If you are using a dowel rod, experiment with wider and narrower grips, as well as internally and externally rotated shoulders. (Figure 11.04)
- Perform 2-4 sets of 5 slow controlled reps.

Each rep of the pullover exercise can take as long as you want it to. You can pause at your first resistance point and take a breath, then with an exhalation, try to sink into a slightly deeper range.

For those who found asymmetry in shoulder flexion during the movement screen: When performing this bilateral pullover, focus on keeping the upper back on the side with limited shoulder flexion on the ground as you perform the exercise. Asymmetries in shoulder flexion can be one cause of twisting in the snatch. If this is you, you may find that you also want to twist during the pullover. Again, focus on keeping both sides of your upper back on the ground. A unilateral focus can also be achieved by simply

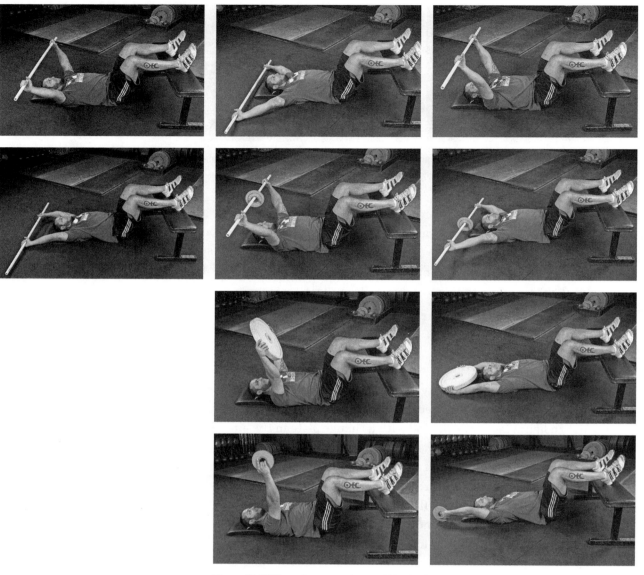

Figure 11.04 The pullover exercise to add load to low-level overhead mobility work. Several variations can be used, including a weighted PVC pipe, a plate, or single-arm. Experiment with narrower and wider grips when using a PVC pipe.

holding a light change plate in your hand and performing the movement with one arm, as outlined above.

To increase the trunk stability demands a bit, the drill can be performed in the exact position (supine squat) as above, but without the wall to support the feet so the legs are being held in the air by the hip and core musculature.

Movement Cluster Options

- Alternate with SMR for bouts of approximately 20 seconds to the lats/underside of the shoulder area to inhibit perceived tightness that would limit overhead movement.

Mobilization: Sidelying Scapular Facilitation

This and the previous drills are great complements to one another with respect to helping a lifter feel a "stacked" shoulder versus not. The "golf ball on tee" analogy, in reference to the shoulder joint, really applies here in the sidelying position and it will help you feel the position you'll try to recreate in an overhead squat position.

Starting Position

- Assume a sidelying squat position with a foam roller between the knees.
- Set your ribcage with an inhalation followed by a full exhalation through the mouth. Then breathe comfortably in this lightly braced position.

Execution

- Lift your top arm up to the ceiling with the palm pointed forward.
  - › Reach as long as you can with the top arm. Reach through the shoulder blade as you did previously.
  - › Now pack your shoulder blade down and back.
  - › The optimal shoulder blade position to receive the barbell will likely be somewhere in between these two extremes. (Figure 11.05)
- Now you can explore what it feels like to pop your shoulder forward versus pulling it back. With rolling the shoulder forward, think of this as moving the "golf ball forward on the

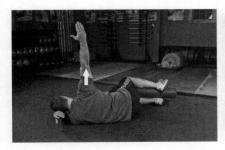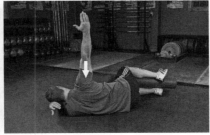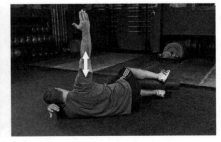

Figure 11.05 In the Sidelying Scapular Facilitation mobilization, explore various shoulder blade positions to mimic what you'll do overhead. Reach up to the ceiling completely, then pull the shoulder back down completely—then move to the approximate mid-point between these two extremes to find what should be the optimal position.

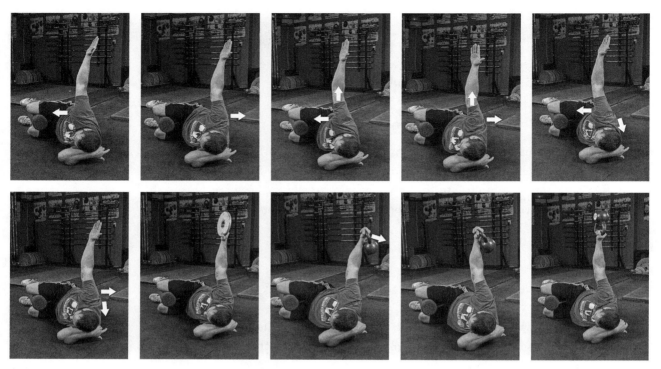

Figure 11.06 Experimenting with the position of the humeral head (golf ball) will clue you in on which positions feel "stacked" and stable. Adding load will provide immediate feedback as to what positions feel strong and sustainable. Typically, the lifter will feel more comfortable when the load is stacked in line with shoulder, which is supported by the trunk.

tee." For some, increased forward translation of the humeral head (golf ball) may sacrifice your "stacked" position. Now pull the humeral head back to a position that is flush with your pec muscle. You can monitor with the opposite hand. Think of it as "sucking the front of the shoulder back into the socket."

- Combine anterior and posterior translation of the humeral head (golf ball) with reaching the arm long or pinching the shoulder blade back. We are building some powerful awareness of shoulder position here, and this is low-threshold focused experimentation. (Figure 11.06)
    › If you are unsure of which position would be most stable, imagine someone putting a 50lb (or whatever is relatively heavy for you) dumbbell in your hand, and think about if you would feel comfortable supporting it.
    › Likewise, you can hold a light kettlebell, dumbbell or plate in your hand to add a bit of load to the position.
- When the most comfortable and stable position is identified, you can hold statically for 5 breaths to "lock it in," then move through partial ranges of adduction and abduction while maintaining this shoulder congruency for 8-10 reps each side (Figure 11.07).

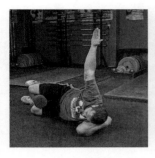 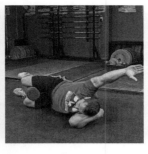 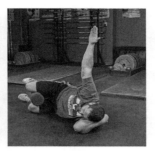

Figure 11.07 Here you focus on maintaining the "ball on tee" position as you move back and forth through overhead range in the Sidelying Scapular Facilitation mobilization.

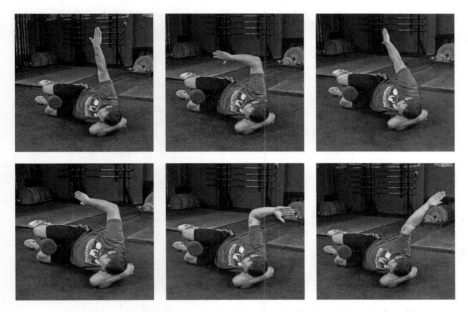

Figure 11.08 Mimicking the snatch bar path with the position that has been determined to allow you full, comfortable range in the Sidelying Scapular Facilitation mobilization.

- Finally, move through a range that mimics the transition to receiving position, all while maintaining this shoulder congruency for 8-10 reps each side (Figure 11.08). Keep the elbows locked out actively, just as you would with a snatch.

Mobilization: Standing Back to Wall Scaption

Here we are putting the previous two drills together in standing to create a stacked shoulder position that will be sustainable and comfortable under load. The word *scaption* is slang in the therapy and rehab world, and my professors would probably be disappointed that I am using it. It denotes the "Y" position that we can move our shoulders into. This particular angle is in direct line with how the scapula is oriented on the ribcage—its movement plane. So, when we move in this scapular plane, we can call it *scaption* for short. We will use it to mimic the snatch receiving position.

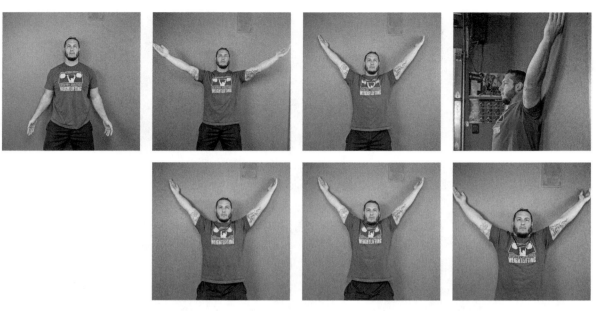

Figure 11.09 The Standing Back to Wall Scaption mobilization, mimicking the snatch angle. Maintain a consistent relationship with the wall.

Starting Position

- Same starting position as previous Back to Wall drills.
- Set the trunk position with an exhalation. The relationship between the spine and wall should not change as the athlete performs the exercise.

Execution

- With the palms facing each other, but angled out slightly, move the arms overhead in a "Y" pattern (scaption) until you reach the wall or until maximum range is attained without moving through the low back or ribcage. The width of the finished position should be comparable to your normal snatch grip, and shoulder position should be similar to where it was in the Supine Scapular Facilitation drill above, although it's recommended to experiment with hand widths to find what positions are more mobile. (Figure 11.09)
- Exhaling as you raise the arms can ensure that the trunk stays neutral, and inhaling at the top may help you gain more mobility.
- At the top of the movement, you can incorporate an active "reach" to maximize range (Figure 11.10). Keep in mind it's not a large excursion of movement—it should come from the shoulders blades pushing up slightly.
- Perform 1-3 sets of 5-8 reps, focusing on dissociating movement through the shoulders from the lower back.

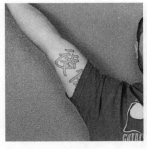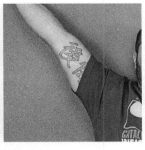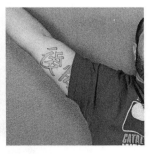

Figure 11.10 Incorporating an active reach at the top of the movement can solidify the position and may allow more range for some. Note the difference in strategies. The second picture shows a subtle "push" up, but the stacking of the shoulder remains constant. The third picture shows the lifter popping the humeral forward. This is commonly seen, but for some lifters may not be the most stable position to support load.

Movement Cluster Options

- Alternate Standing Back to Wall Scaption with 20-second bouts of foam rolling to the underside of the shoulder/lats and/or the upper back.

Mobilization: Standing Front to Wall Scaption with Liftoff

The premise of this drill is similar to the Back to Wall variation; however, now we are facing the wall, teaching the athlete to maintain a consistent trunk position while standing. The wall, in this case, provides a cue for the scapula and facilitation of the upward rotators of the shoulder blades bilaterally. And again, the motion that the lifter moves through (scaption) mimics the receiving position of the snatch. The last portion of the drill will aid in gaining some active upper thoracic extension over top of a relatively motionless low back and pelvis.

Starting Position

- Stand facing a wall with the feet roughly 8-12 inches away and knees slightly bent
- Place the forearms flush on the wall with the palms facing each other and shoulders externally rotated about 35 degrees.
- Slightly tuck the tailbone underneath so that low back is still lordotic, but not excessively so.
- Exhale fully to set the rib position. (Figure 11.11)

Execution

- Slightly protract the shoulder blades and press the forearms into the wall.

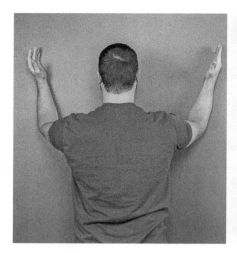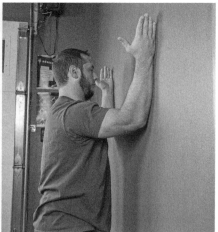

Figure 11.11 Starting position of the Standing Front to Wall Scaption with Liftoff drill to teach overhead mechanics

- Slide the forearms up the wall following the 35-degree angle of the forearms, maintaining them flush, and maintaining the elbow reach into the wall.
- Do not alter your pelvis or low back position.
- At the point at which you can no longer keep your elbows on the wall, pause and perform 1-2 full breath cycles. From here, you can reset to the starting position or continue to slide up, maintaining an active reach through your fingers. (Figure 11.12)
- A slight shrug and activation of the upper trap is normal for proper upward rotation of the shoulder blades. This likely will happen naturally.
- Reaching long while keeping your low back neutral should also facilitate the upper thoracic spine extension that we desire.
- Lastly, if you are able to maintain position, lift your hands off the wall 1 inch in the plane of the snatch. This will further encourage upper thoracic extension. (Figure 11.12)
- Perform 1-2 sets of 5-8 repetitions, or as needed.

Notes If performed strictly, you should feel a point where your lats and other shoulder depressors are restricting your wall slide. Simply work within your limits. Improvements in range will come.

Movement Cluster Options

- Alternate with 20-second bouts of foam rolling to the underside of the shoulder/lats and/or the upper back.

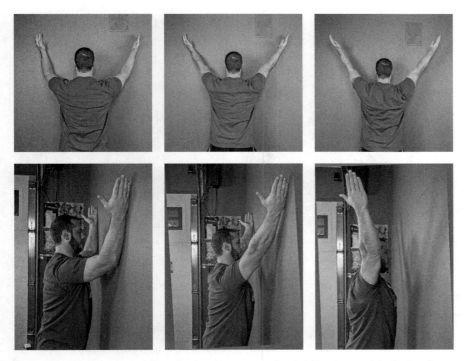

Figure 11.12 Moving into the full overhead position at an angle mimicking the snatch in the Standing Front to Wall Scaption with Liftoff drill. Notice the torso position remains constant. The liftoff will facilitate natural upper T-spine extension.

Stabilization: Kneeling Scapular Facilitation & Behind the Neck Press

Half Kneeling We return to our half kneeling position, but now as a tool to practice the overhead position. For this drill, we will elevate the front foot, which will help "lock in" the lumbar spine and pelvis, isolating movement at the shoulders. It also provides a light mobilization to the hips. The drill can be done just as well without front foot elevation. We are working to recreate the shoulder positions of the previous drills with a pressing/ loading component.

Starting Position

- Half kneeling with the front foot elevated.
  - › Orient the down leg into straight line from knee to hip to shoulder to ear.
  - › Tuck the toes under the back foot—try to touch the balls of the foot to the ground.
- Set the rib position with an exhalation, and slightly tuck your tailbone so that your pelvis is underneath you. You may feel a stretch in the front of the down leg.
- Shoulder slightly internally rotated across the body, shoulder blade protracted, forearm pronated. (Figure 11.13)

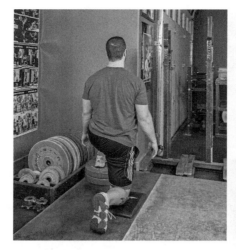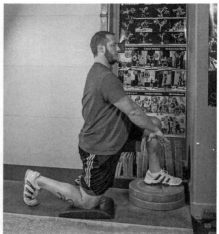

Figure 11.13 Starting position for the Kneeling Scapular Facilitation drill

Diagonals Execution

- Begin the arm movement by pulling the shoulder blade back to mid range and externally rotating the arm as you move through the range.
- Maintain the shoulder blade in mid range and *reach* long through the fingertips, finishing with shoulder external rotation, forearm supination and wrist extension. (Figure 11.14)
- Maintain ribcage and low back position throughout movement.
- Perform 1-2 sets of 6-8 controlled reps.

Notes If you feel a pinch in the front or top of your shoulder when beginning the movement, reposition so that you are not starting with your arm so far across your body—pull the shoulder blade back more to start, or simply begin with the shoulder externally rotated. Load this with a small plate if you are able.

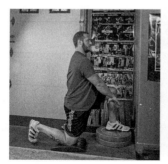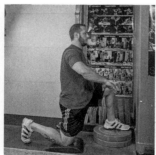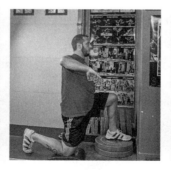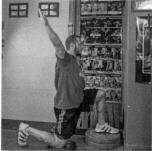

Caption 11.14 Kneeling Scapular Facilitation Diagonals. Begin by tilting the shoulder blade back. Then move from shoulder internal to external rotation, ending in a position mimicking a snatch.

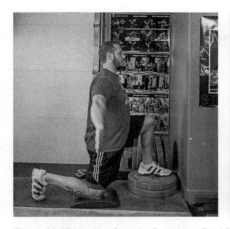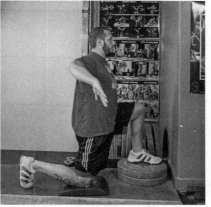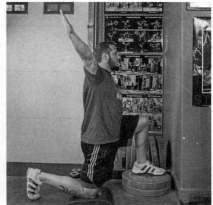

Figure 11.15 Kneeling Scapular Facilitation Third Pull: Begin with the arm abducted to the side and mimic the third pull of the snatch. The emphasis will be recreating a stacked shoulder position at the top.

Third Pull Execution

- To further simulate the bar path of a snatch, the lifter can keep the arm abducted to the side, as opposed to across the body, when moving from internal to external shoulder rotation and overhead (Figure 11.15).

Ribcage Lock Execution

- To create stability through the core, the off arm can be pressed against the top knee or into the wall. This will further lock down the position, to isolate movement at the shoulder. (Figure 11.16)
- Load can be added to this exercise with use of lighter change plates, with the focus of increasing muscle activity and maintaining the exact same positions (Figure 11.17). The load here is not meant to build brute strength, it's simply there to reinforce the movement.
- The drill can be transitioned into a strict press as well (Figure 11.18).

Behind the Neck Press Execution

- Hold a PVC pipe, dowel or light training bar behind the neck in a snatch grip. Tuck the elbows under the dowel or bar as well as possible.
- Set the ribcage position with a forceful exhalation and inhale into that position to reinforce. Breathe comfortably after this point without altering trunk position.

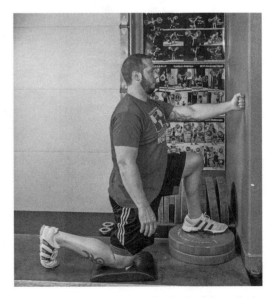

Figure 11.16 Kneeling Scapular Facilitation Ribcage Lock: Actively pushing the off arm into the wall or front knee can create more stability through the trunk.

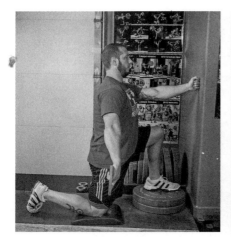
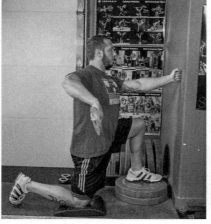
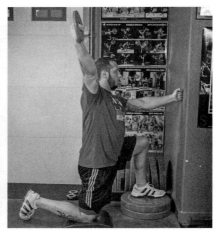

Figure 11.17 Light load can be added to reinforce positions in the Kneeling Scapular Facilitation drill.

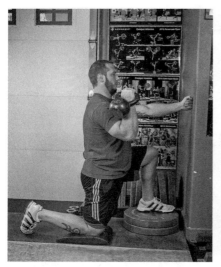
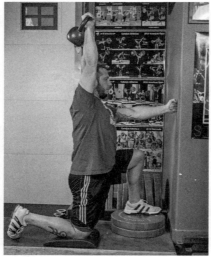
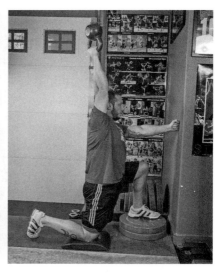

Figure 11.18 The loaded Kneeling Scapular Facilitation drill can be transitioned to a strict press. Push straight up without altering position of the rest of the body. This can also be done with a kettlebell in the bottom-up position.

- Without altering the trunk position, press the bar overhead, ending over the back of the head directly over the shoulders (Figure 11.19).
  - › A behind the neck press can be a challenging move for some. If it is uncomfortable or you do not feel you can attain an adequate position, return to previous drills instead.
  - › If you can attain the starting position comfortably, focus on a straight bar path and consistent force all the way through the press. A behind the neck press is not inherently dangerous and can be a great tool for a lifter to learn to stack the bar over the upper back.

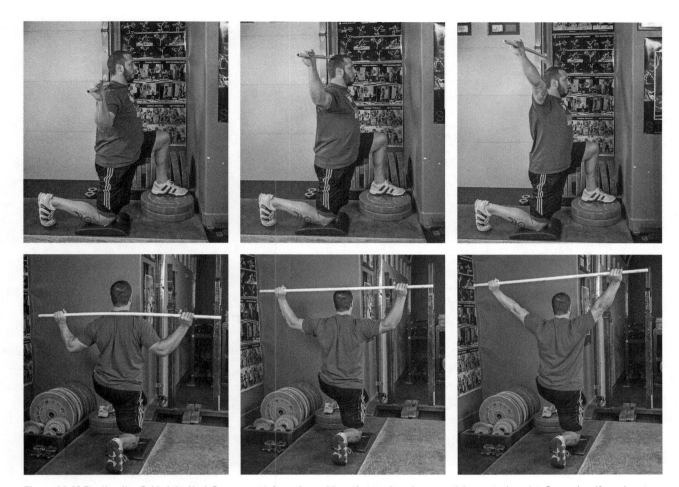

Figure 11.19 The Kneeling Behind the Neck Press can reinforce the positions that you have been practicing up to the point. Remember, if you do not tolerate this position, perform an earlier variation.

- Perform 1-2 sets of 5-8 reps.
- This drill can be performed in standing as well.

Tall Kneeling Variation All of the above variations can also be done in tall kneeling (Figure 11.20). It is more challenging to maintain pelvis and low back position and also better resembles the bilateral stance position of a snatch. A helpful cue here is to maintain an active "tail bone tuck", as that will keep the pelvis and ribcage stacked.

Movement Cluster Options

- Alternate Supine Squat with Scapular Facilitation with plate loaded scapular facilitation for 2-3 rounds or as desired.
- Alternate Supine Squat with Scapular Facilitation with behind the neck press for 2-3 rounds for 2-3 rounds or as desired.
- Alternate the above mentioned with 20-second bouts of SMR to lats and/or upper back.

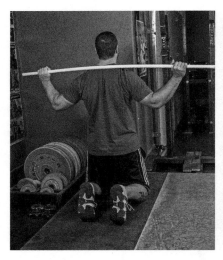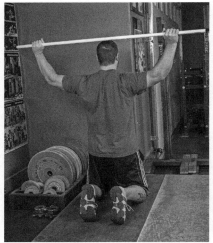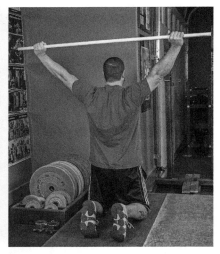

Figure 11.20 Tall kneeling variation of the behind the neck press. Tall kneeling variations put more emphasis on active hip extension.

Integration: Snatch Grip Push Press

By now, you have established where your overhead position is most comfortable in a snatch grip. The snatch grip push press is a good exercise to reinforce this position, as well as to gain valuable practice controlling the trunk and ribcage when overhead, before we add a squatting component.

Starting Position

- Before getting under the bar and unracking it, we want to establish a solid positional foundation first.
- Establish your grip with arms outstretched.
- Perform a partial exhalation to set a neutral position as you are reaching into the barbell.
- Inhale into that position partially to reinforce it. You should be able to breathe in and out over top of this newly established position. The goal is to create a scenario in which your body is stacked from ankles to hips to shoulders in order to support the weight that will be on your shoulders.
- As you bring your body under the bar in preparation to unrack it, this is a GREAT time to incorporate the concept that you have learned of attaining upper T-spine extension.
- In preparation for the dip and drive, perform one last inhalation, pushing the air down and ultimately filling your upper back. This will put the finishing touches on establishing a robust platform for the bar to be supported on.

Execution

- On the dip and drive, we want equal pressure in the middle of both heels. This is not necessarily something that you want to consciously be thinking about during such a dynamic movement; however, it may be beneficial to practice 2-3 dips and partial drives as practice. During these reps, you can focus on even foot pressure from left to right.

■ Think of the dip as an unlocking of the hips and knees—straight down, straight up—with equal foot pressure throughout (Figure 11.21).

> Again, the athlete can perform the dip for repetitions, experimenting with depth of the dip and foot width, to find where they feel they can create the most drive into the ground and up into the barbell.

> If performing for reps as practice, incorporate a pause at the bottom. A helpful cue is to learn to "put the breaks on." One common error is drifting during the transition of the dip and drive, which may leak power. Work on a distinct transition from dip to drive. This will also help maximize utilization of the barbell oscillation.

■ As you extend and drive up, the goal is for the trunk position that you established previously to change as little as possible (Figure 11.22).

> There will likely be a change during the bar's transition overhead, as the legs generate great force with extension that will likely cause a natural, slight increase in lordosis of the lower back. What's most important is that the stacked position of the ribcage and pelvis is re-established when the weight is locked out overhead.

■ The overhead position should be comfortable and very familiar now, since you have drilled it in several different positions previously. Reach up on the bar actively at the top while keeping the bar stacked over the upper back.

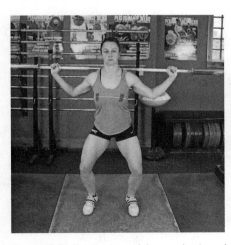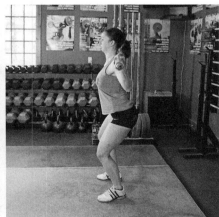

Figure 11.21 The dip phase of the snatch grip push press

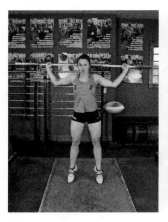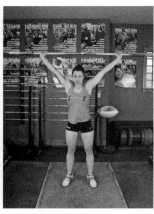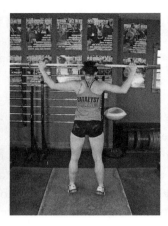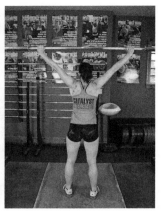

Figure 11.22 The drive phase of the snatch grip push press

- Sets and reps of this drill will depend on the goal of the current program, since this is an exercise that can illicit strength adaptation. Sets of 3-5 are common.

Movement Cluster Options

- Alternate Snatch Grip Push Press with Kneeling Scapular Facilitation during lighter barbell sets.

Squat Position

Achieving an adequate bottom position in a full snatch obviously requires the athlete to be able to squat with a relative amount of comfort. Here we will work to restore the movement variability of the pelvis and hip joints, and then use that mobility to groove the squatting pattern.

Since we have already addressed ankle dorsiflexion mobility in Chapter 7, we will not repeat that info here—just keep in mind that those drills and clusters can be a part of your squat prep if ankle dorsiflexion is limited.

Mobilization: Supine Squatting with Hip Internal Rotation

If there was perceived restriction in the hip internal rotation test, or you felt restriction deep in the front of the hip socket during the squat screening and assessment, this may be an effective strategy for you to improve hip comfort in the bottom.

Individual anatomy will dictate the amount of movement in this drill to a degree. The goal is to mobilize within *your* comfortable range of motion, without feelings of impingement in the front of the hip.

Starting Position

- Lie supine with the feet flat on a wall with the toes straight up and 3 points of contact—big toe, little toe and heel.

- Bend the hips and knees to 90 degrees each.
- Hold a foam roller between the knees to stabilize the pelvis.
- Place the hands on the lower ribs.
- Keep the shoulders relaxed.
- Keep the chin tucked slightly so that the back of the neck is long. Have something under your head to keep from straining your neck backwards. (Figure 11.22)

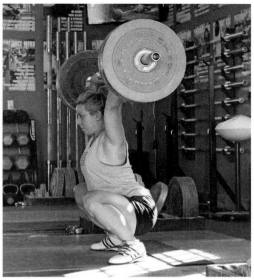

Figure 11.21 The snatch receiving position

Execution

- *Fully exhale* through your mouth to set the ribs down and turn the abs on.
- Gently dig your heels down into the wall, pulling your tailbone off the floor slightly, just like in the supine squatting drill. You can also use a bench under the heels. The posterior pelvic tilt will aid to clear a little bit of space in the font of your hip with which to attain a bit more flexion + internal rotation.
- Maintaining the pelvic lift, walk the feet out to the sides slightly, putting the hips into internal rotation. You should feel the inner hamstrings engage slightly.
- After 5 breaths, lower the hips and scoot closer to the wall (maybe even a half-inch—use small increments). (Figure 11.23)
- You can gently oscillate side to side, or perform one leg at a time.
- Repeat for a total of 3 sets of 5 breaths (You can do more sets if desired).

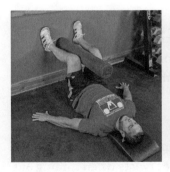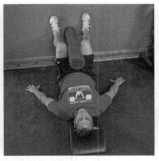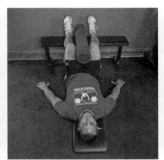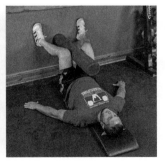

Figure 11.22 The Supine Squatting with Hip Internal Rotation mobilization is a variation of the Supine Squatting drill, in which we look to mobilize the internal rotation capacity of the hips. Can be done with or without a bench under the heels.

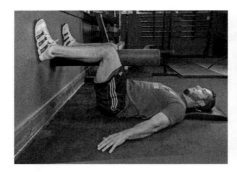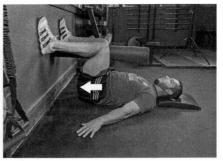

Figure 11.23 Scooting slightly closer to the wall each set can increase the mobility demands of the Supine Squatting with Hip Internal Rotation. Remember, you should not feel impingement/pinching in the hip crease.

Cues

- Relaxed neck.
- Exhale fully until the ribs disappear, then pause for 3 seconds before your next inhalation.
- Relax the abs enough to fully inhale, filling the low back and then upper back with air.
- Hamstrings are activated.
- If you feel a pinchy or cramping sensation in the front or outside of either hip, adjust your position by squeezing the roller a little harder, posteriorly tilting the pelvis more, using a longer, more forceful exhalation to facilitate the abdominals, and/or scooting away from the wall.

Tension Adding a higher tension exhalation and subsequent abdominal contraction can further inhibit feelings of tightness in the front of the hips here. To facilitate this, incorporate a plate press to give some leverage. (Figure 11.24)

Movement Cluster Options

- Alternate Supine Squatting with Hip Internal Rotation with 20-second bouts of SMR to the hip flexor area in the front/side of the hip joint around the area of the TFL muscle.

Mobilization: Sidelying Hip Series

This drill is a compliment to the drill above. It can be helpful for lifters who want to correct noticeable shifts in their squats or twists when coming out of the hole in the snatch. It helps with this by moving the athlete through several planes of motion in the pelvis and hips, with a goal of creating symmetry in hip flexion + rotation mobility.

We can manipulate the sagittal plane by altering how close we are to the wall and by tilting the pelvis anteriorly or posteriorly, the frontal plane by altering foot width, and the transverse plane by externally or internally rotating the hips and shifting the pelvis forward and backward. It's femur on pelvis and pelvis on femur movement in all three planes—movement variability gold.

Starting Position

- From the supine squat position in the previous drill, simply roll over to one side, maintaining the same angles at the hips and knees. Bring the feet back to hip width.
- This drill can be done with or without a foam roller between the knees. You may feel different muscles activate in each version (lateral glute/hip with no roller, inner thigh with roller). One is not necessarily better than the other. Explore both, then retest your air squat to determine which version you feel inhibits tension in the hips most effectively. (Figure 11.25)

Execution

- Exhale fully to set the ribcage, perform a slight tailbone tuck and maintain this position throughout the drill. Again, this aids in maximizing the mobility that we can find in our hips and minimizes feelings of impingement. It also takes the lower back out of the equation.
- Squeeze the roller slightly (if you are using one), and shift the top knee forward and backward within a controlled range of motion that is coming from the pelvis. With this movement, we are shifting in and out of each hip. (Figure 11.26)
- Perform 8-10 reps on each side.
- Make note of any asymmetries you feel.
- Then, move the top foot up the wall so that it's higher than the knee. This puts the top hip into internal rotation.

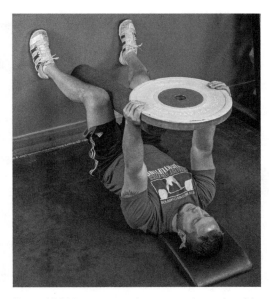

Figure 11.24 Incorporate a plate press and more forceful exhalation/breath cycles to increase facilitation to the abs and hip musculature and inhibit perceived tightness in the front of the hip in the Supine Squatting with Hip Internal Rotation mobilization.

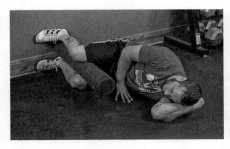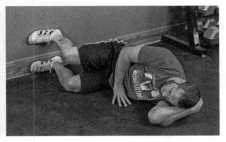

Figure 11.25 Sidelying Hip Series starting position. These drills can be done with or without a foam roller between the knees.

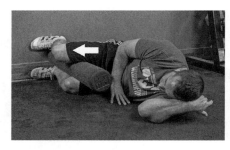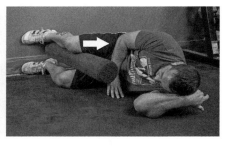

Figure 11.26 Sidelying Hip Series execution. Shift the top knee forward and backward within a controlled range of motion coming from the pelvis.

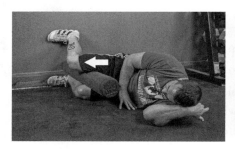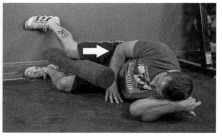

Figure 11.27 Elevating the top foot increases hip internal rotation mobility. Shift the top knee forward and backward the same way you did previously.

- Perform the same hip shifting forward and backward while continuing to breathe and maintain the slight squeeze of the roller and tailbone tuck (Figure 11.27).
  - › We have now established a femur on pelvis position with internal rotation, while creating pelvis on femur motion, which can be effective to mobilize the hip.
- Perform 6-8 reps on each side.
- Return the top foot back to the starting position and lift the bottom foot toward the top foot. This externally rotates the bottom leg, facilitating the glutes on that side. You can experiment with shifting the top leg either forward or backward to certain degrees while you externally rotate the bottom hip, with or without a roller between the knees. (Figure 11.28)
- Perform 6-8 reps on each side.

You have several options here as far as where to position yourself and what body parts to move, so experiment. No TFL/side hip cramping or pinching allowed. If this is happening:

- Posteriorly tilt the pelvis more.
- Squeeze the roller a little more.
- Exhale forcefully to facilitate the abdominals.
- Move farther away from the wall.

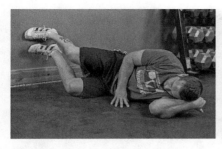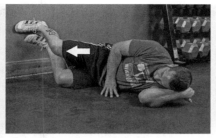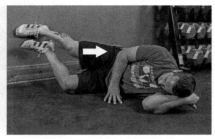

Figure 11.28 Experimenting with different positions in the Sidelying Hip Series. Lift the lower foot up toward the top foot and shift the top knee forward and backward as you did previously.

Movement Cluster Options

- Alternate with Supine Squatting Hip Internal Rotation drill.
- Alternate with 20-second bouts of SMR to TFL/hip flexor area.

Mobilization: Quadruped Squatting

The two above drills should have done the job of preparing your hips for flexion and rotation. This quadruped squatting drill will now allow you to use the benefits we just described in a squatting pattern. Use this drill to smoothly explore your hip range of motion and experiment with different positions to figure out where your hips are most mobile and comfortable, very similar to what we did in our basic quadruped squatting drill and in our squatting screen.

Starting Position

- On the hands and knees with the knees and feet spread to a width similar to the athlete's normal squatting stance
- Set the spine in neutral curvature. (Figure 11.29)

Execution

- Gently rock back and forth from the starting position to past 90 degrees of hip flexion while keeping the spine neutral. Use your hands as leverage, and exhale through your mouth fully as you rock back. Practice pausing in the bottom and taking a deep breath in through your nose, pushing the air down to expand your trunk 360 degrees. (Figure 11.30)
    > High-tension breathing and bracing can be utilized here to solidify the position, or low-tension, more relaxed strategies to facilitate mobility in the position.
- No rep and set recommendations here. Spend a minute or two exploring your movement or however much time you need, especially if the bottom position of a squat is troublesome for you.

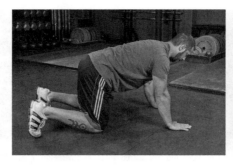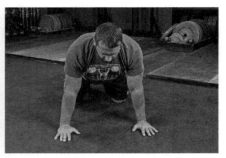

Figure 11.29 The starting position for the Quadruped Squat Mobilization drill

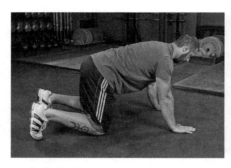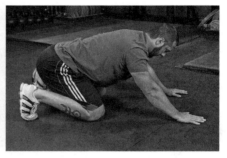

Figure 11.30 Gently move in and out of the quadruped squat, exploring your hip range of motion.

Stance Width Variation Widen your knees and feet and explore your quadruped squatting range in this new position. Pause periodically to fully inhale and exhale in the bottom position. You may find that a full exhalation allows you a deeper squat. (Figure 11.31)

Hip Flexion Variation Drop down to your forearms in order to increase the amount of hip flexion required. This position is nearly identical to the amount of torso angle appropriate for a squat when you are standing. Spread your fingers and create as much ground contact as possible. Utilize forceful exhalations as you push your hips back into a squat. (Figure 11.32)

Hip Rotation Variation Experiment with wider knees and narrower feet (hip external rotation), and wider feet with narrower knees (hip internal rotation) to gain more awareness of your hip function. Rotational hip capacity is key in squatting, and this is a great way to gain access to it, especially after the Hip Internal Rotation drill described earlier. Stay in comfortable ranges, utilizing pauses and high-tension breathing and bracing strategies to reinforce the position. Use this variation in conjunction with any of the Quadruped Squatting variations described above. (Figure 11.33)

Pelvic Tilt Variation In the bottom of your quadruped squat, tilt your pelvis back and forth anteriorly and posteriorly, gently discovering the limits in each direction (Figure 11.34). This mobilizes your hips by moving the pelvis around the hips instead of the other way around.

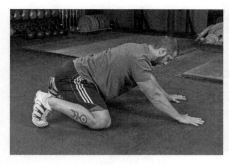
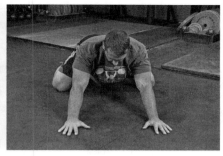

Figure 11.31 Use a wider position of the hips and feet to mimic a wider squat and explore your ranges here. Rock in and out of the squat, allowing range of motion to improve naturally.

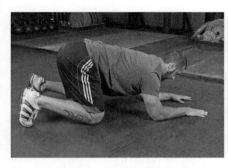
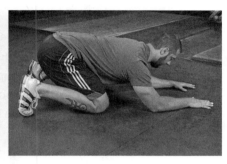

Figure 11.32 Dropping down to the forearms increases the amount of hip flexion, so now you are really exploring the squatting pattern.

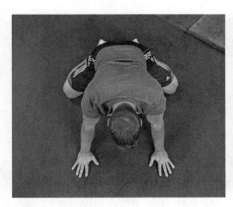
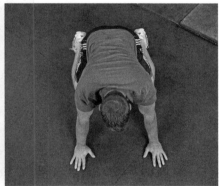

Figure 11.33 Widening the knees outside the plane of the foot biases more hip external rotation as you flex back. Widening the feet even with or outside the plane of the knees biases hip internal rotation. Perform the Quadruped Squatting drill experimenting with these variations.

This variation is especially good for those who have trouble keeping the low back relatively neutral when squatting. If you have to round your low back a bit to even get into the quadruped squat, that is OK, but see if you can anteriorly tilt the pelvis at the bottom.

This may be the most uncomfortable of all the variations if you tend to feel restricted in your hips during a squat, so work through the range slowly. Commonly, a little more hip external rotation and a slight posterior pelvic tilt will allow for a deeper quadruped squat; once you're down there, you can attempt to anteriorly tilt the pelvis and reverse the curve of the spine back to lordosis.

Arm Lifts: Adding a Light Stabilization Component This drill moves the Quadruped Squatting drill to a position of less ground contact and inherently less external stability, but still mimics the position of an overhead squat.

Starting Position

- Same as Quadruped Squatting

Execution

- Rock the hips back slightly past 90 degrees.
- Walk the hands back until they are 2-4 inches in front of the knees without moving the hips back any farther.
- Without moving any other body part, lift an arm up slowly in the scapular plane. Exhale forcefully as you do this. At this point, you should feel your abs reflexively fire to keep you from falling on your face. (Figure 11.35)
  - > If you do not feel your abs, shift forward slightly. You should be teetering on the edge of a broken face, with only your breath and abs to rely on. Exhale forcefully with high bracing tension to hold the position.
- Perform 1-2 sets of 5-6 reps with each arm.

Notes on Quadruped Squatting Do not jam into range you do not have. Instead, just move smoothly and comfortably. Explore, rock in and out of a squat, oscillate at different depths, breathe, etc. Range of motion will come over time.

Also use this time to really sense what a squat (triple flexion) feels like. In quadruped when you are in a very deep squat and everything seems to work as it should, pretend that you are standing. Burn into your brain what that pattern feels like.

Use your arms and forearms as leverage. Try to actively push into the ground.

Movement Cluster Options

- Alternate with the Sidelying Hip Series drill for 2-4 rounds.
- Alternate with the 90-90 Supine Squatting with Hip Internal Rotation drill for 2-4 rounds.
- Alternate with the above and/or 20-second bouts of SMR to glutes, low back or hip flexor area.

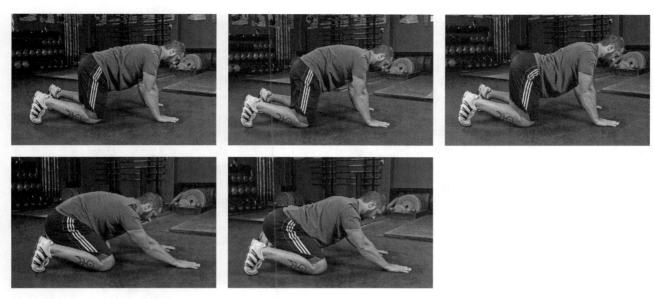

Figure 11.34 Using pelvic tilt is another way to mobilize your hips. Anterior pelvic tilt puts your lower back in lordosis, while posterior tilt causes your lower back to round. Move through both gently back and forth.

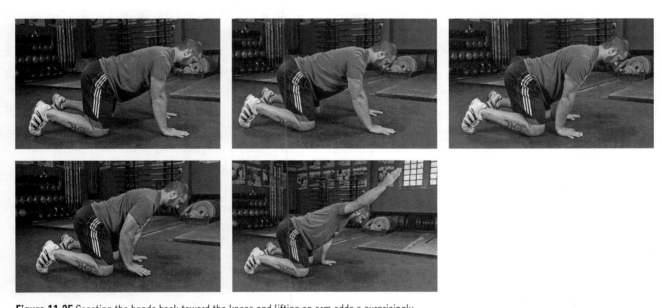

Figure 11.35 Scooting the hands back toward the knees and lifting an arm adds a surprisingly difficult challenge for the athlete to maintain position.

Mobilization: Hip Flexion with Manual Downward Glide

This drill aids in restoring the perceived roll and glide of the ball of the femur into the socket when the hip is in deep flexion, with mobilization to the inferior and posterior direction, and aids in improving comfort in the bottom position of the snatch or clean.

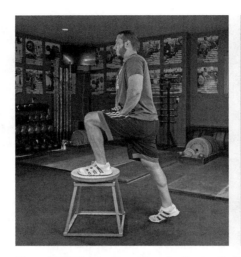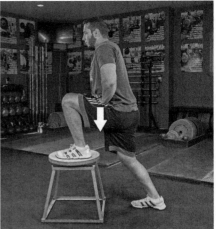

Figure 11.36 The direction of force for the standing hip mobilization is down and back.

Starting Position

- Stand with one foot up on a box that is at least knee height.
- Allow a slight bend in the opposite knee.
- Place your hands deep in the crease of the hip of the up leg.

Execution

- Leverage your body weight forward.
- Provide a downward force with the arms to the femur angled slightly back. You should feel the femur glide down. (Figure 11.36)
- Maintaining this glide, "roll" your pelvis over the top by anteriorly rotating. You should have the sensation that head of the femur (ball) is deeply seated in the socket (Figure 11.37).
- You can keep your hands in the hip crease and oscillate at end range, or you can move your hands to your knee and pull back to create a force that further drives the femur back into the socket (Figure 11.38).
- With the hands at the knee, perform small circles while continuing to roll the pelvis over the top of the ball of the femur (Figure 11.39).
- Grab a PVC pipe or barbell and perform behind the neck presses with your hip joint seated to simulate the bottom position of the snatch for 1-2 sets of 6-8 reps each side (Figure 11.40).

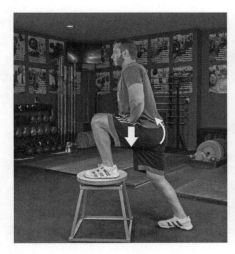
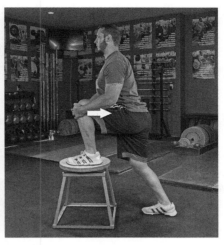

Figure 11.37 An anterior pelvic tilt while maintaining downward pressure can further "seat" the ball and socket.

Figure 11.38 Adding a posterior glide may improve the perceived benefits of the mobilization.

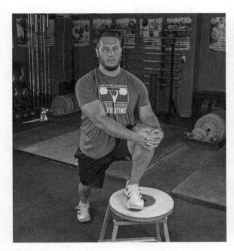
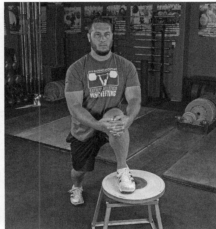

Figure 11.39 Add small rotations for subtle mobilization within the joint.

Notes

- Perform for 1-2 bouts of 20-30 seconds for any of the mobilization variations.
- This is very similar to the ankle mobility drill in Chapter 7 and can be combined with it.
- If you feel a distinct pinch in the front of your hip, you are impinging the joint and not mobilizing it desirably. Try to reposition the hip or pelvis to take the pinch away, similar to what you did in quadruped squatting. If you cannot, then discontinue the drill.
  - › It may be beneficial to add a band around the hip joint to create a distractive force if you feel impingement.

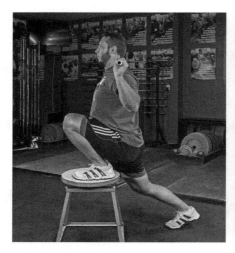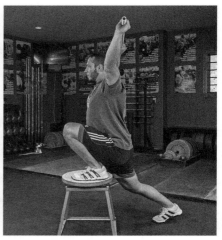

Figure 11.40 Add a behind the neck press to simulate the snatch.

However, if you can create the mobilization without a band, this is preferred. We need a hip joint that can sit in the socket with compressive forces acting on it, not distractive forces. There is no band pulling on our hip while on the competition platform.

Movement Cluster Options

- Alternate with the Quadruped Squatting drill and/or 20-second bouts of SMR to hip flexors or glutes for 2-4 rounds.

Stabilization: Squat Pattern Reinforcement

If you had trouble performing squatting type movements during the screening and assessment, this will be an important stop for you, as previous drills have set the foundation for what we will discuss. If you are someone who can slam into the bottom of a squat, but cannot stabilize any substantial weight, this is equally important for you. If you have a great squat and you are strong as an ox, hopefully you still pick up a few cues that can further enhance your movement.

To start, we have a couple of very simple rules for the squat:

- Motionless (relatively), stable pelvis and spinal column throughout the movement, from beginning to end.
- Motionless, stable foot position (3 points of contact) throughout the movement, from beginning to end.

If these two guidelines are followed to the athlete's or coach's standard, squatting becomes very simple—stable spine and foot and natural hinging of the hip, knee and ankle. Triple flexion. Sit down, stand up. Boom. There are, of course, body positions and cues that make our guidelines for the squat easier or more difficult to follow. These will be discussed.

Movement Discussion: Pelvic Tilt Another hot topic: pelvic position in the squat. Anterior tilt, posterior tilt, neutral, etc. I will qualify this with the fact that individual structure and preference plays a role in the pelvic position that lifters use to squat comfortably and support weight overhead. Understand that one athlete's comfortable pelvic position (degree of anterior or posterior tilt) may not be what works for another. With that said, we will discuss pelvic tilt from a biomechanical standpoint, and leave it up to you to experiment with different positions to find what works best for you.

A posterior pelvic tilt relative to neutral (Figure 11.41), which causes flexion of the lumbar spine, is probably not a sustainable position for most to support substantial weight, considering the dynamic nature of the snatch and clean & jerk. It is more likely your spine will fold under the load and lose the weight.

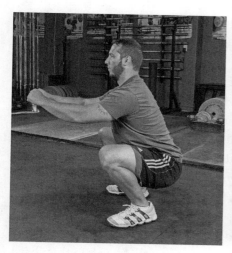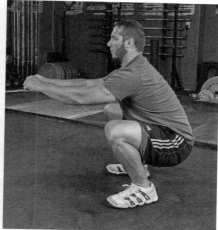

Figure 11.41 Posterior pelvic tilt with lumbar flexion in a squat

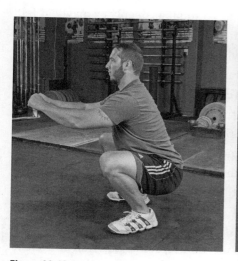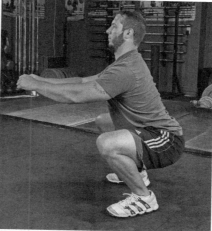

Figure 11.42 Anterior pelvic tilt with lumbar extension (lordosis) in a squat

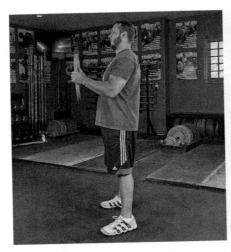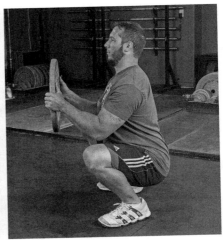

Figure 11.43 Counterbalance squat with a neutral pelvis

A relative anterior pelvic tilt (Figure 11.42) will restore the natural lordotic curve of the lumbar spine, and likely be a more sustainable position to support load for most lifters compared to a relative posterior pelvic tilt past neutral.

What has also been shown in the literature about anterior pelvic tilt is that as it increases, hip flexion and internal rotation range of motion *decreases* to an extent, which are two planes of motion that are useful for a deep squat position. You can feel this yourself with a simple demonstration. Grab a 5 or 10kg plate and hold it in front of you for a counterbalance. Perform a squat as you normally would, without consciously altering your pelvis (Figure 11.43). Perform a few reps and monitor how this feels in your hips.

Then, anteriorly tilt your pelvis to a point that is past your norm. This will increase the lordosis in your lumbar spine as well. Maintain this "hard arch" and squat down as deeply as you can. (Figure 11.44)

Many of you were probably not able to squat as deeply or maybe it felt a little more "crowded" in the hips. An anterior pelvic tilt already sets your hips into relative flexion, meaning with that hard arch, you are basically quarter squatting before you even start the actual descent—you just end up running out of room in the hips. (Figure 11.45)

Perform the same test, only this time, posteriorly tilt your pelvis more than you typically would (Figure 11.46). Think about tucking your tailbone under "pooping dog" style. This may not even put you in actual lower back flexion, but it will certainly change the orientation of your hip sockets in the other direction. Test your squat. For many of you, this will allow a deeper squat position.

The moral of the story is simply to understand that pelvic tilt can have implications with respect to your hip mechanics, spinal position and squat position. If during the squatting screen you discovered that your hips do

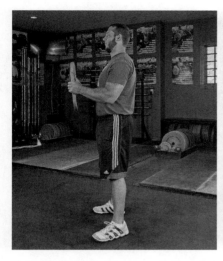
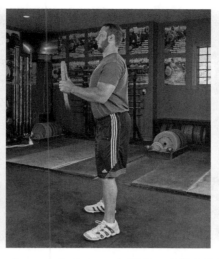
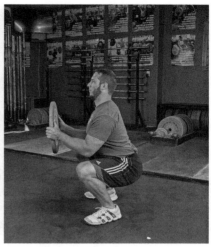

Figure 11.44 Counterbalance squat with an increased amount of anterior pelvic tilt. You will likely find you are unable to squat as deeply than you did with a neutral pelvis.

not possess a great amount of internal rotation capacity, do not be surprised if a hard low back arch and anterior pelvic tilt restricts you from hitting the squat depth that you would like, or that it requires you to turn your feet out a little more than you're used to in order to hit your desired depth. Again, there is not necessarily a *right* or *wrong*. Each lifter will be different, so find the position that allows our two guidelines to be met.

This leads into a conversation about the dreaded *butt wink*, which is characterized by an uncontrolled posterior pelvic tilt in the bottom of the squat. Since we know that increased anterior pelvic tilt results in a decrease in end range hip flexion and internal rotation, a posterior pelvic tilt (butt wink) may, in some cases, be due to a significant degree of *anterior* pelvic tilt earlier in the movement. The pelvis is dumped forward, the hips hit their end range, and in order for the athlete to squat deeper, the entire pelvis must rotate backward to accommodate.

For example, let's take an athlete that has difficulty achieving a below parallel squat position, or exhibits an uncontrolled posterior pelvic tilt (butt wink) that is deemed to be problematic. We must look at the strategy that the athlete uses to begin the movement first before considering the end result. Commonly, this same athlete descends into the squat with a pelvis and low back that begins to unnecessarily anteriorly tilt and extend on the way down. We know that increased anterior pelvic tilt results in a decrease in end range hip flexion and internal rotation, so a subsequent posterior pelvic tilt (butt wink) may just be the lifter's way of compensating in the other direction (Figure 11.47). Go back to our hip screening tests. If an athlete can rock his or her hips back in quadruped

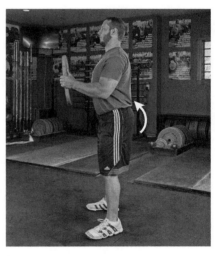

Figure 11.45 With an excessive anterior pelvic tilt, your hips are already partially closing before you even begin to squat.

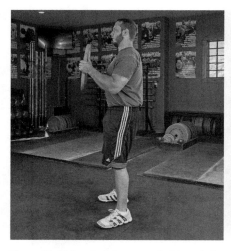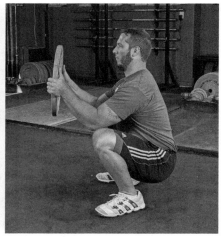

Figure 11.46 Counterbalance squat with a relative posterior pelvic tilt

while keeping a neutral spine, but cannot in standing, the mobility is there but motor control may be a factor.

Of important note is that a *relative* amount of posterior pelvic tilt is actually a *normal* finding in a deep squat position and has been deemed "unavoidable" in some literature, even with high-level lifters. Of course, the question is *how much is too much?* That is ultimately up to the discretion of the coach and athlete. We will give some basic guidelines going forward. In general, if you observe what you would describe as a butt wink in a lifter, have him or her pause in the bottom of the squat and note the low back position. Sometimes what appears to be an obvious change in pelvic or spinal position is simply the athlete going from hyperextension of the lower back to less extension, while still remaining lordotic. In other, cases, the "wink" is such that when the athlete pauses in the bottom of the squat, they are truly in observable lumbar flexion, at which point we would likely intervene. Refer back to the squatting assessment for individual squatting stance. Make note of how altering stance affects the lifter's ability to maintain a relatively motionless spinal column and pelvis. (Figure 11.48)

Important Points Regarding "Butt Wink"

- Be sure to consider where the pelvis *starts* as opposed to only where it finishes.
- Posterior pelvic tilt is likely a normal, unavoidable occurrence in a deep squat. *How much is too much?* is context-dependent.
- There needs to be a balance between what pelvic position affords the deepest squat, and what position maintains a spinal position that can support load and performance.
- Be sure to combine pelvic position (anterior-posterior tilt) with experimentation of stance width and hip rotation (toes in/out) to truly optimize your individual position.

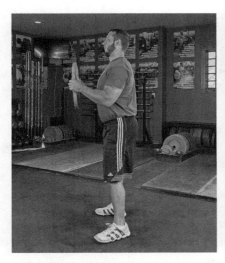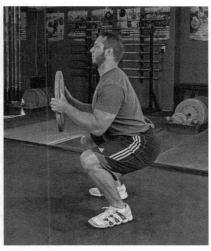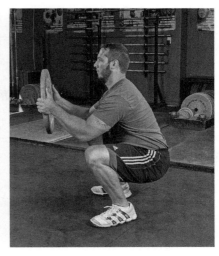

Figure 11.47 There are times when a "butt wink" is simply the only place the pelvis has to go because it has been excessively anteriorly rotated during or before the descent.

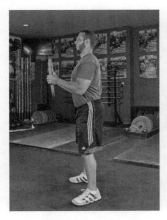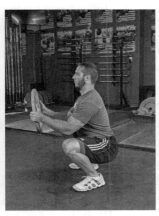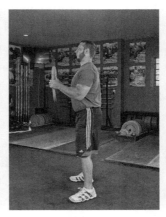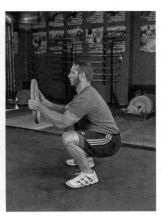

Figure 11.48 In the first sequence, you observe less anterior pelvic tilt in the athlete's squat than in standing; however the low back is still in relative neutral. In the second sequence, the athlete appears to be in true flexion of the lumbar spine in the squat. This would probably indicate a greater need to correct in order to achieve positions that can more effectively support load.

- Spinal extension and anterior pelvic tilt is typically desirable for lifters, but we also want to be able to control it.

In any drills to follow, I will make a distinction between a posterior pelvic *tilt* which actually puts your lumbar spine into flexion, and posterior pelvic *tilting* which means going from a certain degree of anterior tilt to less anterior tilt, but still within a neutral range.

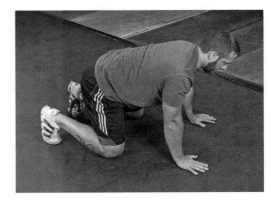

Figure 11.49 Starting position for Quadruped Squatting to Counterbalance Squat

Stabilization: Quadruped Squatting to Counter Balance Squat

This drill takes the previous, in which the lifter became acquainted with his or her hip mobility in quadruped, and transitions to a standing squat.

Starting Position

- In quadruped with a neutral spine.
- Feet widened out to your squatting stance.
- Place a weight between your feet. (Figure 11.49)

Execution

- Rock the hips back past 90 degrees, keeping the spine neutral (as well as possible—some rounding may occur).
- Walk the hands back and roll onto your feet, placing yourself into the bottom of a squat.
    - › Try to keep your back flat as you do this.
    - › If you find that your feet end up too narrow or in an awkward position to squat from, return back to quadruped and reposition your knees and feet in order to better mimic your squat stance.
- Grab the weight and let it balance you in the deep bottom position you just found. Hang out for a breath or two and fight for a vertical upper back. (Figure 11.50)
- You can repeat this sequence, moving from quadruped to the bottom of the squat and back, for several reps, until it feels comfortable down there, without ever standing up. Don't be in a rush. Think of this as building the squat position from the bottom up as opposed to top down.
- Utilize full exhalations to sink deeper into the squat. Utilize high-tension breathing and bracing strategies to reinforce the position and increase muscle activation there.
- Then you can stand up and squat back down using the weight as a counterbalance. Perform for 2-4 sets of 6-8 controlled reps. (Figure 11.51)
    - › It will likely be easier to find your bottom position because you were just spending significant time there already.

Removing the Counterbalance To truly "own" the position, losing the counterbalance is a great progression. After all, you obviously have the mobility to get into the position.

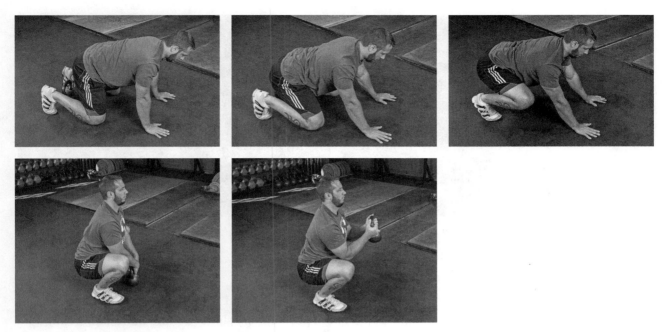

Figure 11.50 Push the hips back until you are in a squat, then grab the weight for counterbalance.

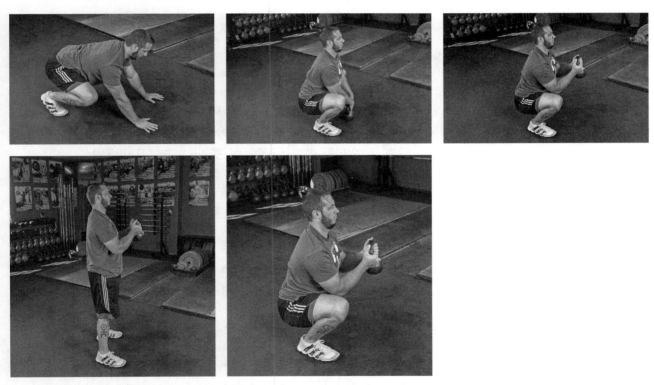

Figure 11.51 After performing repetitions moving from the quadruped to squatting position, squat for repetitions trying to recreate a consistent bottom position.

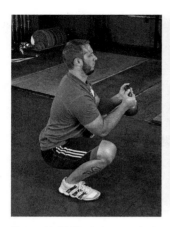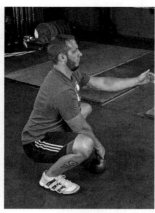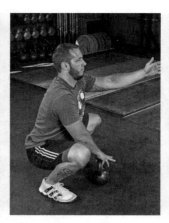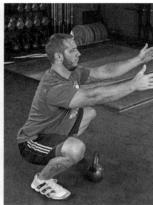

Figure 11.52 Slowly lower and take your hands off of the weight to solidify the position.

Execution

- After you have used the weight to settle into a deep and comfortable bottom position, try slowly setting down and letting go of the weight while maintaining your exact squat position (Figure 11.52). This will put the onus on the core and hips to act as your counterbalance.
- Don't be in a rush here. If you have to take your hands off literally one finger at a time, that's fine. If you feel yourself starting to lose your balance backward, utilize bracing strategies with enough tension to bring your stability back where it needs to be to hold the position. Just try to maintain a steady breathing pattern as opposed to holding your breath and becoming overly rigid. After all, we are trying to improve your comfort down there.
- Perform 1-3 sets of 3-4 reps of moving from the quadruped squat to counterbalance squat and releasing the weight.

Movement Cluster Options

- Alternate with Quadruped Squatting for 2-4 rounds and/or 20-30-second bouts of SMR to glutes or hip flexor area.

For the Counterbalance Squat as a Standalone Remember, as long as you are able to follow the two guidelines we outlined above (stable spine, stable foot), it is less important that everyone have a narrow stance with feet straight ahead. However, if you want to experiment with a narrow stance and toes forward now that you have a counterbalance, that's cool too.

Starting Position

- Pick your toes up, spread them, and plant them down *flat* (not scrunched) to attain three points of contact—big toe, little toe and heel (Figure 11.53).
- Keep a slight bend in the knees.
- Pull the pelvis into neutral.
- Exhale to set the lower ribs down and flush with the abdomen, but stay tall.
  - › This will ensure that your pelvic floor and diaphragm are facing each other, but you are staying extended through your upper back.
- Hold a plate, kettlebell, dumbbell or other weight roughly 8 inches away from your body to give you a counterbalance.

Execution

- While holding the weight out in front, set the hips back slightly without breaking at the pelvis, low back or foot.
- From there, sit *straight down* into a squat as deep as is comfortable, while maintaining our two guidelines and allowing your hips, knees and ankles to hinge naturally. (Figure 11.54)
  - › Keep your toes (especially your big toe) actively planted down the entire time.
  - › Allow the knees to hinge naturally and track over the second toe or middle of the foot.
  - › Keep the upper back tall.
- Then stand *straight up*.
  - › LET YOUR KNEES COME FORWARD. Maintaining a flat, stable foot and allowing the hips, knees and ankles to hinge naturally will distribute forces throughout your legs safely, and teach you to push with your legs. We are not

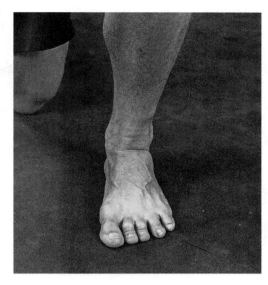

Figure 11.53 The foot is our base, so we are looking for it to be broad, as opposed to scrunched and rolled to the outside. Actively press the toes down, but keep them flat.

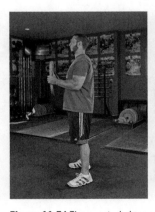 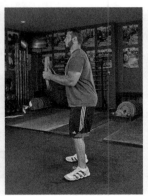 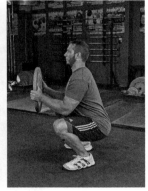

Figure 11.54 The counterbalance squat is a great tool for teaching squat depth and position.

concerned with terms like *hip dominant, knee dominant,* etc. During this drill, you are simply focused on keeping your hips underneath you and using your legs: LEG DOMINANT.

> The knees should hinge naturally and generally track over the middle of the foot. If the knees collapse into significant valgus, most likely the outside of the foot (pinky toe) will lose its stable contact with the ground. This violates one of our two guidelines for squatting. *How much is too much?* in regards to knee valgus is similar to the *butt wink* discussion—it depends on context. For the purposes of simplicity, keep the feet broad and motionless during the movement, and allow the knee to hinge naturally over the middle of the foot. In general, if both knees are tracking in symmetrical planes throughout the movement, without observable deviations in the path, and are in the vicinity of the first or second toe, there is usually not a concern. If you see a change in the path of the knee during the squatting motion that puts the entire kneecap on one or both sides entirely inside the big toe, then by all means, let's correct. It's beneficial to spin the reasoning for such intervention for performance enhancement, rather than injury prevention, to avoid fear mongering or *nocebos* (a benign stimulus becoming problematic). In this instance, a simple cue can do the trick to correct positioning. *Keep your knee over your foot. Keep your knee over the middle of your foot. Keep your knee over your second toe.* You get the idea. The rationale for these cues can then be something like, *If your knee is stacked over your foot, then you have better leverage to push into the ground and create more force* as opposed to *If you're knee goes in, you'll hurt yourself.*

> You have probably seen pictures or videos of even experienced lifters demonstrating some observable form of inward knee movement during a squat. Many times, it's an inward movement of the knees when reversing directions and coming out of the bottom of the squat. There are a few theories as to why this happens, none of which (to my knowledge) have been "proven," but it's always a fun discussion. Here are some thoughts:

1. An inward movement of the knees when reversing the bottom of the squat is a mechanism of the powerful muscle group adductor magnus. Adductor magnus becomes a decently powerful hip extender at the bottom

of the squat, but is obviously also a hip adductor, so those two actions may be what we are seeing.

2. An inward movement of the knees is a reflexive way for the body to put a stretch reflex on the glutes. Femur internal rotation + flexion would put a stretch on the glute, perhaps creating some type of elastic recoil for femur external rotation and extension.

3. An inward motion of the knees creates a combination of femur flexion + adduction + internal rotation, which will likely decrease mobility in the hip joint. So, essentially, the hip reflexively impinges itself to create structural stability (form closure) in the moment.

> Excessively pushing the knees outward over the pinky toe or even past the plane of the foot is also an unnatural and awkward scenario. (Figure 11.55)

■ Such a position will likely result in the athlete lifting the big toe or rolling to the outside edge of the foot, which opposes our guideline of a stable, balanced foot. This position is also not realistic or sustainable for most in a dynamic movement such as the snatch or clean. The knees will likely just default to their natural path, which is simply hinging over the middle of the foot the way they are designed. In regard to the hip musculature's role, think of it as *resisting* forces that would cause the knee to track unnaturally rather than actively creating motion in the transverse plane. Lastly, such a position may put an odd rotational force through the knee, as the tibia (shin bone) and femur (thigh bone) are no longer tracking in the same plane. Again, simply allow your hips, knees and ankles to hinge naturally.

■ Ankle Integration

> Just as we did with the Split Squat and Half Kneeling Ankle Rocker in the Pulling Stance section, we can focus on ankle motion by first anchoring the foot. Lift the toes to create a stable midfoot and spread the toes as you place them *flat* back down. Of course, if you are wearing weightlifting shoes, you will not be able to spread the toes; however, you can still focus on actively pressing the big toe into the floor throughout the duration of the squat.

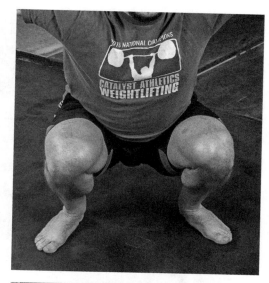

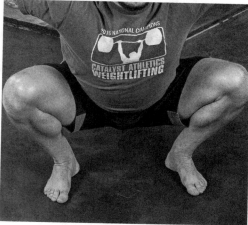

Figure 11.55 The first picture shows a valgus knee position, in which the lifter loses contact with the outside edge of foot. Such a position makes it more difficult to create force down into the floor with the legs. The second picture shows a varus knee position, in which the lifter loses contact with the inside edge of the foot. Such a position is not sustainable under loads, puts unnatural rotational force through the knee, and has no evidence of superiority in the literature. A natural squatting position should allow the knees to hinge over the middle of the foot.

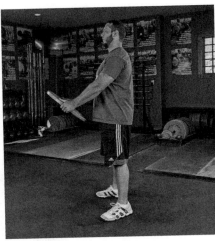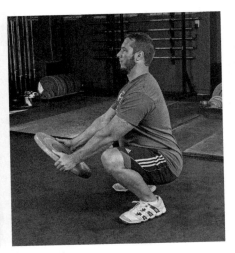

Figure 11.56 Holding the weight at a downward angle can be a slightly easier variation for a lifter focused simply on depth.

> As well as keeping your big toe grounded, feel your entire heel against the floor, including the inside of it.

- The athlete can also hold the weight at a downward angle to take some of the burden off of the shoulders and upper back (Figure 11.56).
- Perform 1-3 sets of 5-8 reps, or as needed to work on position. Progress to a *lighter* weight in which your abs have to act more as your counter balance.
- Get comfortable in the bottom. Hang out there for a second or two. Take a couple deep, forceful breaths.

Added Scapular Facilitation Here we incorporate an overhead component to the counterbalance squat to integrate the overhead drills performed previously into an actual squat.

Execution

- Establish a stable foot with three points of contact and perform a counterbalance squat, in which you let your hips, knees and ankles comfortably hinge.
- In the bottom of the squat, work to attain upper thoracic extension by exhaling simultaneously as you try to create a "tall" spine. Pretend that a string is being pulled from the top of your head.
- Slowly transfer the weight to one side while maintaining the exact same squat position. This frees one arm up for movement.
- Perform scapular diagonals mimicking your snatch receiving position (Figure 11.57).

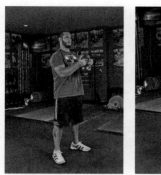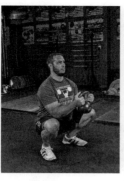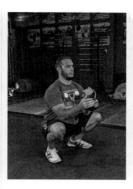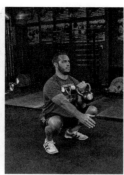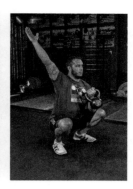

Figure 11.57 Counterbalance squat with scapular facilitation

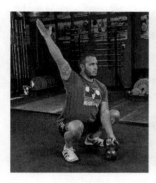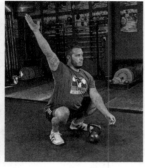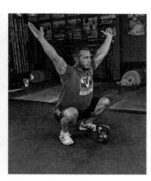

Figure 11.58 Counterbalance squat with scapular facilitation without the counterbalance

- Repeat on the opposite side.
- Establish your bottom position with one arm free once more.
- Perform the arm movement described above.
- Then *slowly* lower the weight to the floor while maintaining your exact body position. You're going to have to really fight here to stay tall. If possible, take your hand off the bell one finger at a time until you are able to control position.
- Then attempt to perform the same arm movement while in your deep bottom position with the other arm. (Figure 11.58)
- Repeat this for 1-2 sets of 5-6 reps on each side.

Key Points

- If performed under strict control, these drills can be very demanding on the abs and upper T-spine extensors. With a pelvis and ribcage that is inherently locked in place with such a deep squat position, the upper back and scapular musculature has nowhere to hide.

Movement Cluster Options

- Alternate with Quadruped Squatting for 2-4 rounds and/or 20-30-second bouts of SMR to the glutes or hip flexors.

- Alternate with 90-90 Supine Scapular Facilitation and/or 20-30-second bouts of SMR to the lats or T-spine for 2-4 rounds.

Overhead Squat

Taking concepts from both the overhead and squatting portion of this Receiving Position section, we now begin to incorporate both halves of the body in order to stabilize the mobility positions that we have created for integration into the snatch.

Integration: Overhead Squat with or without Elevated Heels

The previous drills transition nicely to our talks now about refining a lifter's overhead squat position. The Overhead Squat can be initiated with the exact sequence that we outlined for the Snatch Grip Push Press. At this point, with the weight overhead, we have some key concepts:

- The torso and shoulders when in the *standing* overhead position should look as similar as possible to the torso and shoulders when in the *squatting* position. Put another way, if a picture was taken of a lifter in a snatch grip overhead position and it was cut off from the ribcage up, you should not be able to tell whether the athlete is standing or squatting—the positions should look the same. The only things moving in an overhead squat are the hips, knees and ankles—at least that is what you are striving for. The shoulders are not rolling forward or backward, the bar is not being pushed forward or backward, the angle of the torso should change very little, and the spinal curves remain relatively the same. (Figure 11.59)

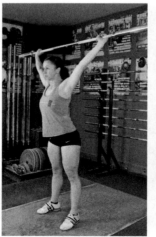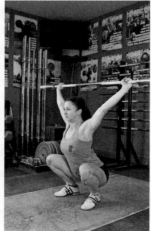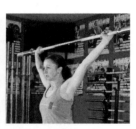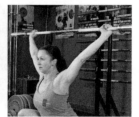

Figure 11.59 The torso and shoulder position should look the same in standing and squatting.

- The guidelines above are important to the movement patterns to receive a snatch in the desired position. It takes tedious focus and practice and is very difficult for many, considering the overhead squat requires an extreme balance of mobility and stability at multiple joint locations.
  - › This is why an athlete or coach should not hesitate to incorporate heel lifts when teaching the overhead squat. It gives the athlete a counterbalance and decreases the significance of any lower extremity joint limitation so that the mechanics and positions can be drilled and practiced over and over. This goes for barefoot practice as well as with weightlifting shoes. It simply gives the lifter a little slack from which to work. Obviously, the idea is to wean the athlete off of an extra heel lift as he or she becomes more adept at achieving the desired positions.
- As the athlete descends into the overhead squat, he or she should continue actively reaching up into the bar enough to maintain the exact position that was established in standing.
- Whether in weightlifting shoes or barefoot, maintain floor pressure through the middle of the heel and big toe.
- Along with trunk and shoulder position, neck position should not change as the athlete descends.

Movement Discussion: How Much Upper Trap is Too Much in Overhead Movement? This question comes up a lot. I will address it by simply explaining the scapular mechanics of overhead movement, and describe a simple drill that should help you figure out the right muscular balance.

When going overhead with a normal, healthy shoulder, the arm (humerus) begins to elevate first. From anywhere between 90-120 degrees, the shoulder blade begins to protract, elevate, upwardly rotate and posteriorly tilt to accommodate for the 60-80 degrees of elevation left to go. This scapular motion is important for achieving a full overhead position. Do not concern yourself with attempting to measure these motions, or trying to determine if the shoulder blade moves at just the right time. The evidence shows that we are unreliable attempting to measure or even eyeball such things, and there is not an established right, wrong or optimal gold standard in the first place.

I'll follow that by saying that we are not huge fans of using one magic cue for shoulder position, as athletes can respond differently to the same cue. Nor do we often refer to specific muscles in regard to the shoulder joint or scapula. It's a complex, three-dimensional system in which several muscles rely on each other for opposition and support. Talking about one individually may add to confusion.

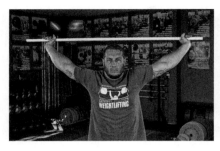
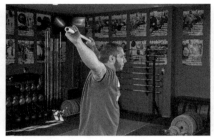
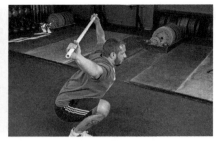

Figure 11.60 Here the athlete is popping the front of the shoulder forward and pushing the bar back, which is a position that may be less stable for many.

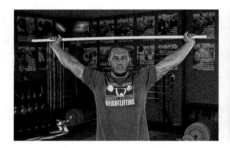
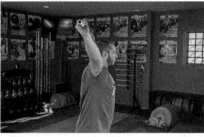
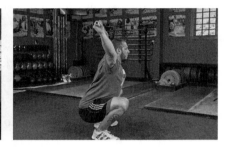

Figure 11.61 Here the athlete stacks the shoulder in line with the ribcage and reaches on the bar through the shoulder blade.

Nonetheless, the upper trap is probably the most discussed (and demonized) of them all, so it's a relevant talking point. I'll put it simply—the upper trap HAS to fire in an overhead position. As in, it's not wrong—it's just what happens. It's all part part of that 3D system just mentioned to assist the shoulder blade into protraction, elevation, upward rotation and posterior tilt. In fact, it's been shown that movements in the scapular plane (similar to everyone's favorite *lower* trap exercise, the Y), that the upper trap is "maximally activated," which is funny considering the common thought process is that we do our Y exercises to train the lower trap, and often cue athletes to avoid any degree of shrug or upper trap recruitment.

Now, having said all of this, we do believe there are positions that are more effective in supporting load overhead than others, but pointing to specific muscles as problematic creates confusion considering those same muscles will be firing just as much in the positions that we desire.

A common overhead strategy that we tend to steer lifters away from is shown in Figure 11.66. The cue of an *active shoulder* is misconstrued by translating the humeral head forward and upward and pushing the bar back past the plane of the body. During the descent of the squat, the torso drifts forward to accommodate the bar position. As you can see in Figure 11.60, the bar ends up over the midfoot, which is what we teach; however, these compromised levers make it very difficult to support load overhead and rely on passive structures for support ("Hanging on your ligaments").

Now compare Figure 11.60 with Figure 11.61. In Figure 11.61, there *is* an active shrug up and use of the upper traps. However, this looks much

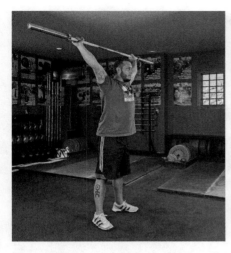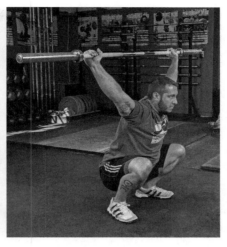

Figure 11.62 Not maintaining a consistent overhead position, with what appears to be an internal rotation compensation.

different than Figure 11.60 picture in the previous series. There is little forward translation of the humeral head, and the bar is stacked over the upper back, hips and midfoot and remains so during the squat. This is how we coach *active shoulder*. It's certainly an active lengthening, reach, shrug (whatever you want to call it) through the plane of the shoulder blade and humerus, but the humeral head stays flush with the front of the shoulder. The golf ball stays on the tee. Refer back to Sidelying Scapular Facilitation for another demonstration of this in a regressed position.

Consciously achieving a perfect balance of all the muscles involved during facilitation drills, or worse yet, during dynamic barbell training, is not really possible. Consider position over individual muscles by exploring and practicing the overhead drills outlined in this chapter.

Movement Discussion: Internal Rotation This is a similar discussion as the one above regarding the shrug. We cannot demonize shoulder internal rotation as inherently "bad" without context. What is thought of as an isolated shoulder internal rotation fault during the overhead squat may again be a result of global suboptimal positioning and stacking of the shoulder and bar. Figure 11.62 illustrates what we commonly see.

In this example, the standing overhead position and squatting overhead position are vastly different. The second picture is not simply a matter of internal rotation of the shoulder. It's a global suboptimal position through the shoulder and trunk as a way for the body to find a passive counterbalance, many times in an effort to attain a deeper squat position. When learning the lifts and positions in a training environment, a lifter does not want to sacrifice shoulder position in order to attain a deeper squat position. It doesn't do you much good to break parallel in your squat if your shoulders are not in a position to support a load.

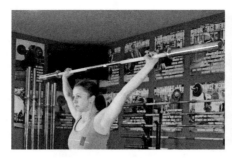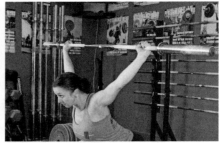

Figure 11.63 Can you tell in which picture the lifter standing and in which the lifter is squatting? Probably pretty easy to tell.

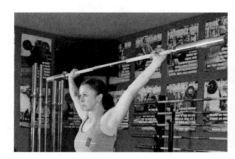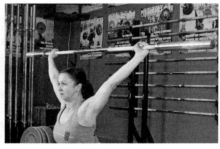

Figure 11.64 Can you tell in which picture the lifter standing and in which the lifter is squatting now?

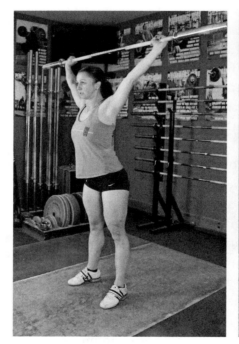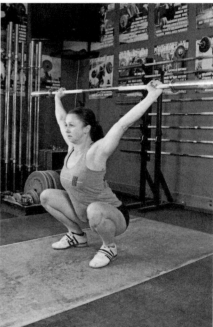

Figure 11.65 There should be minimal change between the overhead position in standing and the bottom of the squat as shown here.

We have found it much easier to address humeral head and bar position as we did in our Upper Trap discussion than to cue and crank a lifter into an exaggerated amount of shoulder external rotation. Again, experiment with various overhead positions as we have done and adhere to the guideline of maintaining the exact overhead position from start to finish. (Figures 11.63—11.65)

Integration: Pressing Snatch Balance with or without Elevated Heels

Snatch balance variations are a great way to work on the receiving position of the snatch. They take the pulling portion of the snatch out of the equation so that on each rep the athlete can practice exactly where they want to be when receiving the bar. If a lifter is still developing his or her movement patterns, it can be beneficial to slow portions of the lift down for even more focused practice. The pressing snatch balance is one such drill.

Starting Position

- Assume your squat stance.
- With a barbell or dowel on your back, set your torso position in the way that you did with the overhead squat—a slight exhalation to set a neutral position and to get the hips stacked underneath the shoulders. The bottom of the ribcage and top of the pelvis should more or less face each other. Inhale to reinforce this position, in which the air is pushed down into the low and upper back.

Execution

- Slowly press your body down under the bar, maintaining the torso angle and position that you started with (Figure 11.66).
- The tendency here is for athletes to begin hyperextending at the T/L junction as they press down, and/or excessively popping the front of the shoulders forward.
- The bar should stay right over the back of the ears and the spinal curves should remain constant.
- The elbows should lock out at the same time that the lifter reaches the bottom of the squat. Focus on pushing the body down as opposed to pushing the bar up. The level of the bar should remain relatively constant.
- Experiment with exhaling forcefully on the way down or inhaling and holding on the way down. Learn to manipulate your breath to give you the right balance of mobility and stability for the positions that you desire.

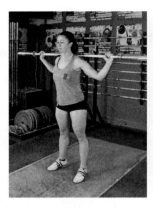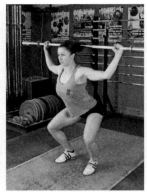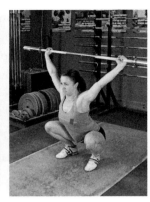

Figure 11.66 The pressing snatch balance

- Utilize plates under the heels (even if you already have shoes on) if you need some slack to get into comfortable positions. Remember, this drill is about MSA and focused practice. Elevated heels are very beneficial for a novice in this case.

Integration: Heaving & Standard Snatch Balance

Now that we have worked to carefully control the optimal position to receive a snatch, we progress to layering on dynamic elements and speed, while beginning to make the movement more automatic and reflexive.

Heaving Snatch Balance with or without Elevated Heels This variation is next in our progression because it adds a dynamic dip and drive but the athlete keeps the feet stationary to minimize any errors in footwork.

Starting Position
- Place the feet in your established squatting stance.
- Hold the bar with a snatch grip behind the neck.

Execution
- Perform a dip and drive in the exact way that we did with the snatch push press. However, the focus is not pushing the bar up, but pushing the body down like in the previous drill.
- Push down against the bar with the arms to sit into the bottom of an overhead squat.
- You should be able to hit the same bottom position that you achieved during the overhead squat and pressing snatch balance. (Figure 11.67)

Standard Snatch Balance This variation now requires that the athlete find in a reflexive manner both the overhead and squat stance that we have repeatedly drilled.

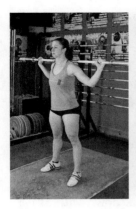 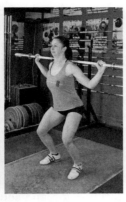 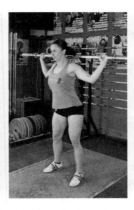 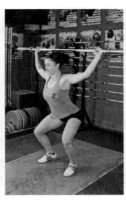 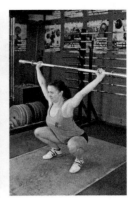

Figure 11.67 The heaving snatch balance adds a dip and drive for a dynamic element.

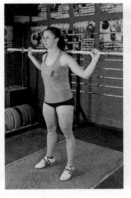 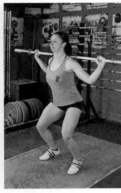 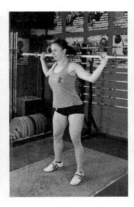 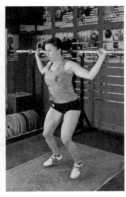 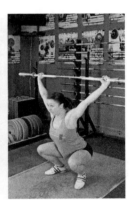

Figure 11.68 The snatch balance adds to the speed of the heaving snatch balance the movement of the feet from the pulling stance to the squatting stance.

Starting Position

- Start with the feet in the established *pulling* stance.
- Hold the bar with a snatch grip behind the neck.

Execution

- Dip and drive and punch under the bar just like the heaving snatch balance.
- Lift and move the feet out to the squatting stance to receive the bar.
- The elbows should lock out at the same time that the feet hit the floor, just like in a full snatch.
- A common mistake is turning this into a push press + overhead squat. That defeats the purpose of the drill, and if you are unable to punch under with confidence, then perform the previous variations until you are able.
- Your feet should land in the stance that you have established as optimal for you based on previous testing and drilling. (Figure 11.68)

Integration: Snatch Grip Behind the Neck Press with or without Elevated Heels

We have placed this variation last because pressing from the bottom of a squat properly is an advanced movement, and elevating the heels is certainly warranted here. To perform this exercise, position your elbows under the bar without losing a full grip. If the lifter is comfortable with that, this particular movement can really drive the last little bit of upper thoracic extension. If that is not comfortable or attainable, return to the thoracic spine drills.

Assume your established squat position and squat down with as vertical a torso as you can while limiting hyperextension of the lower back, even though that's what the tendency will be because the athlete anticipates the subsequent press. However, we will leverage the bar for extension once you are down there. For the squat, attempt to mimic the triple flexion pattern you practiced during the Counterbalance Squat sequence.

Starting Position

- Sit into the bottom of your squat and make sure you are comfortable.
- Hips, knees and ankles should hinge symmetrically and you should be able to feel the middle of both feet equally.
- A short, forceful exhalation will further set your position. Inhale into your lower abdomen, as this will create a very stable platform from which to press.
- The full squat position makes it more difficult to hinge at the T/L junction, so we will take advantage of this by now trying to be as tall through the upper back as possible. Tuck your elbows under the bar at the same time that you pretend there is a string pulling the top of your head up. Exhaling at the same time will ensure the extension is coming from where we want it. This should stack the barbell and your shoulders right over your hips.

Execution

- Inhale deeply and press into the same shoulder position you attained with a standing snatch grip push press.
- If you are unable to attain the same pressing position, then you are not ready for this exercise. Elevating the heels can be a great tool to get the benefits while working back down to the ground over time. (Figure 11.69)

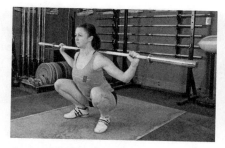 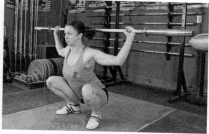 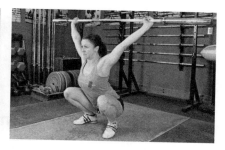

Figure 11.69 The Snatch Grip Behind the Neck Press is an advanced movement.

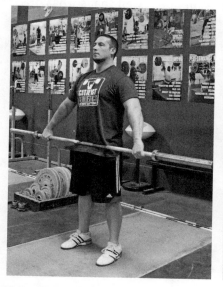 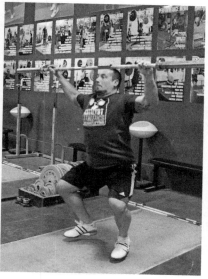 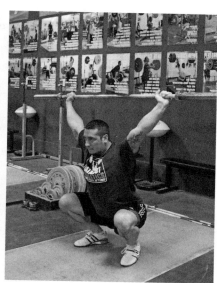

Figure 11.70 The Tall Snatch teaches the lifter to keep the elbows up and out while pulling under the bar and to establish a squatting stance quickly after full hip extension.

Integration: Tall Snatch

Whereas the snatch balance adds a speed element with the weight on the lifter's back, the tall snatch requires and develops significant speed under the bar with the barbell beginning where it will be during the full lift—in front of the lifter. This drill happens fast, and is not meant to be performed with significant weights. The idea is to reinforce balance in all phases of the lift.

Starting Position

- Hold the barbell at arms' length in an erect standing position using the established pulling stance and snatch grip.

Execution

- Initiating with a shrug, pull under the barbell with no countermovement of the hips, knees or ankles.

- Land in your established squatting stance while receiving the bar in your established overhead position.
- Stand with the bar overhead.
- Perform sets of 3-5 reps. (Figure 11.70)

Integration: Snatch

Now it's time to train. You should have the tools and understanding to work toward hitting all of the necessary positions for the full snatch lift. Putting them together and improving technique… well that's what practice is for.

CHAPTER 12

Summary of The Snatch

What is great about "corrective exercise" is that the options are endless as long as you understand the concepts. This is by no means an exhaustive list of what an athlete can do to improve snatch positioning, and we could brainstorm countless variations of what was outlined. That's what we want! Use your screen and assessment to guide you to what needs to be improved, and then use the concepts we discussed regarding stance, squat mechanics, overhead mechanics, and ribcage and pelvis position to practice what you struggle with.

The idea is that you always integrate it in a way that carries over to the snatch. We don't perform drills just to do them. We do them with the purpose of creating patterns specific to the snatch and clean & jerk. So, if you are lying on your back and trying to learn how to lift your arm over your head without popping your ribs up, that's great! But be sure that whatever the focus is, it's ultimately integrated into the barbell lifts.

The corrective strategies have been laid out in bottom-up format. Meaning, we presented them in a ground-based to barbell or low-level to high-level format. We did this for logistical purposes and flow of reading. However, it is recommended, especially for lifters with experience, that you utilize a top-down approach whenever possible—perform the most challenging position or variation in which you can attain the desired position. Remember, the easier or lower level the exercise, the less the adaptation. The regressions are there when you need them.

■ The Clean

We will begin most of our discussion regarding correction of the clean at the moment the lifter receives the bar in the front rack position. The concepts of movement from the beginning of the clean to the point of receiving the bar are very similar to the corresponding movements of the snatch.

One obvious difference to note is the width of the hands on the bar. The narrower clean grip may alter the starting position such that the hips are higher in relation to the knees than they were in the snatch. However, this does not change the movement principles, and they can be extrapolated to the clean pull.

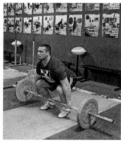 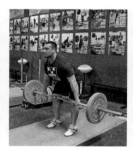 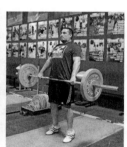 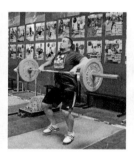 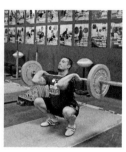

The Clean

■ CHAPTER 13

Clean Receiving Position

The receiving position of the clean, also called the *front rack*, clearly has different characteristics than that of the snatch receiving position. Although shoulder elevation of the front rack is half or less than that of the snatch, there is a shoulder external rotation component that winds up surrounding tissues and can be challenging for some to attain.

The anterior placement of the bar requires that the abovementioned position be maintained through the completion of the clean, or else the lift becomes very difficult to complete successfully. This differs somewhat in the snatch, as the overhead position allows some room for error. We see this as a lifter whose torso dives forward or shoulders collapse inward upon receipt of the bar, but is able to save the snatch successfully. In the clean, because the weight is anterior to the lifter's center of mass and the shoulders are wound in a relatively fixed position, forward tilt of the torso or flexion of the upper back often leads to the weight being lost forward, or in some cases, the athlete putting excessive strain on the wrists and elbows in an attempt to save the lift.

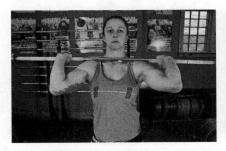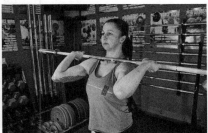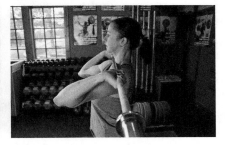

Figure 13.01 The receiving position for the clean, also known as the front rack.

Wrist & Elbow

Like the ankle often being the scapegoat of the squat, the wrist is frequently blamed for a poor front rack position in the clean. We mentioned before that this joint is often a victim of shoulder and torso position, and if a lifter is having difficulty or discomfort at the wrist, it is important to address shoulder and trunk position as a whole. The front rack and over-head jerk position certainly require a certain amount of wrist mobility to attain comfortably, but once that mobility is established we must then optimize torso and shoulder position.

Mobilization: Quadruped Wrist Extension

Starting Position

- On the hands and knees with the hands underneath the shoulders and the knees underneath the hips.
- Fingers straight and outstretched.

Execution

- Rock forward to gently mobilize the flexor muscles of the forearm and the wrist joint (Figure 13.02).
- Alter the angle of the wrist in and out to change the angle of the stretch, and rotate the wrist and hand in and out (Figure 13.03).
- Oscillate gently at end range for 1-2 sets of 30 seconds or as needed.

Notes

- If you feel a distinct "pinching" or "jamming" feeling in the crease of the wrist, reposition or do not go so far into range.

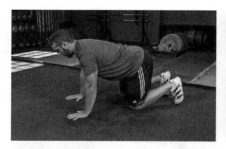 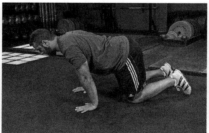 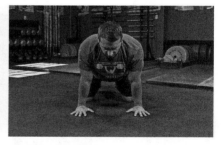

Figure 13.02 Quadruped Wrist Extension mobilization. Create a broad contact area with the hand and rock forward to mobilize the wrist into extension.

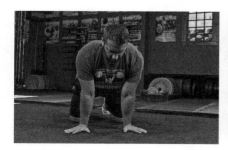 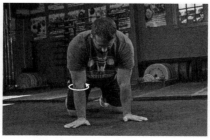 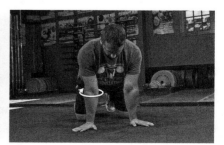

Figure 13.03 Alter the angle of the wrist to mobilize different areas, and try rotating the forearms.

What would be a more common feeling is a stretch in the forearm musculature.

- Actively spreading the fingers wide as you perform the mobilization will enhance the perceived effectiveness, as a lifter's hands are typically spent in a clenched fist.

Movement Cluster Options

- Return to your front rack or overhead position in between sets of the mobilization and gauge any change in comfort or range of motion felt while holding the barbell.

Elbow Flexion Screen

In terms of the elbow, a significant amount of flexion is required to attain the front rack, but again, most lifters possess adequate elbow flexion. Here is a quick screen to see where you stand, but those with thicker builds up top may be limited no matter what due to soft tissue approximation (body parts squishing together).

Execution

- With the arm outstretched and palm facing inward, bend at the elbow and try to touch the thumb to the shoulder. Provide over pressure with the opposite hand in an attempt to touch the thumb knuckle to the shoulder. (Figure 13.04)
- If you can do this without a problem and do not have a history of elbow issues, you likely possess adequate elbow flexion for the front rack position, and that will not be a primary mobility focus.
- If you cannot, it could be for a few reasons:
  > The tissue of your forearm and upper arm approximate, making it impossible to bend the elbow any further. This

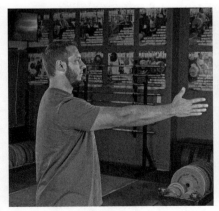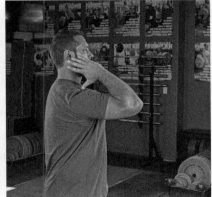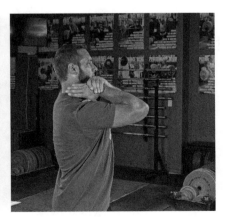

Figure 13.04 Elbow flexion screen. We are looking for the thumb to touch the shoulder.

is not a red flag, it just is what it is. If it feels symmetrical and you do not have history of elbow issue, there is little concern.

> Your triceps (the muscles on the backs of your arms) are resistant to stretch and limit the ability to flex the elbow (rare in my experience).

> There is some type of mechanical block in the joint, which is likely out of the scope of this book. In this case, you won't feel a stretch in the back of the upper arm, you will just feel the joint stop, which may or may not be associated with pain. If that's the case, you should probably get checked out by a professional to see if performance of a movement like a clean is a good idea.

Thoracic Spine & Shoulder

Upper thoracic spine extension (or a strong anti-flexion force) is very useful now, as flexion through the upper back can cause the lifter to dump a clean forward and lose the lift... or grind out a pooping-dog-Quasimodo clean that leaves nothing in the tank for the jerk.

As we did with the snatch, we will teach the lifter to move the thoracic spine through its entire sagittal plane range of motion to maximize mobility, and then learn how to fire the thoracic extensors and stack the torso in order to stabilize and use that mobility.

Also a focus will be positioning the shoulder to support a barbell in the front rack, which opposes large muscle groups such as the lats and pecs.

Mobilization: Quadruped Thoracic Series

We are going to return to a couple of drills that were outlined previously, add some tweaks, and put them together as an alternating series. The goals are to:

- Create upper back expansion for general T-spine mobility.
- Maintain congruency between the shoulder blade and ribcage.
- Generate sagittal plane thoracic spine active motion.
- Gently mobilize the hips into flexion (mimicking a front squat).
- Oppose the muscles and soft tissue that act to prohibit a comfortable front rack.
  > Let's use the latissumus dorsi (lat) for an example, as it is one of the muscles that will oppose a front rack position. Based on the lats' attachment sites, if we somehow caused an isolated spontaneous contraction of this muscle, it

would move the arms into the position illustrated in Figure 13.05.

> You can see how the front rack position would challenge this, since our elbows are up and shoulders externally rotated. The quadruped position allows for a nice adjunct mobilization to the front rack.

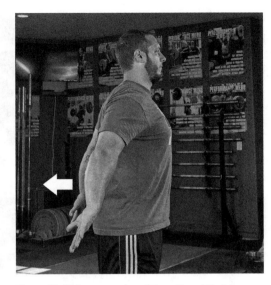

Figure 13.05 Demonstration of the action of the lat muscle—it's clear that this opposes the position of the front rack.

Starting Position

- From on the hands and knees, rock the hips back toward the heels, letting the lower back comfortably relax.
- Drop the chest so that the forearms rest on the ground with the elbows underneath the shoulders.
- Spread the fingers, creating as much ground contact as possible.
- Keep the head and neck relaxed in mid-range.

Execution

- Inhale through the nose with a relaxed neck while maintaining your position, filling your upper back with air.
- Exhale *fully* through the mouth, *reaching* lightly through elbows and forearms, spreading the shoulder blades apart (protracting) and rounding the upper back.
- Maintain this new position as you inhale again, filling upper back with air. (Figure 13.06)
- Exhale and repeat this reaching sequence for 3-4 breaths.
- This can be performed on the hands if the rockback position is not tolerable.
- Arm Elevation
  > Maintaining the scapular reach, walk your fingertips forward, creating length (perceived inhibition) through the lats. Go to the point of first resistance and hold for 3-4 breaths. (Figure 13.07)

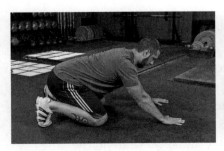
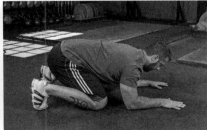
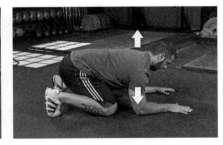

Figure 13.06 Restoring the normal curve of the upper back by reaching through the shoulder blades as a starting position for T-spine and shoulder mobility.

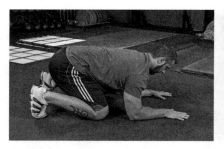
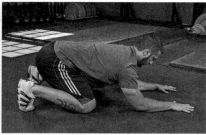
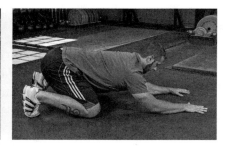

Figure 13.07 Quadruped Thoracic Series: Walking the hands out to inhibit perceived lat tension.

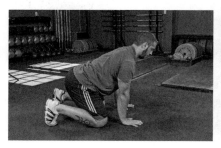
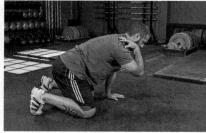
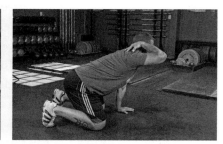
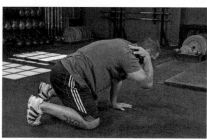
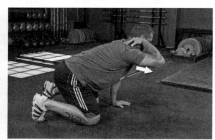

Figure 13.08 Quadruped Thoracic Series: Active thoracic extension in a position that mimics the front rack.

- The difference between this a more traditional yoga-type stretch is that we are maintaining ground contact with the forearms, and maintaining active scapular protraction. As discussed previously, learning how to reach the shoulder complex and create a large excursion of shoulder blade motion independent of the ribcage is useful for full, free shoulder range of motion, a comfortable front rack, etc.
  › Repeat for 1-2 more sets.
- Front Rack Extension & Rotation
  › This can be done either on forearms or hands (pictured).
  › With the elbows back underneath the shoulders and scapular reach maintained, place one hand on the back of the same shoulder, mimicking a front rack position. Maintaining an active reach straight down with the other hand, perform reps in which you flex and extend the thoracic spine, using the up hand as a guide.

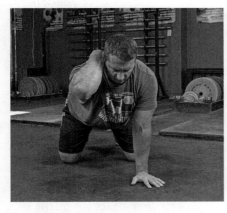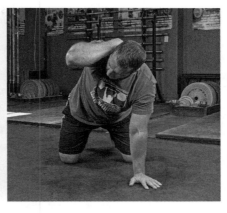

Figure 13.09 Quadruped Thoracic Series: Adding a rotational component to thoracic spine mobility.

> As you flex and extend, perform full breath cycles as you hold in various degrees of flexion or extension. (Figure 13.08)
>   - The low back remains motionless.
>   - You will notice here that thoracic extension is not actually a large excursion of movement.
> Now, with the same hand position as above and maintaining an active reach straight down with the bottom arm for leverage, perform a thoracic rotation toward the elevated arm. This can be done on hands or forearms. Attempt to maintain the same pseudo front rack position as you use the muscles of the upper back to rotate. (Figure 13.09)
>   - As before, cycle through entire breath cycles in which you hold a position and perform a full inhalation through the nose, then a full exhalation through the mouth as you attempt to move further.
>   - You can also experiment with rotating from a flexed thoracic spine position and an extended thoracic spine position. Think *cat/cow* with a rotational component.
>   - Some may wonder why we are adding a thoracic rotation component when the sport of weightlifting does not have such a plane of movement inherent to it. This is a valid thought process, and you will notice that most of what we do in this book is done in the sagittal plane for specificity to the snatch and clean & jerk. However, we humans often have subtle asymmetries that add an element of rotation to our bodies, whether this is readily observable or not. If you had an asymmetry during the Apley Scratch Test in Chapter 4 *and* have noticed observable twisting with overhead movement or in the front rack, there may be a rotational

asymmetry through the ribcage and/or thoracic spine. When restoring range of motion, we look to restore sagittal plane function (flexion/extension) before the transverse plane (rotation). In the rotational component of the series, some may notice that there is an asymmetry from side to side in regard to range of motion, ease and comfort of movement, etc. These asymmetries may or may not correlate to things such as elbow level being uneven in the front rack, one collar bone that gets more beat up than the other, an observable twist of the upper torso in the front rack or during the dip and drive of the jerk, among other things. If you are a lifter who has difficulty with the front rack position, it can be beneficial for you to spend time here to improve controlled range of motion, but also in terms of being able to breathe and expand the ribcage in different positions. Then, integrating shoulder motion is often easier to implement.

Cues

- Try to push air into your upper back when inhaling without losing position.
- Try to keep the shoulders relatively relaxed
- For some, breathing in this position may be difficult, as it forces the athlete to expand his or her ribs. If this is you, the tendency may be to come out of the rockback position as you breath in. Don't let this happen. Stay rocked back and let the air flow in as it may without straining.

Movement Cluster Options

- Alternate with Supine Overhead Wall Press and/or 20-second bouts of SMR to the lats or upper back for 2-4 rounds.
- Alternate with Standing Wall Press and/or 20-second bouts of SMR to the lats or upper back for 2-4 rounds.
- Alternate with Front Rack Holds.

Mobilization: Squatting Lat Stretch

Up to this point, we have not outlined a significant amount of static muscle lengthening strategies; however targeting the lat in this manner can certainly augment the previous drills and aid in making the front rack position more comfortable and achievable.

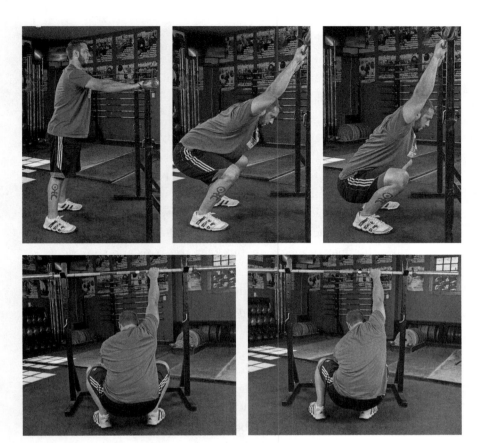

Figure 13.10 Squatting Lat Stretch. Sit back and down to stretch both sides, and side bend with one arm to increase the intensity.

Starting Position

- Grab a barbell, rack, doorway or other implement that is about chest height with both hands.
- Walk back while bending at the waist and letting the lower back comfortably round.
- Sit into a deep squat that is comfortable for you. (Figure 13.10)

Execution

- Reach long through your arms and take deep breaths in through your nose, trying to fill the sides of your chest with air. This will increase the stretch.
- Exhale through the mouth fully and reach longer.
- This can be performed with one arm or both (Figure 13.10).
- To increase the stretch on the internal rotators, you can flip your grip (palms facing up).
- This stretch can be performed in a partial squat as well.
- Perform 1-3 sets of 5 full breaths or as needed.

Notes

- Inhaling into the space you are trying to lengthen will increase the stretch from the inside out. Rather than cranking on the shoulder with more force, simply take in a fuller breath.
- Allowing your lower back to round slightly increases the stretch on the lat due to its attachment to the thoracolumbar fascia. It is safe to round here, as we are not loaded, and are focused on mobility rather than training motor patterns.
- When reaching long with your arms, allow the shoulder blades to passively glide upward as well. When you exhale fully, pull the ribcage down, but keep the arms and shoulder blades where they are.
- If using one arm, side bending toward the arm being stretched can increase the intensity.

Movement Cluster Options

- Alternate with Supine Overhead Wall Press and/or 20-second bouts of SMR to the lats or upper back for 2-4 rounds.
- Alternate with Standing Wall Press and/or 20-second bouts of SMR to the lats or upper back for 2-4 rounds.
- Alternate with Front Rack Holds.

Mobilization: Standing Wall Squat

Here we begin to integrate the previous concepts into the standing position. Don't hesitate to elevate the heels during any variation of this drill to maximize the vertical torso position.

Starting Position

- Assume your established squatting stance with your back facing a wall or squat rack (pictured) approximately 8-10 inches away.
- Perform an air squat with focus on a neutral lumbar spine. A slight tailbone tuck will suffice here to ensure a small, but not excessive, amount of lordosis.
- The distance away from the wall should be such that the lifter is supported by the wall but is not totally relying on it for balance, making this much different than a traditional wall sit. If the wall or rack were suddenly taken away, the lifter would not immediately fall over. (Figure 13.11)

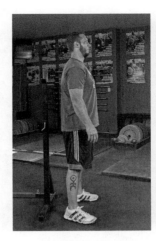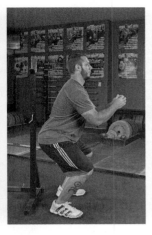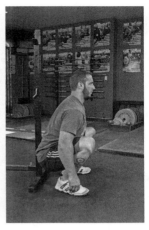

Figure 13.11 Starting position of Standing Wall Squat for thoracic mobility in the front rack (pictured using a squat rack)

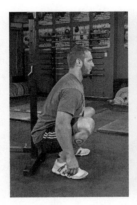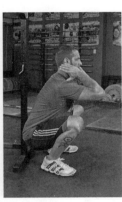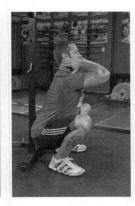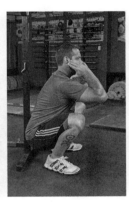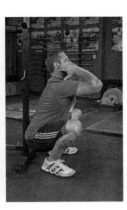

Figure 13.12 In the Standing Wall Squat, the wall or rack helps hold the pelvis in place so that we can isolate movement at the thoracic spine and shoulders.

Execution

- With the minimal support of the wall or rack, the athlete can focus on attaining mid- to upper-thoracic spine extension by first reaching long through both arms forward, then placing both hands on the backs of the shoulders, just as in the Quadruped Thoracic Series previously.
- Breathe in through the nose, exhale through the mouth and arch/extend the upper back by leading with the elbows, which are reaching forward and up. Pause, inhale into the new position, and exhale again, attempting to gain new range through the thoracic spine.
- You should feel the muscles of the upper thoracic spine light up. (Figure 13.12)

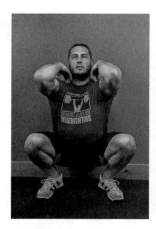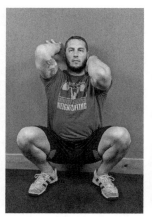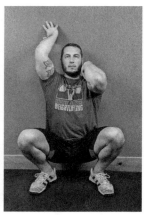

Figure 13.13 Incorporating increased shoulder flexion with a fingertip wall walk on one side in the Standing Wall Squat to further improve mobility requirements of the front rack.

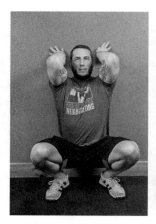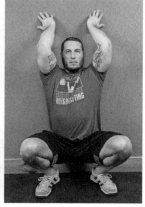

Figure 13.14 Incorporating a fingertip wall walk with both hands simultaneously in the Standing Wall Squat to increase mobility and stability demands. Maintain the forward reach of the elbows.

Fingertip Wall Walk Variation Place the fingertips of one hand on the wall behind you and slowly begin to walk your fingertips up it. Continue to reach long and forward with the elbow—do not let it flare out. The opposite arm can remain on the back of the shoulder or reaching forward for a counterbalance. (Figure 13.13)

If you want to get really saucy, walk the fingertips of both hands up the wall. Keep the neck neutral. If you've never felt your mid and upper back erector muscles before, this may be the ticket. (Figure 13.14)

Progress the range of motion slowly here. No one is winning the fingertip wall walk trophy, so if just getting your hand back to the wall is challenging enough, stay there and take a few breaths instead of trying to walk up higher.

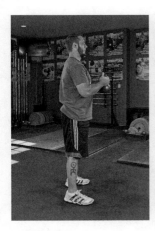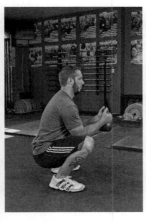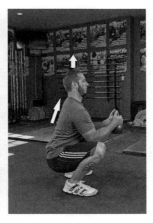

Figure 13.15 Use the counterbalance to create a "tall" spine and upper thoracic extension. Use a forceful exhalation while creating length through the top of the head.

Movement Cluster Options

- Alternate with Supine Overhead Wall Press for 2-4 rounds.
- Alternate with Quadruped T-spine Series for 2-4 rounds.
- Alternate with Standing Wall Press and/or 20-second bouts of SMR to lats or upper back for 2-4 rounds.
- Alternate with Front Rack Holds and/or slow eccentric front squats.
- Alternate with 20-second bouts of SMR to the lats or upper back for 2-4 rounds.

Stabilization: Counterbalance Squat Half Rack

This drill uses a similar concept as the previous, but with no wall for support.

Execution

- Establish a stable foot with three points of contact and perform a counterbalance squat in which you let your hips, knees and ankles comfortably hinge as we did in Chapter 11.
- In the bottom of the squat, work to attain upper thoracic extension by exhaling and pulling the front ribs down while simultaneously trying to create a "tall" spine. Pretend that a string is being pulled from the top of your head. (Figure 13.15)
- Slowly transfer the weight to one side while maintaining the exact same squat position. This frees one arm up for movement.
- Place the free hand behind the shoulder. Placing the elbow straight forward, reach long and up with it, just as you did with the Standing Wall Squat previously (Figure 13.16).

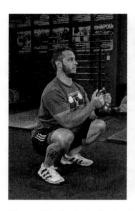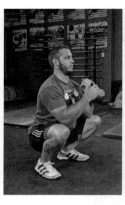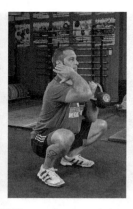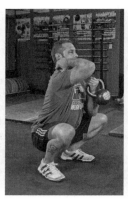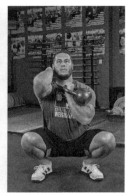

Figure 13.16 Mimic the front rack and isolate the T-spine with the use of a counterbalance.

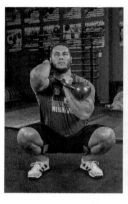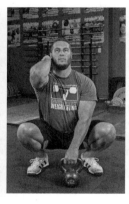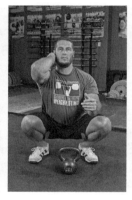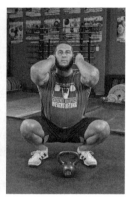

Figure 13.17 Truly "owning" the front squat position without a counterbalance

- Repeat on the opposite side.
- Establish your bottom position with one arm free again.
  - ❯ Perform the movement described above with one arm.
  - ❯ Then *slowly* lower the weight to the floor while maintaining your exact body position. You're going to have to really fight here to stay tall.
  - ❯ Attempt to perform the same movement with the second arm while in your deep bottom position. (Figure 13.17)
  - ❯ Repeat this for 1-2 sets on each side.
  - ❯ For all variations, weightlifting shoes or a heel lift can be used to assist in positioning.
  - ❯ When you begin to feel yourself lose position, utilize a high-tension breathing and bracing strategy to reestablish control.

Movement Cluster Options

- Alternate with Supine Overhead Wall Press.
- Alternate with 20-second bouts of SMR to the lats or upper back for 2-4 rounds.

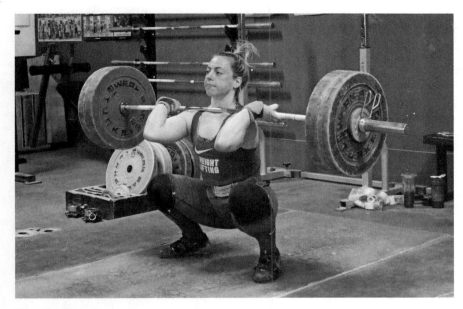

Figure 13.18 The front squat

- Alternate with Quadruped T-spine Series for 2-4 rounds.
- Alternate with Standing Wall Press and/or 20-second bouts of SMR to the lats or upper back for 2-4 rounds.
- Alternate with Standing Wall Squat for 2-4 rounds.
- Alternate with Front Rack Holds and/or slow eccentric front squats.

Integration: Front Squat

Hopefully at this point the athlete is ready to integrate all of the mobility and stability concepts previously established into the front squat movement. As with the overhead squat, elevating the heels (even if already wearing weightlifting shoes) can be beneficial for the novice lifter when learning the front squat, or for an experienced lifter who is re-appraising his or her movement and working to attain a more vertical torso.

Breathing & Bracing for the Front Squat For lighter weights, the sequence of breathing and bracing may be of less consequence. However, it is of greater significance for stability when the weights get heavy, so practicing habits with lighter weight can be beneficial.

There are no one-size-fits-all rules for how to set up your position and breathe for a front squat. Having said this, we will outline a couple sequences that have worked well for many lifters.

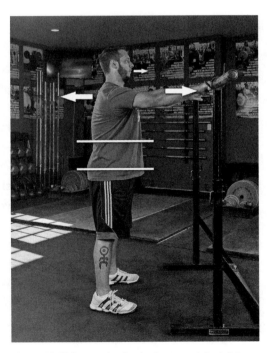

Figure 13.19 Preparation for the front squat. Push into the bar slightly while performing a short, forceful exhalation. This exhalation should aid in setting a neutral trunk.

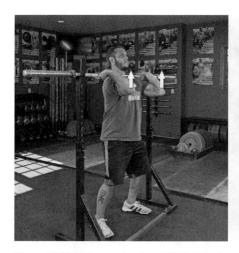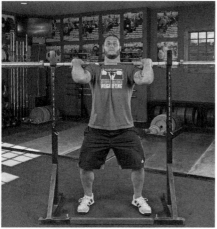

Figure 13.20 With your already established trunk position, pull under the bar, rolling your elbows forward and up until the bar is sitting on your shoulders. The elbow position will provide reinforcement for the upper thoracic extension.

Sequence 1

- After establishing the grip on the bar with the arms outstretched, forcefully exhale to set an abdominal brace. This will *not* be a complete exhalation as we have performed in previous drills, but enough to pull the ribs down and cue the abdominals—setting position. (Figure 13.19)
  - ❯ The exhalation, combined with the arms outstretched and pushing into the bar, will re-establish a neutral upper back position and subsequent fixing of the scapula to the ribcage (this is a good thing).
- Next, inhale down into this position to reinforce it. This will *not* be a *maximal* inhalation—it's just enough to expand your torso and create some pressure for the barbell to rest on and reinforce the position. At this point, your torso position is set, and you can breathe shallowly over top of it.
- Pull under the bar with the hips stacked underneath the shoulders and the elbows reaching forward and up just like your practiced in previous drills. With your torso already stable and pressurized, the elbow position will aid in keeping your upper back tall. Maintain as full of a grip on the bar as possible. (Figure 13.20)
- Walk the weight out to your established squatting stance, breathing shallowly if needed but maintaining the torso position that you set even before the bar was on your shoulders. Use as few steps as possible to establish your stance. At this point, you should know where your preferred squat stance is.

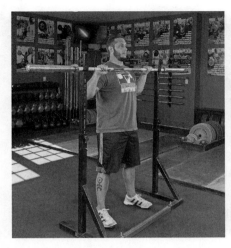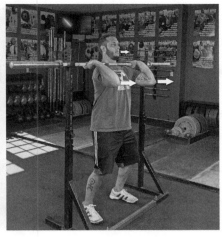

Figure 13.21 Perform a short, forceful exhalation as you reach the elbows forward and up into the front rack.

- Now comes the last inhalation. Initiate the breath in through the nose, pushing the air down forcefully, until it drives into your upper back. With significant percentages of one-rep max, it may be necessary to finish the inhalation through the mouth to maximize airflow and pressure.
- As you attain full depth in the squat and then drive up, pressure and air may be released naturally and as needed, but any exhalation should be performed forcefully with pressure behind it so as not to "deflate" under heavy load.

Sequence 2

- Pull under the bar with the hips under the shoulders.
- Exhale forcefully as the elbows are pulled forward and up. As before, this will not be a full exhalation, but enough to pull the lower ribs down and set the abs. Stay tall through the upper back as you do this. (Figure 13.21)
- Inhale into this position by pushing the air down into the lower back until it fills the upper back and expands the torso 360 degrees. As before, this is not a maximal inhalation. You should be able to breath shallowly over top of this position.
- Unrack the bar and repeat the rest of Sequence 1.
- The difference between this and Sequence 1 is that we are setting and reinforcing trunk position while in the front rack instead of with outstretched arms before moving under the bar.

Again, these are simply suggestions of how to sequence your breathing and bracing when squatting heavy. Experimentation of what works best is needed, and the lifter may develop his or her own unique sequence.

Elbow, Hand, Shoulder & Upper Back Position in the Front Rack

By now, you probably get the idea of what we recommend in regard to elbow position. We want the lifter to reach forward and up through the elbows for the duration of the lift. This will aid in reinforcing the upright torso that carries over to receiving a clean. This also protracts the shoulder blades slightly, stabilizing them to the ribcage, and creating a nice shelf for the bar to rest on.

Of course, lifters will have individual preferences that vary from this. One such tweak is elevating the shoulders once the bar position has been established to create a deeper "slot" for the bar to rest in. We have recommended against such a position when the arms are overhead, but in the front rack, it can be beneficial and comfortable for some. (Figure 13.22)

The lifter should be actively fighting to keep the upper back "tall" during the descent of the front squat. Pretend that a string is pulling straight up from the top of your head. You will see many high level lifters use a certain degree of neck hyperextension during a heavy squat, especially when driving out of the hole or through a sticking point. This is a natural reflex of the body that increases neural drive to the extensor muscles for a transient increase in output. It is driving extensor tone and is a very effective maneuver for increasing performance in that moment. Something like this should come reflexively and is not necessarily a technique that would be coached. The body will do it if it feels that it's stuck, and then return the head to a more neutral position once through the struggle. For the purposes of general biomechanics and tissue longevity, we will encourage

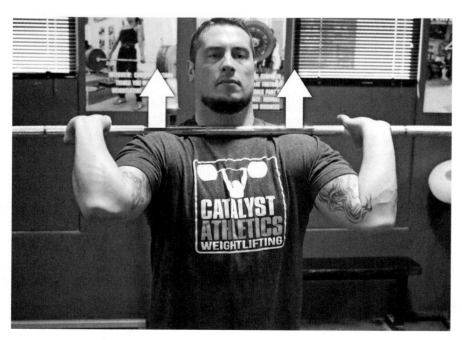

Figure 13.22 Elevating the shoulder blade complex slightly in the front rack can create some space for the bar to rest in.

a neutral neck position, in which the back of the neck is long, for our default position. (Figure 13.23)

If possible, it is ideal to have your whole hand around the bar. This will aid in maximal control of the shoulder girdle and upper back, and also takes pressure off of the wrist. Many lifters will not be able to attain this, but can still strive for the cues that we have established for the elbows and upper back to optimize positioning.

Hip, Knee & Foot Position in the Front Squat If the above mentioned breathing and bracing sequences are practiced, lifters should find themselves in a balanced position in which they can simply sit straight down into the squat, allowing the hips, knees and ankles to hinge naturally. The weight is centered over the ankle joint, and pelvis is stacked under the shoulders. It is common to see lifters' shoulders hanging back behind the hips as they prepare to front squat (Figure 13.24). This can make it difficult to stay pressurized and stable through the core.

For some, especially those with limited ankle dorsiflexion, it may be difficult to simply "sit straight down" into the squat, as they max out forward tibial translation prematurely. Again, this can be a product of restricted ankle dorsiflexion range of motion, a lack of motor control, or from having picked up the habit of being pulled forward

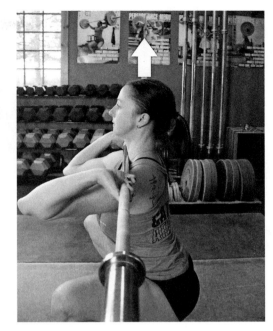

Figure 13.23 As we did in our counterbalance sequence, create a "tall" spine for upper back extension. Incorporating pauses and forceful exhalations as you extend the upper back can be helpful.

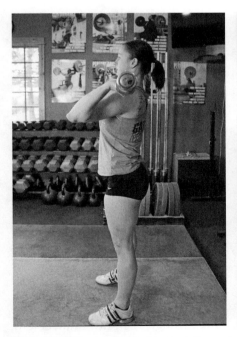 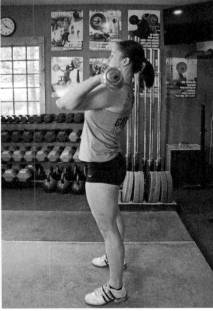

Figure 13.24 We want the shoulders and ribcage stacked over the hips as shown in the first picture, rather than allowing the shoulders to hang behind the hips as shown in the second picture.

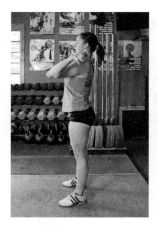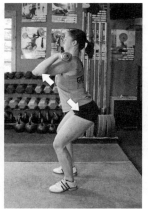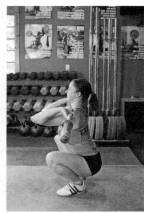

Figure 13.25 "Setting" the hips means a slight down and back motion to initiate the squat.

through the torso during lifts. One such maneuver to correct this is to "set" the hips upon initiation of the front squat. This is done by simultaneously reaching the elbows forward and up while sitting the pelvis down and back SLIGHTLY, as we still want to maintain balance through the midfoot. A subtle break at the hips, when coupled with the elbow position being maintained, creates a nice counterbalance over the ankle. The front squat is *initiated* with this movement during the first eighth of the descent, then the lifter sits straight down to perform the rest of the squat. (Figure 13.25)

When coming out of the hole of a front squat, it is common for a lifter to allow the hips to shoot back, which causes the upper back and torso to dump forward. This is not what we want in terms of translating to the positions of our clean. Be sure to establish a stance width that allows you to sit straight down and stand straight up without substantial changes in torso angle. A stance that is too narrow for the lifter's comfort can cause the lifter to feel "crowded" at the bottom, which can make the movement slow and awkward, preventing any type of elastic rebound out of the bottom. A stance that is too wide for the lifter's comfort may cause him or her to lose tension through the core when changing directions.

The weight distribution of the feet should be balanced between the big toe, little toe and heel. Being rocked back so far on your heels that your toes are coming up demonstrates an unbalanced position. Keep the big toe actively planted down into your shoe and make sure to feel the middle to inside edge of the heel during the entirety of the movement. This will ensure you are "sitting in between your feet" evenly during the lift. Actively pressing your big toe down into your shoe will minimize chances of midfoot collapse.

Performing pause squats with strict focus on a controlled descent in which your torso angle remains constant through the entire movement is also beneficial to reinforce position. 3-5 second pauses are usually recommended.

Tempo squats can be utilized for similar goals of reinforcing position. Slow the descent down to a deliberate 3-5 seconds before exploding up out of the hole. A failed front squat is rarely, if ever, caused by a lack of leg strength, as front squat weights will typically always be lighter than one's best back squat. The focus of a front squat should be about maintaining posture, position and balance over the foot. Tempo squats are very effective at teaching this.

Integration: Barbell Front Rack Mobilization & Holds

Now that we have discussed front rack mechanics, nothing will help your front rack position more than getting in the front rack position.

Starting Position

- Standing with the bar in a squat rack at about shoulder height.
- Grab the bar with your typical front rack grip (the grip you clean with, or that you and your coach feel you front squat best with).
- The bar should be loaded with a heavy weight so that it remains stationary.

Execution

- Keeping your entire hand around the bar, assume your front rack position.
- Balance yourself so that the bar is over your midfoot.
- Maintain a stacked torso as we have discussed and practiced.
- Protract your shoulder blades by *reaching* long and up through your elbows.
  - > Think about touching the wall in front of you with your elbows.
- With your lower back locked in neutral and your elbows actively reaching forward, work to extend your upper back.
  - > Remember, do not change your lumbar position, and keep your hands around the bar.
- Inhale through your nose and try to push the air into your upper back. Exhale through your mouth and reach your elbows long and up. Use high-tension exhalations in an effort to inhibit perceived tightness that limits the position.
- Put upward pressure into the barbell as if you were going to lift it off the rack and hold. (Figure 13.26)

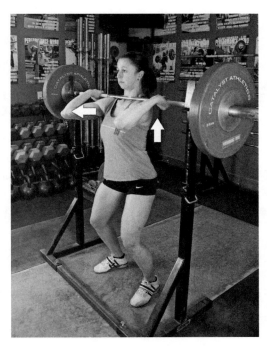

Figure 13.26 Solidify the front rack position with holds using a heavy barbell in a squat rack.

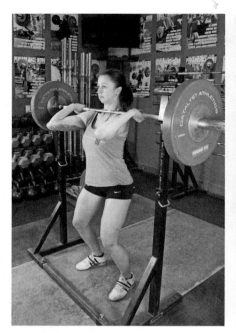
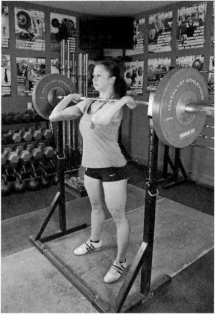

Figure 13.27 Use front rack support holds to strengthen the position.

- Perform 2-4 sets of 5-15-second bouts. The number of sets and duration of each can increase as the comfort of the position improves. For those who struggle with the front rack position, this may be a pretty significant stretch. Be easy, and do not force what you do not have. It will come with consistent work.
- Finally, using a weight that is manageable, you can lift the bar straight up out of the rack and hold, maintaining the same position as above. This will allow you to feel comfortable and learn to breathe under heavy loads with the correct torso position, as this can be loaded at or past the lifter's maximum clean. (Figure 13.27)

Movement Cluster Options
- Alternate with 20-second bouts of SMR to the lats and T-spine.
- Alternate with 20-second bouts of deep Squatting Lat Stretch.
- Alternate with Standing Wall Squat or Counterbalance Front Squat.

Integration: Sots Press

This lift is commonly mistaken for being performed behind the neck. A true Sots press is done from the front rack... unfortunately. We take the

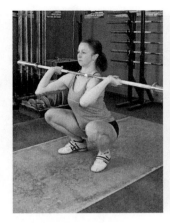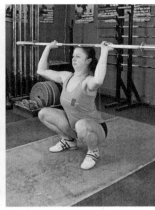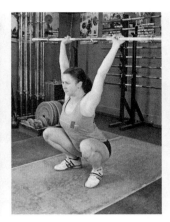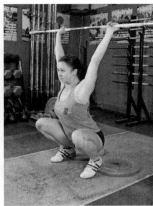

Figure 13.28 The Sots press. Be sure to establish a squat stance that provides you with a base to push from. Utilize a heel lift until you can lock out a press while maintaining a full-depth squat position.

pause front squat mentioned above and add a press—the ultimate opposition of any tissues that restrict the front rack position.

Do not be the athlete who performs ugly, half-squat Sots presses just for the sake of saying you did it. Use these as the powerful movement tool that they can be to improve your positioning in the clean. Remember the Standing Wall Squat with double arm Fingertip Walks and the Wall Press Squat? Very similar positioning here.

Starting Position

- Sit in the bottom of a front squat with your established stance.
- Utilize elevated heels if you are not completely comfortable pressing from the bottom of a front squat.

Execution

- From the bottom of the squat, simply press straight up on the barbell. Think about pressing the bar up while you are pushing your body down. Use the weight of the bar on your shoulders and possible heel lift as leverage to attain as vertical a torso as possible. Being in a full squat will help minimize hyperextension through the lumbar spine, so we can focus on gaining as much extension in that position as possible. (Figure 13.28)
- Perform anywhere from 1-5 reps here, but position is the name of the game.

Movement Cluster Options

- Alternate with 20-second bouts of SMR to the lats and T-spine.

- Alternate with 20-second bouts of deep Squatting Lat Stretch.
- Alternate with Standing Wall Squat or Counterbalance Front Squat.
- Alternate with Barbell Front Rack Holds.

Integration: Tall Clean

To finish our talks on clean positioning, we'll outline a drill that allows the lifter to take every concept learned in this chapter and apply it to the lift in a dynamic fashion.

Starting Position

- Pull a barbell to an erect standing position using the your established pulling stance.

Execution

- Initiating with a shrug, pull under the barbell with no countermovement of the hips, knees or ankles.
- Land in your established squatting stance while receiving the bar in your established front rack position. Stand and repeat. (Figure 13.29)
- Perform sets of 3-5 reps.
- This drill happens fast and is not meant to be performed with significant weights. The idea is to reinforce balance in all phases of the lift.

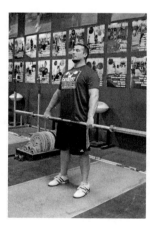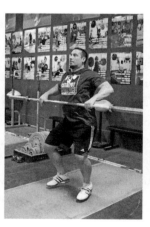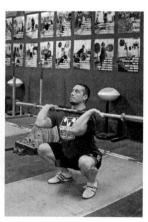

Figure 13.29 The Tall Clean. This drills teaches the lifter to get the elbows around the bar and establish a squatting stance quickly after full hip extension.

CHAPTER 14

Summary of The Clean

_____

For clean pull corrections, simply refer to those outlined in Chapters 7-9 for the snatch. The barbell integration drills for the snatch can be used just as easily for the clean, but obviously using your clean grip and ending with the bar at the shoulders as opposed to overhead. Again, use a top-down approach with your corrective strategies whenever possible to maximize time efficiency and adaptation.

We focused on the front squat and rack position thoroughly in the context of the clean, as that will set you up nicely for what wins or loses the meet for many lifters—the jerk.

■ The Jerk

The jerk is the most commonly missed lift in weightlifting. Many factors contribute to this, including technical and motor control errors and movement deficiencies. We will spend most time discussing the most common jerk variation—the split jerk.

From a mobility standpoint, the requirements for a front rack position discussed in the previous chapter still hold true here, since that is our starting position. The narrower jerk grip (compared to a snatch) requires more elevation range of motion of the shoulder joints to attain the overhead position. From a lower body perspective, hip extension will be of great significance for the jerk drive (similar to the pull) and split receiving position (for the back leg). The hip flexion required for the front leg is typically well within a lifter's mobility capacity.

What is of utmost importance is possessing the motor control and stability to integrate these mobility needs with well-timed movement and relative stiffness through the trunk during the entirety of the split jerk process.

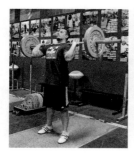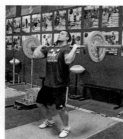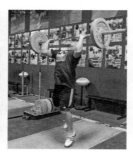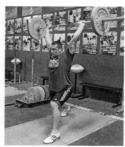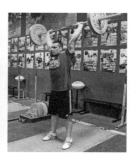

The split jerk

■ CHAPTER 15

Jerk Front Rack

I recommend returning to Chapter 13 for the bulk of discussion regarding the development of a proficient front rack position. For the jerk, many coaches will cue their lifters to reposition the hands (when coming up from the clean) so that the bar rests deeper in the palm. This may also lead to a repositioning of the elbows to point more downward and slightly out relative to the front squat or clean front rack position. (Figure 15.01) This makes intuitive sense, since we are looking to drive the bar up and slightly back, so repositioning the elbows more under the bar will theoretically facilitate this.

Regardless of your preference, what is most important is that you find a position in which the bar can rest on your shoulders that is relatively comfortable and that you can breathe in. THIS is where many jerks are lost, even before the start of the dip and drive. Many lifters (inexperienced ones especially) fail to establish a comfortable jerk front rack after coming out of the clean. Doing so has a couple beneficial effects:

- The lifter can breathe sufficiently under the bar, resulting in an ability to re-create a pressurized system through the trunk and subsequent core stability. This will help to combat rounding of the upper back during the dip (and dropping of the elbows), or hyperextension (unstacked torso) of the lower back in the receiving position.

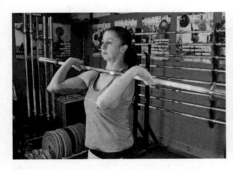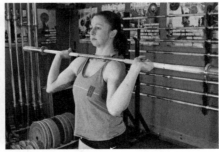

Figure 15.01 Elbows down and out is a common teaching in preparation for the jerk, although some lifters may prefer a higher elbow position.

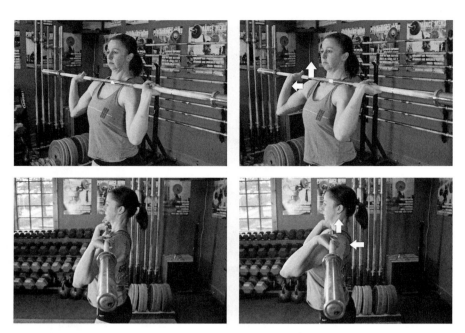

Figure 15.02 Utilizing relative amounts of scapular protraction and/or elevation can help to seat the bar comfortably in the front rack.

- The lifter can stay with the dip and drive as needed. Many lifters will rush the dip and drive as a result of being uncomfortable in the front rack, so of course they are going to want to get out of that position as fast as possible. However, we want to stay patient with our dip and drive in order to impart maximal force to the barbell in the upward direction. As with the pull, cutting the extension at the top of the drive short will reduce the height of the bar.

The athlete needs to experiment and establish his or her optimal jerk front rack position. For heavier weights, utilizing jerk blocks is great for this because you do not have to clean the weight up or step back from a rack. You simply quarter squat the weight up and try out various shoulder and trunk positions.

The bar should rest in a nook, valley, groove, crevice (however you want to word it) between your shoulders and collarbones. This should not cause pain or feel like the bar is resting directly on the collarbone, and the lifter should be able to breathe in and out without obstruction in this position. These criteria should not change just because there is heavy weight on the bar—what changes is simply the perceived general pressure that you feel from the weight.

We understand that not all lifters will be able to grasp an empty barbell or lightly loaded barbell with a full hand, but strive to attain as much hand contact as possible. This does not mean gripping the bar tightly—it means getting as much hand underneath the bar that you can.

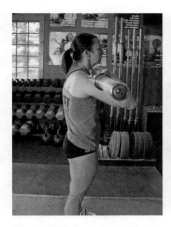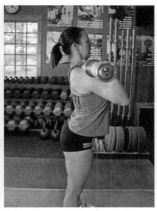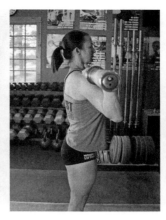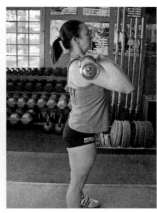

Figure 15.03 First picture: Upper back flexion makes it difficult to support heavy load in the front rack and to create upward drive on the bar. Second picture: "Pseudo" T-spine extension in which the athlete extends excessively from the T/L junction to achieve the overall extended position. This is not a stacked position. Third picture: Upper T-spine extension and stacked torso, which is what we are striving for. Fourth picture: A strategy using slightly more spinal extension than the previous picture, but still a sustainable position to dip and drive from.

From here, alter your shoulder blade position:

Protraction

- By now, you should have a grasp on how to protract your scapulae. Perform this movement with the bar in the front rack. For many lifters, this will provide a groove for the bar to rest in. There will be an optimal amount, however, as maximally protracting may set the bar uncomfortably on the collarbone. (Figure 15.02)
  > To remedy this, one can add an element of slight shoulder elevation at this point to raise the bar off of the collarbones if that is an issue.
- At this point, we cannot forget about our upper back. We want our thoracic spine to remain tall through this process so that our trunk stays vertical during the dip. The abovementioned elbow and scapular positioning will put many lifters in the correct upper back position naturally without much extra focus in that area. For others who struggle with attaining upper thoracic extension, a little extra "chest puff" can be beneficial here to give the barbell a robust platform to rest on. This can be done as the lifter is inhaling a final time before the dip and drive. I would have hesitated to give the cue of a "chest puff" before discussing all of our previous points about spinal position, because this is often misconstrued by athletes as a cue to hinge at the T/L junction. The lower back and pelvic position remains relatively constant throughout this process, as we are attempting to isolate motion in the upper back. (Figure 15.03)

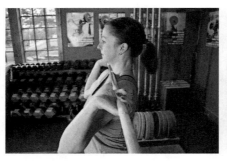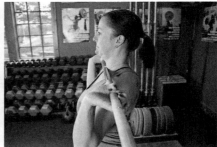

Figure 15.04 Experiment with both positions of protraction (first picture) and retraction (second picture) in order to find the most comfortable combination.

Retraction

- Try the exact same protocol above with an element of scapular retraction—instead of reaching long and forward with the elbows and shoulder blades, pin them back together. (Figure 15.04)
- We are not going to deem this right or wrong. What we want, instead, is for the lifter to try the extremes of protraction and retraction in the front rack position in order to find whatever "middle ground" position works best for them. Remember, it needs to be relatively comfortable and you need to be able to breathe. *Comfort* is certainly relative here, but to put it in context: You should be able to rest in that position with 70% or more of your best jerk (That number is made up and arbitrary, but it conveys the point) for 6-10 seconds without suffocating, passing out, or feeling like your collarbone is going to snap or shoulder is going rip off. You might get a little tired, but that would be normal.

Foot pressure is also of importance before initiating the jerk dip. We want our weight (plus the weight of the barbell) to be evenly distributed from left to right. If a lifter is favoring one side over the other to start the dip, he or she will likely continue to favor or even favor that leg more during the drive, leading to the lifter being off balance when he or she receives the jerk. As a cue, focus on feeling the big toes and middle to inside half of the heels on both feet. If you feel the inside of one heel, but the outside of another, you may be leaning towards the outside heel (this can be very subtle). If you do not have a problem with balance in your jerk, then this may be a non-issue (don't chase ghosts); but if you do, focus on even foot pressure.

Breathing

A final element of importance before moving on to the dip and drive is the breathing sequence for the jerk. If using jerk blocks or taking the bar from a rack, you can essentially use the identical breathing and bracing sequences that we outlined in for the front squat. When coming up out of a clean, it can be common to reflexively exhale *slightly,* as a result of the exertion of the squat. This, however, is not a full exhalation, as we certainly do not want to deflate ourselves under load. Think of it more as a short, forceful burst through pursed lips. The goal is to maintain as much air and internal pressure as is comfortable.

After standing up from the clean, it will be beneficial to attain your established jerk position as quickly as possible. Many lifters will utilize the momentum of coming out of the squat to pop the bar off the chest just enough to establish the jerk position. Other lifters can do this without popping the bar off the chest, but this is more rare.

Whether the lifter is coming out of the clean or taking the bar from blocks or a rack, one final inhalation before initiating the dip and drive can be beneficial in reinforcing relative stability through the trunk and creating as broad a platform to support the bar as possible. Go back to our breathing and bracing practice drills in Chapter 2. The cue to initiate the inhalation in the jerk by pushing the air down toward the lower back is helpful to expand the lower abdomen 360 degrees and establish lumbar stability. This also helps the lifter to keep the neck and shoulders relatively relaxed. Then, finish the inhalation by filling the upper back with air. Think about it like this: if your head were cut off, the air would fill your torso in the same way that water would fill it if it were poured into your empty carcass. This creates that robust "can of stability" that we need, and should all be done while attempting to keep the hands and neck *relatively* relaxed.

Important Note We are obviously discussing some very fine details in regard to movement and positioning for these lifts. Please remember that when it is time to go heavy in training and on the competition platform, you are not focusing on these subtle things. They should come automatically at that point. However, in order for that to happen, we must put in conscious practice with submaximal loads.

CHAPTER 16

Jerk Dip

The dip phase of the jerk sets us up for the explosive drive phase, so it's very influential in the subsequent trajectory and height of the bar.

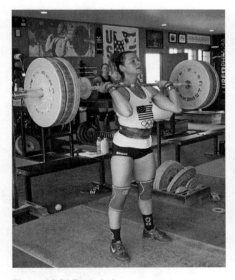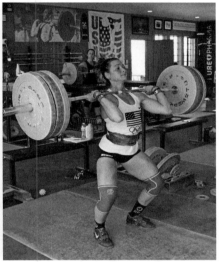

Figure 16.01 The jerk dip

Elbows & Upper Back

The position of the elbows should remain relatively constant during the dip. The tendency will be for the lifter to drop them prematurely in preparation for the drive phase. A drop of the elbows will certainly occur as the lifter transitions from the bottom of the dip to the drive in order to gain better overhead leverage; however, a noticeable drop of the elbows should not occur during the descent of the dip.

For many lifters, this can cause a subsequent upper back rounding, the bar sliding down the chest (creating a longer distance the bar now has to move), and/or a premature forward weight shift toward the toes. To combat this, actively push forward and slightly up with the elbows as you are performing the dip. You are creating an active "chest puff" as you do.

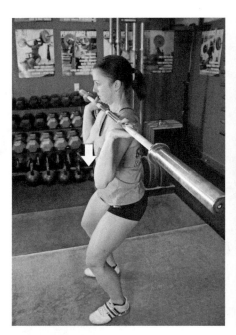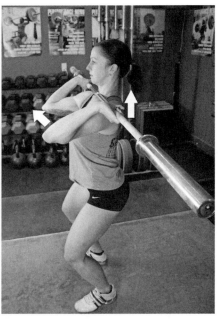

Figure 16.02 The first picture shows a jerk dip in which the lifter has allowed the elbows to drop and the T-spine to flex. The second picture shows a jerk dip in which the lifter has pushed the elbows out and up slightly during the descent, facilitating continued T-spine extension.

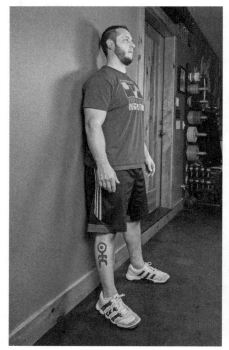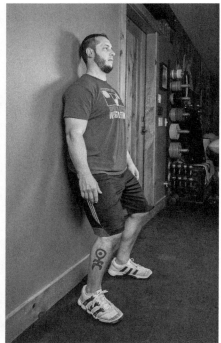

Figure 16.03 A common drill to practice the jerk dip—standing against a wall and keeping the back in contact through the dip movement.

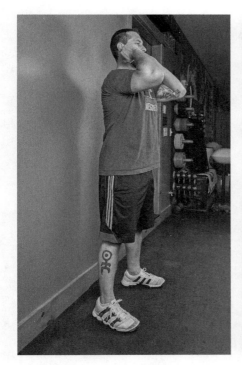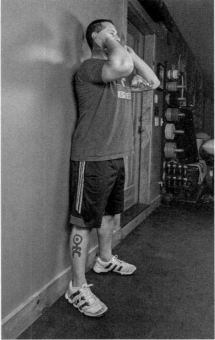

Figure 16.04 Perform a forceful exhalation to stack the ribcage over the pelvis. Scoot gradually closer to the wall while maintaining this torso position and stop when your glutes touch the wall. The shoulders and head will likely not be touching.

By doing so, you resist the forces trying to pull you into thoracic flexion. (Figure 16.02)

A common drill is for the lifter to stand with his or her back against a wall or rack and practice sliding up and down, mimicking the dip and drive. This practice certainly has merit and is helpful for teaching the athlete to maintain a constant torso position during the dip. (Figure 16.03)

However, if the lifter has any ass at all, it's difficult to get the shoulders back to the wall without hyperextending the lower back. To remedy this, one might tuck the tailbone to flatten the lower back and/or walk the feet away from the wall. The problem with those corrections is they don't mimic the real life position of the jerk, with the lifter's weight shifted so posteriorly or a degree of posterior pelvic tilt (flattening against the wall) that wouldn't be cued otherwise. Here is a little tweak that may provide better carry over:

- Stand about a foot away from a wall or enough to be able to stand erect without the glutes touching the wall.
- With the hands on the lower ribs, perform an exhalation *while* continuing to remain tall. This will set the torso position, and the athlete can just breathe comfortably from there.

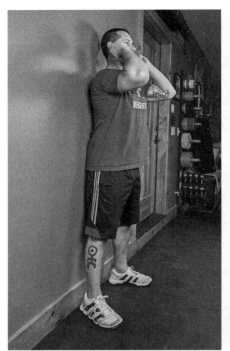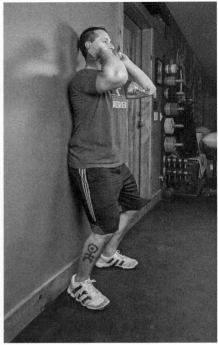

Figure 16.05 Replicate the jerk dip motion by sliding the glutes down the wall while maintaining a constant stacked torso position and proper balance over the feet.

- With the shoulders stacked directly over the hips, scoot the feet back inch by inch until the glutes touch the wall and stop there. (Figure 16.04)
- Maintaining light glute contact, readjust your feet (if needed) so that you feel balanced on both of your heels. For many, the shoulders will not be touching the wall.
- From here, bend at the knees to slide the glutes up and down the wall, mimicking the dip and drive of the jerk. Concentrate on maintaining heel contact and constant position through the trunk. The wall is still the proprioceptive cue, but the athlete is now required to actively participate a little bit more to maintain a position that more closely resembles how weight will be supported during the dip. (Figure 16.05)

Hips, Knees, Ankles & Feet

Theoretically, the hips and pelvis stay directly underneath the shoulders during the dip as the lifter's torso travels straight down and straight up (as in the drill above). What may happen as the lift is actually executed, however, is that the hip and pelvis go back slightly as the lifter fights to maintain an upright torso. Essentially, this is a counterbalance: as the lifter descends, the elbows travel up and forward slightly (to maintain upright

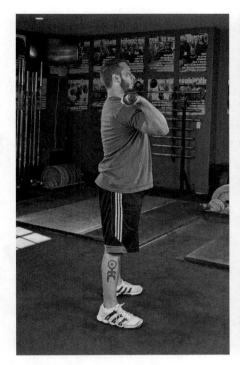
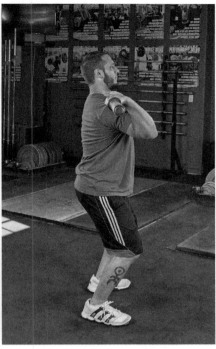

Figure 16.06 Setting the hips, similar to what we did with the front squat, is a technique used by some lifters to maintain balance over the center of the foot. This is a very subtle movement, however, and should not cause the torso to dip forward.

torso) and pelvis goes back slightly. This should keep the lifter's weight centered over the ankle joint. The key word here is *slightly*. These deviations are very subtle and happen naturally. Use the wall drill described above to experiment. A deliberate cueing of the athlete to sit the hips back during the dip may cause a subsequent dropping of the torso and forward trajectory of the bar (what we don't want). One can use the wall or rack and perform the drill with push press of the barbell, dumbbells or kettlebells, then step away from the wall and push press again, trying to recreate the same dip and drive positions. (Figure 16.06)

Knee position in the dip is a commonly debated topic. Allowing the knees to hinge naturally and track in line with the second toe is commonly sufficient. For many lifters, when simply focusing on "knees over feet" as the cue for the dip, a slight toe out will allow them to hinge at the hips, knees and ankles naturally (Figure 16.07).

Mobility of the ankle joint is a less common issue with regard to performing the dip phase of the jerk than it is for a movement like the squat. If one can stand with his or her foot against a wall and touch the wall with the kneecap without the heel coming up, there is generally enough ankle

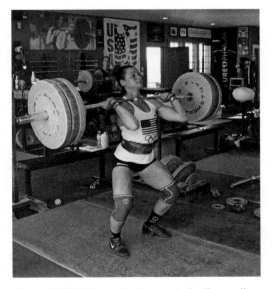

Figure 16.07 Utilizing a slight toe out in the dip can allow the lifter to sit evenly between the hips.

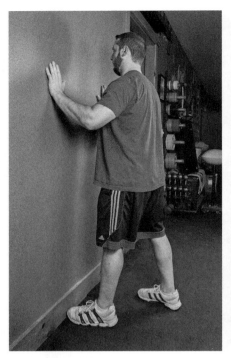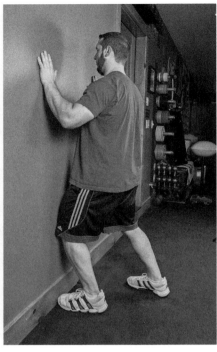

Figure 16.08 A quick screen for ankle dorsiflexion for the jerk. The pictured range of motion is likely sufficient for the dip.

dorsiflexion to perform a jerk considering the added ankle motion that weightlifting shoes will afford (Figure 16.08).

In regard to foot pressure, ideally we want to be balanced from left to right. For most, favoring one side by putting more weight through it can lead to an observable lateral shift during the jerk and subsequent instability when receiving the weight. The "tripod" foot that we established when squatting by maintaining three points of contact (big toe, little toe and heel) applies here as well. However, it is difficult to focus on such minute detail during the jerk because it happens very quickly, and the more time you spend with the bar on your chest thinking about your position, the less of a chance you have to complete a heavy lift. We will simplify this by cueing the lifter to maintain pressure through the middle to inside edges of both heels throughout the dip, just as we did with the front squat.

Some lifters prefer to have the feet pointed forward during the jerk. This is neither right nor wrong as long as certain criteria are followed. It's a little easier for the knees to continue travelling forward, resulting in a seemingly "never ending dip" in which the athlete cannot find the tension to change directions in order to drive up. This can result in the heels being pulled off of the floor prematurely, upper back rounding, and forward trajectory of the bar. (Figure 16.09)

A common remedy for this is the cue to push the knees over the outside edge of the foot slightly, during the dip phase. Contrary to our squat

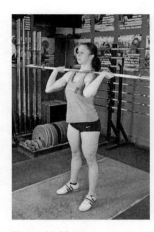 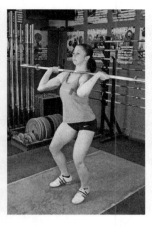 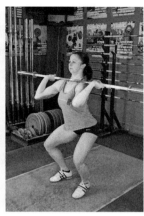

Figure 16.09 It is common to see some lifters sink deeper and deeper into the dip, commonly resulting their weight shifting forward prematurely.

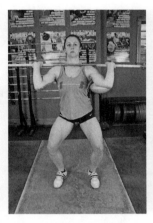 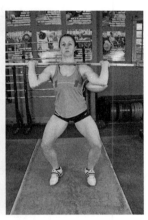

Figure 16.10 If utilizing a slight knee-out position, be sure to maintain pressure through the entire foot (first picture) instead of allowing the feet to roll to the outside edges (second picture).

discussion regarding such a technique, there is merit to this as a way to maintain tension in the legs in order to keep the dip short and the change of direction abrupt. With this cue to push the knees toward the fourth or fifth toe, foot pressure is an important consideration. If the lifter pushes the knees outward but also allows the inside edge of the foot to lift (rolling to the outside of edge of the foot) then tension created at the hips is less useful because it cannot be transmitted through the ground. The lifter must maintain foot pressure with the big toe and middle to inside edge of the heel *while* they are pushing the knees outward *slightly*. This will also limit any exaggeration of a knees-out position that will have limited benefit to creating upward force of the barbell. (Figure 16.10)

Practicing loaded paused dips are a great way to experiment with and reinforce the concepts and positions discussed above. There are several things for the lifter to dial in:

- Maintaining the proper elbow and torso position during the dip.
- Maintaining balanced pressure between both feet.
- Determining the preferred foot and knee angles.
- Determining the preferred depth for the dip.

All of these things can be worked on by incorporating some focused work in which the lifter dips and pauses just before changing direction to reinforce the preferred positions.

Overloading such a drill is not necessarily the focus. The focus is on controlled posture and position, so intensities up to the 70-85% range with pauses in the 3-second range will provide the desired benefit. Work with an empty bar and lower intensities can be included in warm-ups.

■ CHAPTER 17

Jerk Drive

The importance of the drive phase of the jerk cannot be overstated. This is where the lifter imparts the energy, force and trajectory of the bar in order to create height and receive it successfully.

From a movement standpoint, hip and knee extension are the most important elements here, as they were with the finish position of the snatch and clean pull. Driving up to full hip and knee extension will impart maximal force on the bar. An athlete who shorts the extension because of motor control and/or mobility restrictions will not impart the same upward drive to the bar. Return to Chapter 9 for reminders on hip extension testing and options for corrections.

The finished, extended position of the jerk drive is different than that of the snatch or clean pull. This is not because of the hips themselves, as bilateral hip extension is bilateral hip extension. It is due the position of the upper extremities and barbell:

- As discussed previously, with the arms in the front rack position, the lat musculature is put on stretch.
- The arms being in a partially elevated position raises the lifter's center of mass and further increases the demands of the core.
- The weight in the front rack versus below the waist (during the pull) puts the lumbar spine in a position to be a fulcrum (i.e. an area of motion, where we don't necessarily want it).

All of these points speak to the fact that the musculature of the trunk is further challenged with regard to its job in maintaining ribcage and pelvic alignment. Maintaining this relative trunk stability is how we will transfer the energy from the ground, through the core, and into the bar. If we have leaks in the form of trunk movement (most commonly in the form of hyperextension of the lumbar spine), then maximal force will not be imparted to the bar. The lifter must learn how to forcefully extend at the hips, dissociating this from spinal movement as much as possible, all while the upper extremities are tied up.

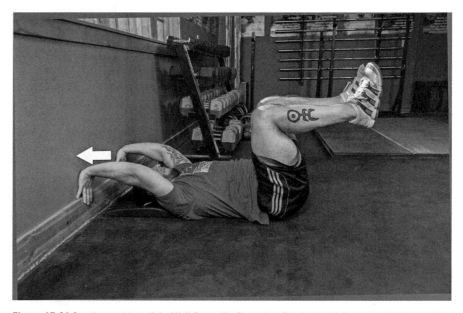

Figure 17.01 Starting position of the Wall Press Hip Extension. Exhale forcefully and push through the wall for leverage, similar to pushing up on the barbell.

Stabilization: Wall Press Hip Extension

This is a progressive variation of the Supine Overhead Wall Press in Chapter 2, and can be helpful in teaching a lifter how to control the core while extending the hips with the arms in a similar position as the front rack.

Starting Position
- Lie on the back with head support and the hands flat against the wall with the arms overhead.
- Keep the hips and knees flexed past 90 degrees, mimicking a squat position. (Figure 17.01)

Execution
- Inhale through the nose to initiate the movement.
- Exhale forcefully through the mouth to pull the lower ribs down.
- As you exhale, push into the wall with the arms for leverage and lift the tailbone straight up off of the floor slightly. Continue to exhale, even when you think you have run out of air. This may give you the "ab shake."
- Inhale through the nose again while maintaining the wall press and tailbone lift.
- Hip Extension (Figure 17.02)
  - ❯ During the next exhalation, tap one heel to the ground while maintaining the wall press and slight tailbone lift.

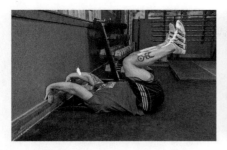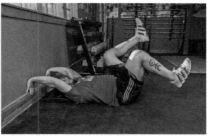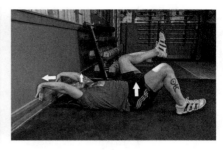

Figure 17.02 Wall Press with Heel Tap to teach hip extension dissociation. Maintain the tailbone lift as you exhale forcefully and lower the heel.

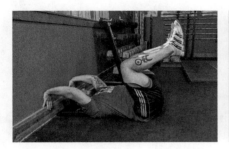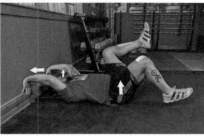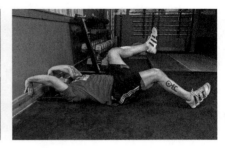

Figure 17.03 Increase hip extension demand and mobility in the Wall Press Hip Extension by sliding the heel out while maintaining all other positions.

Exhale the entire time you are lowering down, even if you run out of air.

- The tendency will be to allow the tailbone to drop as you lower the heel. Don't allow that. This will teach you how to dissociate movement at the hip in relation to the spine.
- Maintain the position of the opposite hip as you lower the heel.
- Inhale and bring the leg back to the starting position.
- If you do not feel your abdominals fighting to hold position, review the cues above, because they should be working.
- Perform 1-2 sets of 3-5 alternating reps each side or until you feel you understand the positions.

> This drill can then be progressed by sliding the heel as far out into hip extension as the lifter can while maintaining position. Continue to exhale forcefully and push into the wall for leverage, keeping the opposite hip flexed past 90 degrees. (Figure 17.03)

> Kicking the leg all of the way out and hovering inches above the ground will provide the hip extension mobility of the previous variation, and add a significant anti-hyperextension stability component. By extending the legs farther, more demand is placed on the trunk musculature

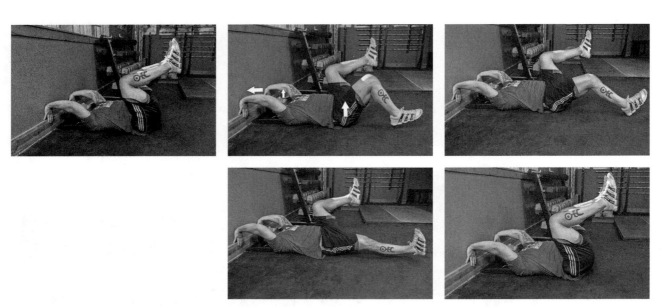

Figure 17.04 Increase the core stability demand in the Wall Press Hip Extension by keeping the foot off of the ground during the hip extension phase.

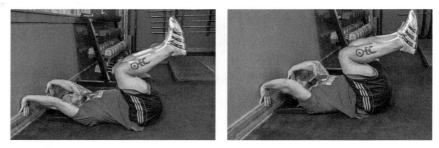

Figure 17.05 Decrease or increase the stability challenge of the Wall Press Hip Extension by moving closer to or farther from the wall, respectively.

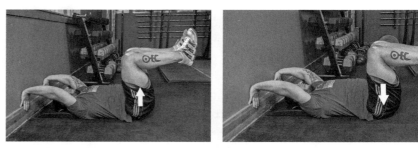

Figure 17.06 Lower the pelvis down, increasing lumbar lordosis, but keep the lower ribs flush with the abdomen.

to maintain trunk position (Figure 17.04). Continue the exhalation all the way through the extension phase. We can then manipulate the overhead position and pelvic tilt to increase carryover to the standing position.

- Manipulating Overhead Position (Figure 17.05)
  - › One can move closer to the wall to make the drill a little easier and decrease the lengthening of muscles such as the lat. This is an option for significantly restricted individuals or those who need to decrease the core demand.
  - › One can also move farther away from the wall to increase the lever the abs have to stabilize and further lengthening the tissues that oppose the front rack. This is a great option for lifters who demonstrated full shoulder range of motion, but could benefit from increased core control. Feel free to experiment here as the athlete.
- Manipulating Pelvic Tilt (Figure 17.06)
  - › We lift the tailbone in the initial variation in order to maximize abdominal recruitment by bringing the top and bottom of our "can of stability" into a parallel relationship and minimizing any unwanted compensation through the low back. However, we can more closely mimic the spinal extension we need for an actual front rack by slowly lowering the tailbone back down to the ground.
    - During the exhalation, slowly roll the tailbone back down flat to the ground.
    - Keep pressure into the wall for leverage, and utilize a forceful exhalation to pull the lower ribs flush with the abdomen. This will ensure that the spinal extension is distributed evenly through the moving segments, as opposed to allowing the lower ribs to flare out and hinge at the T/L junction.
    - Keep the opposite hip flexed slightly past 90 degrees.
    - During the inhalation, you can raise the tailbone back up, and repeat for 3-4 more reps.

Movement Cluster Options

- Alternate with 20-second bouts of SMR to the TFL/hip flexor area.
- Alternate with Option 1 and/or Tall Kneeling Holds.

Integration: Dip & Drive

A very logical way to learn to extend the hips fully in the drive is to simply practice with a barbell. With an empty barbell, and taking into account

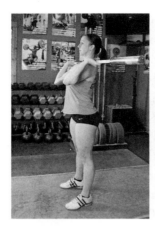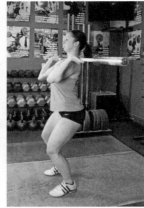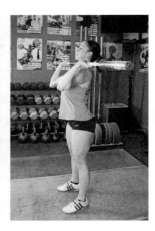

Figure 17.07 First practice the dip and drive with flat heels to maximize focus on hip extension.

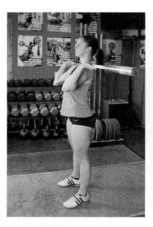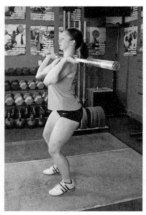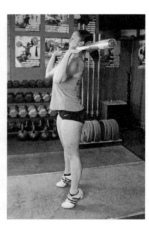

Figure 17.08 Practice the drive with a triple extension movement. Finish through the hips first, then drive through the ankles.

what has been discussed with the dip, perform repetitions in which you dip and drive with a focus on fully extending the hips and knees at the top—*open the hips, squeeze the glutes*, however you want to word it. Focus on driving through the middle of the foot as you come to a position of full hip and knee extension. You can first do this while keeping the feet flat for 2-4 sets of 3-5 reps (Figure 17.07).

Next, perform the same drill but allow for a triple extension movement. Many coaches do not cue for the lifter to actively push through the ankle of the jerk. To keep this universal, think of it as simply allowing the momentum of maximal hip and knee extension to take you where it takes you in terms of ankle plantarflexion (Figure 17.08).

Movement Cluster Options

- Alternate with 20-second bouts of SMR to the TFL/hip flexor area.
- Alternate with Option 1 and Wall Press Hip Extension.
- Alternate with Option 2 and/or Tall kneeing Holds.

Integration: Push Press

We may be jumping ahead of ourselves here, with much of the overhead corrective work coming later, but the push press is a great tool to learn to transfer upward force from the legs and follow through with the arms. Obviously this exercise can be loaded relatively heavily for training purposes, but we aren't even concerned with that here, and will leave it up to the coach's discretion to program for true strength, hypertrophy, etc. For us, working the push press with the empty barbell or lighter percentages is a helpful reinforcement for the lifter to drill full extension with all of the dip and drive concepts that we have talked about.

Be sure that you are driving fully with the legs before imparting significant force with the arms. The arms transfer the push from the legs into the bar to finish the movement.

The force of the hip extension may naturally send the athlete onto the balls of his or her feet. Some coaches will cue this "jump" deliberately. Some feel that less heel elevation is desired for efficiency. Regardless, the lifter needs to open the hips and extend the knees fully to his or her capacity.

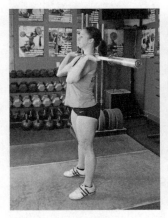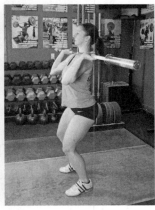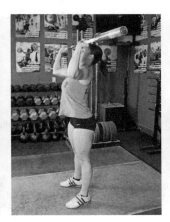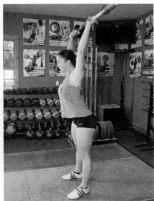

Figure 17.09 Flat-footed push press to isolate maximal hip extension.

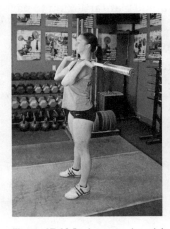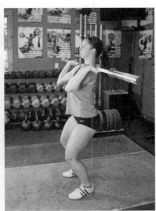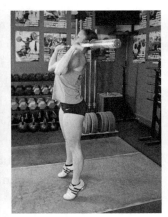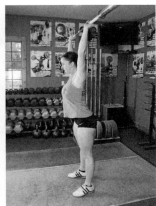

Figure 17.10 Push press using triple extension to impart maximal height on the bar.

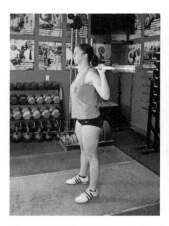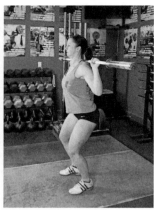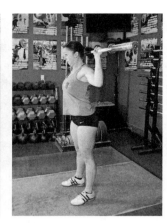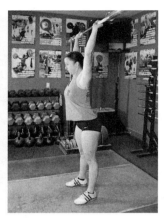

Figure 17.11 Behind the neck flat-footed push press to isolate maximal hip extension.

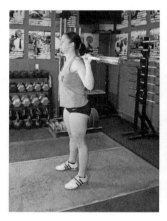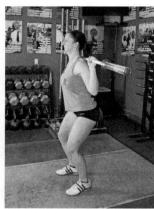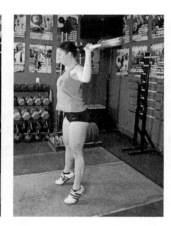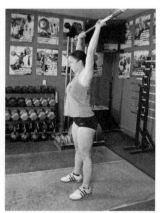

Figure 17.12 Behind the neck push press using triple extension to impart maximal height on the bar

This is why it can be beneficial to practice both flat-footed push presses and push presses in which the athlete rises onto the balls of the feet. The flat-footed push press will ensure that the lifter focuses on driving through the middle of the foot and utilizing the hip and knee drive maximally. Following through with a heel lift can teach the lifter how to properly sequence the transfer of forces: hip and knee extension to ankle plantarflexion to bar leaving the body to arms pushing on the bar. Keep in mind this sequence is happening in fractions of a second. Just think *keep driving through the ground* until the bar is locked out overhead. (Figures 17.09 & 17.10)

Lastly, for any lifter who cannot tolerate the front rack position for any reason, behind the neck push presses using the same principles above is a nice variation. Even for those lifters who can tolerate the front rack position just fine, a behind the neck variation makes it easier to simply focus on leg drive and equal foot pressure since the bar is just going straight up off of the back and not around the face. (Figures 17.11 & 17.12)

Movement Cluster Options

- Alternate with Wall Press Hip Extension.

CHAPTER 18

Jerk Split

The split receiving position is the most common variation of the jerk, as it provides a balance of being able to change levels (high to low) and push the body underneath the bar and an anterior-posterior base of stability compared to the push jerk or squat jerk, which provide medial-lateral stability with the bilateral stance. If we miss a jerk, it's typically forward or backward (as opposed to tipping over to one side), which is why the split jerk tends to feel more stable for most.

As mentioned in Chapter 3, this variation requires the lifter to "split" the hips, in which one hip is stabilized in flexion and the other in extension, all while maintaining reflexive core stability and supporting a barbell overhead. The teaching drills to follow reflect these components and will teach the lifter how to integrate them into the lift.

In regard to the hips, extension is a consideration. Most lifters will have sufficient hip flexion mobility to split jerk. We will first build the jerk overhead position in isolation, as the narrower jerk grip (compared to the snatch) poses more challenges for obtaining it. We will then work to integrate that established overhead position over the top of split hips.

Overhead

Mobilization: Shoulder Flexion Hang

In the two variations below, we use gravity and our own bodyweight to aid in attaining a full overhead position. The focus is isolated range of motion of the shoulder without compensatory movement through the ribcage or low back. If you had limited shoulder flexion during the overhead testing, this can be an effective drill.

Double-Arm Variation This is the basic variation of the Shoulder Flexion Hang mobilization.

Starting Position

- Grab a pull-up bar or barbell in a rack that is a little shorter than arms' reach overhead.
- Your grip can be palms away, palms towards or neutral depending on what you are grabbing. Palms toward you puts the most stretch on the lat, but will be more difficult for some to achieve full shoulder range.
- Put your feet in front of your shoulders either on the floor or on a step, and bend your knees slightly.

Execution

- Push through the floor or step and posteriorly tilt the pelvis slightly. Think *tuck your tailbone under or pull your belt buckle up.*
  > Having the feet on a step allows the athlete to have control of how much bodyweight is being supported through the shoulders.
  > Putting the feet in front aids in maintaining a stacked position between ribcage and pelvis. The relative posterior pelvic tilt (can just be to neutral) also helps with this, and may add extra mobilization to the lat based on its attachment to the thoracolumbar fascia.
- Inhale through the nose, pushing air into your trunk.
- Exhale through the mouth, depressing the entire ribcage, but keeping the arms and shoulder blades reaching long.
- Inhale and fill the chest wall, and then exhale and lower the entire ribcage, reaching long through shoulder complex. (Figure 18.01)
- Perform 2-4 sets of 5 breaths, or as needed.

Notes

- No feelings of impingement on the tops of the shoulders allowed. Reposition or choose another drill if this is what you are feeling. Stay within a comfortable range.
- This is not meant to be a distraction (separation) of the shoulder joint. The entire scapular complex is reaching long, as opposed to trying to create space between the two bones of the shoulder joint. If it's uncomfortable to allow the arms to hang long, add a slight scapular retraction.
- The stretch should be felt along the length of the lateral chest walls as you exhale and depress the ribcage.
- Revisit the Back to Wall or Supine Shoulder Flexion test to gauge change.

Movement Cluster Options

- Alternate with 20-second bouts of SMR to the lats.
- Alternate with 3-5 reps of the Supine Pullover.

Single Arm Variation Some may find the single arm variation easier to perform than the double, especially if they have an asymmetry in shoulder elevation.

Starting Position

- Grab a pull-up bar or barbell in a rack that is a little shorter than arms' reach overhead.
- Your grip can be palm away, palm towards, or neutral, depending on what you are grabbing.
- Bend the knees slightly.
- You can place your opposite hand on your lower ribs to monitor position if needed.

Execution

- Slightly posteriorly tilt the pelvis to a neutral position.
- Inhale through the nose, pushing air into your trunk.
- Exhale through the mouth, depressing the entire ribcage, but keeping the arm and shoulder blade reaching long.
- Inhale and push air down into the chest wall, and then exhale and lower the entire ribcage, reaching long through shoulder complex. (Figure 18.02)
- Perform 1-2 sets of 5 breaths, or as needed.

Movement Cluster Options

- Alternate with 20-second bouts of SMR to the lats.
- Alternate with 3-5 reps of the supine pullover.

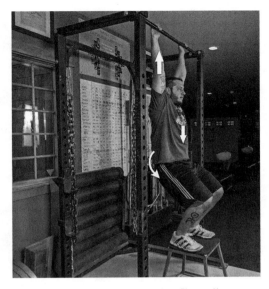

Figure 18.01 The double arm Shoulder Flexion Hang mobilization

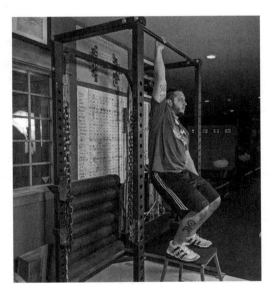

Figure 18.02 The single arm Shoulder Flexion Hang mobilization

Mobilization: Jerk Grip Wall Slides with or without Roller

This is a nice complement to the drill above with a more active component. The setup is very similar to the Standing Front to Wall Scaption with Lift-off in Chapter 11, as we use a roller on the wall for leverage in attaining full overhead mobility.

Starting Position

- Standing facing a wall with the feet roughly 8 inches away and the knees slightly bent.

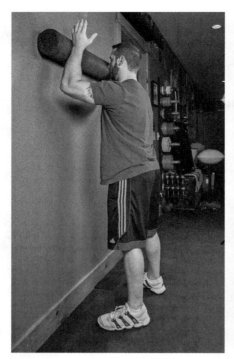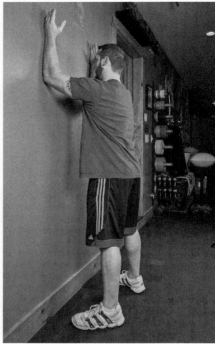

Figure 18.03 Starting position for Jerk Grip Wall Slides

- Press in the forearms against the wall or a roller with the palms facing each other.
- Slightly tuck the tailbone underneath so that the low back is still slightly lordotic, but not excessively so (have the athlete perform a hard anterior pelvic tilt, then a "poop dog" posterior pelvic tilt, and put him or her somewhere in the middle).
- Exhale fully to set the rib position. (Figure 18.03)

Execution

- Protract the shoulder blades and press the forearms into the roller or wall.
- Push the arms up the wall or roller without altering your pelvis or low back position.
- At the point where you feel your limitation in range of motion, pause and take 2-3 full breath cycles and then try to move farther.
- If using a roller, shift your body weight forward and lean toward the wall. Do this without altering your trunk position.
  › The roller plus leaning in with your bodyweight makes a fulcrum right at the shoulder joint, allowing you to leverage more range of motion.
- Pause at the top and take 1-2 full breaths in which you work to expand your side chest walls.

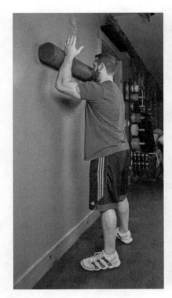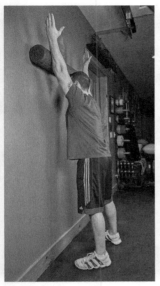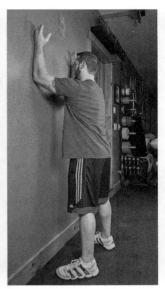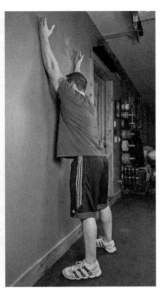

Figure 18.04 Jerk Grip Wall Slide mobilization with and without a foam roller

> The lengthening should be felt underneath the shoulder in the armpit and lat area. Again, if you feel a pinch in the top or back of your shoulder, reposition or choose a different drill

- This can also be performed with one arm at a time.
- Perform 2-4 sets of 5 repetitions, or as needed. (Figure 18.04)

Single Arm Variation The wall allows you to manipulate elbow width and push into the wall for increased activation of scapular musculature.

Starting Position

- Stand at a 45-degree angle from a wall or rack with the forearm flush against the wall.

Execution

- Slide the forearm up as you did in the two-arm wall slide until you hit resistance.
- Once you have achieved maximum range, lean into the wall for leverage as you attempt to shrug and increase range. (Figure 18.05)

Movement Cluster Options

- Alternate with 20-second bouts of SMR to the lats for 2-4 rounds.
- Alternate with Overhead Hang for 2-4 rounds.

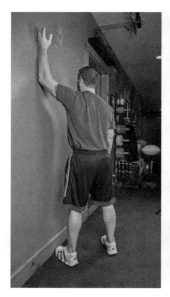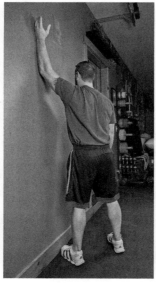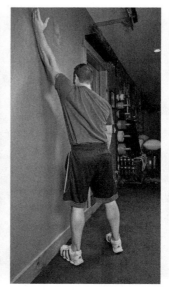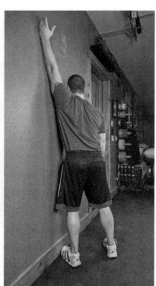

Figure 18.05 Single arm variation of the Jerk Grip Wall Slide

- Alternate with Supine Pullover for 2-4 rounds.

The above wall drills are simple tools that can cue an athlete on how to control his or her trunk when going overhead. They then need to be followed up with a loading strategy to challenge that position.

Movement Discussion: Elbow Lockout Problems Many lifters struggle with locking their elbows out in the jerk. It's common and intuitive to blame the elbow joints themselves for these issues. However, what is often the case in these scenarios is that the lifters can lock out their elbows in the snatch just fine, but not in the jerk. In this case, it's not an elbow joint problem as evidenced by the ability to lock out a snatch.

What is different is that the narrower grip in the jerk requires more mobility at the shoulder. The lifter is unable to achieve this more challenging overhead position due to either mobility or stability limitations, and consequently the elbows bend as a compensatory means to get the weight overhead. It gives the system a little slack. What was seemingly an elbow mobility problem will likely be addressed at the shoulder and trunk.

Another example is a lifter who can lock out light jerks perfectly fine, but has difficulty locking out heavier weights. Again, we are not dealing with an elbow mobility problem. If you have the mobility for lighter weights, then you have it for heavier weights. What changes are the requirements of strength and stability. If this is lacking, then it often manifests as the athlete utilizing a different movement strategy to control the weight. This is why it's beneficial to pay close attention to the positional cues when practicing any correction in this book or any lift in training, as subtle differences in the performance of lift variations can clue you in to what is going on.

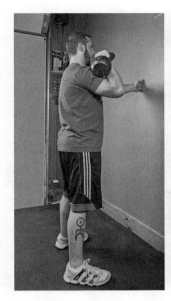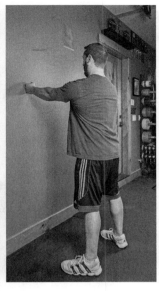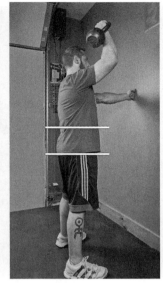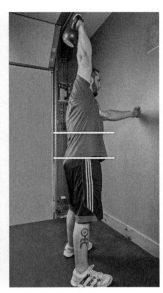

Figure 18.06 The Ribcage Locked Standing Press is used to stabilize newly acquired mobility.

Stabilization: Ribcage Locked Standing Press

After making short-term improvement in overhead mobility and position-ing with the previous drills, we begin to lock it in by introducing load. This drill will teach the lifter how to press a load with the shoulders while stabilizing the trunk.

Starting Position

- Stand at arms' length from a wall with one fist pushing into it.
- Hold a light weight at the shoulder in the other hand.

Execution

- Exhale forcefully to pull the front ribs down while simultane-ously creating a tall spine (string pulling up from the top of the head). At this time, push into the wall with the fist. The arm is reaching into the wall in a way that pushes the ribcage away and stacks it over the hips.
- Inhale through the nose into that position to reinforce it.
- With the pressing elbow at about 45 degrees from the body, press straight up while maintaining the trunk position and leverage with the opposite arm. (Figure 18.06)
- Perform 2-4 sets of 5 on each side.

Notes

- The weight can be a change plate, dumbbell or kettlebell. If using a kettlebell, the "bottoms-up" position works well for a lifter who possesses full overhead shoulder mobility but is seeking a stability challenge. Possessing full overhead mobility certainly does not preclude the athlete from going bottom's-up, but the standard position can actually assist in gaining mobility. The orientation of the weight behind the lifter's arm aids in pulling the load up and back behind the ears (over the upper back).

- In general, the weight should be kept light enough to maintain the positions outlined above, but heavy enough to challenge those positions.
- A common occurrence, especially for those still developing comfort with overhead positions, is an exaggerated jutting forward of the head as the weight is pressed up, in an effort to create a "pseudo" overhead position. A simple cue of keeping the head stacked over the shoulder should suffice here in order to maintain a stacked torso position.
- The elbow angle can be altered to stabilize different positions—narrow to 45 degrees to wider. Experiment here.
- A goal of this drill can be to lose the need for the leverage of the opposite arm into the wall. If the lifter's overhead and trunk positioning is solid, perform a few reps with the ribcage-locked position, then slowly take the opposite fist away from the wall, and finish the set there with the aim to maintain the same trunk and overhead positions.
- If a lifter possesses an asymmetry in mobility, stability or strength from left to right, this drill is a unilateral loading strategy that may address those things.
- This can also be performed in the split position.

Movement Cluster Options
- Alternate with 20-second bouts of SMR to the lats for 2-4 rounds.
- Alternate with Shoulder Flexion Hang for 2-4 rounds.
- Alternate with Supine Pullover.
- Alternate with either of the above and/or a Wall Slide variation.

Integration: Landmine Press

Some, especially those with limited shoulder flexion, may find it very difficult to achieve full shoulder and elbow lock out overhead. In this case, a landmine press is a great option, as the range of motion requirement is less, but will still teach the lifter to dissociate shoulder and trunk motion, and is a nice intermediate shoulder-elevated position.

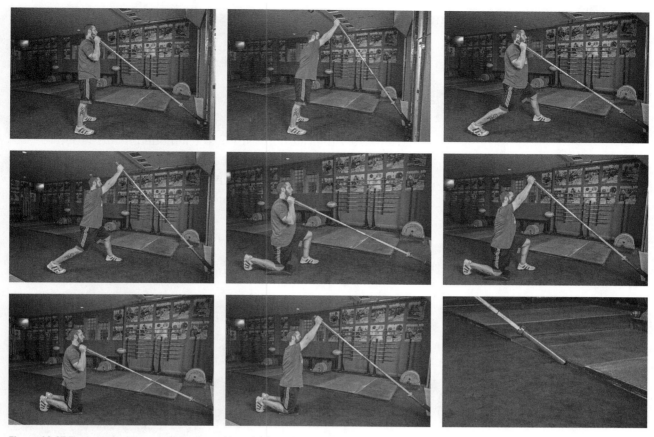

Figure 18.07 The landmine press can be performed in multiple positions such as standing, split position, half kneeling and tall kneeling. If you don't have a landmine base, a barbell can be propped in a corner or against the edge of a platform or base of a wall.

Starting Position

- Hold the end of a barbell in a landmine setup with one arm at the shoulder (one end of the bar fixed in a landmine stand or wedged at the base of a wall or platform)
- The exercise can be performed standing, in a split position, in half kneeling or tall kneeling.

Execution

- Exhale forcefully to pull the front ribs down while simultaneously creating a tall spine (string pulling up from the top of the head).
- Inhale through the nose into that position to reinforce it.
- Press the end of the barbell until the elbow is fully extended without altering the trunk position. (Figure 18.07)
- Perform 2-4 sets of 5 on each side.

Integration: Barbell Strict Press

At this point the athlete should have adequate mobility and motor control and be sufficiently warmed up and prepped for a barbell strict press.

Starting Position

- Before unracking the bar, perform a short, forceful exhalation to set the ribcage position and a moderate inhalation to reinforce that position. You should be able to breathe comfortably over top of this established base.
- Assume your previously established rack position.
- The elbows should be slightly in front of the bar with the whole hand around the bar.
- The knees should be *actively* locked out. Use your muscles.

Execution

- Just as you did in the Ribcage Locked and Landmine presses, press straight up, moving your head back just enough to clear

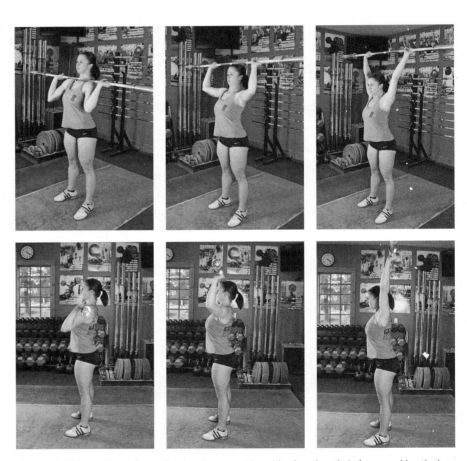

Figure 18.08 Barbell Strict Press. Set the ribcage position with a breath cycle before unracking the bar. The elbows and shoulders should remain stacked under the hands as much as possible, and the torso should stay stacked as it was set in the starting position.

a path for the bar. As soon as the bar is clear of the head, position yourself back under the bar.

- The torso will certainly move back and forward a bit to allow the bar to clear the face, but we are looking to re-establish that stacked torso position upon lockout.
- As with the push press, coaches may program this exercise with heavier weights for strength or hypertrophy. For our purposes, we are using it as preparation for the jerk, so concentrate on position with your empty bar and lighter warm-up set weights before a split jerk session. (Figure 18.08)

Movement Cluster Options

- Alternate with 20-second bouts of SMR to the lats for 2-4 rounds.
- Alternate with Shoulder Flexion Hang for 2-4 rounds.
- Alternate with Supine Pullover for 2-4 rounds.
- Alternate with either option 1 or 2 and/or a wall slide variation.
- Alternate with the Ribcage Locked Press or Landmine Press.

Shoulder & Hip Incorporation

Now we focus on the split portion of the jerk in regard to hip mobility and stability, while integrating an overhead position.

Mobilization: Supine Split Lower

This is exactly the same as our Supine Hip Hinging from Chapter 8, but now we integrate overhead movement, which will further challenge the core musculature in an athlete new to these positions.

Starting Position

- Lie on your back with one leg propped to 90 degrees against a doorway or rack. You may bend the knee of the leg that is on the wall to mimic the position of the front leg of the jerk.
- The opposite hip is flexed with the knee bent to 90 degrees and the foot in the air. Have some head support if at all possible.
- Flex the toes toward you (dorsiflexion) with the feet and kneecaps facing relatively straight.
- Hold the arms outstretched toward the ceiling.

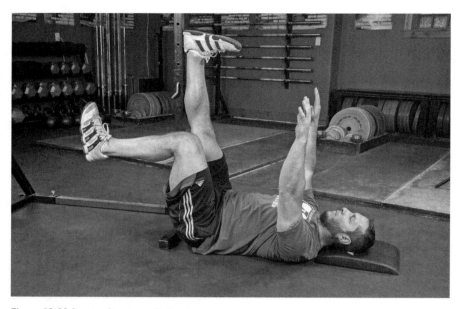

Figure 18.09 Starting Position of Supine Split Lower. The top knee may be bent to mimic the front foot of the jerk and to allow for individual mobility capacities.

- The lower back should be relatively flat to the ground in this position (very slight lordosis). Wherever it starts, it should stay through the movement. (Figure 18.09)

Execution

- Initiate the drill with an inhalation through the nose, pushing the air down into the lower back.
- Exhale through the mouth slowly and forcefully as you slowly lower one heel to the floor without allowing the lower back to arch up off the ground.
- Slide the heel out, which will extend the bottom hip, while maintaining all other positions.
- At the same time, perform shoulder flexion with one or both arms.
- Maintain stability through the trunk as you reach long through the heel and arms. A long, forceful exhalation can help to re-establish trunk position if needed. (Figure 18.10)
- Perform 1-2 sets of 5 on each side.
- To add a bit of internal load to the activity, press the up leg into the door frame or rack as you inhale and bring the opposite leg and arm(s) back to the start position, hold for 3-5 seconds, relax and slide the heel again. Repeat that sequence for the 1-2 sets of 5 reps on each side.
- Remember, you can manipulate the intensity of the mobilization by bending (reduces the intensity) and straightening

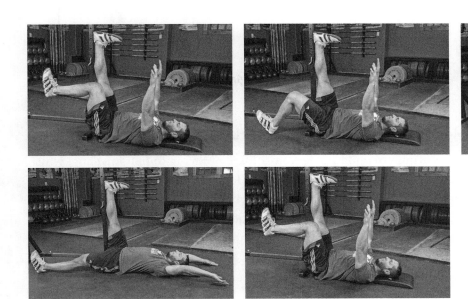

Figure 18.10 Supine Split Lower drill

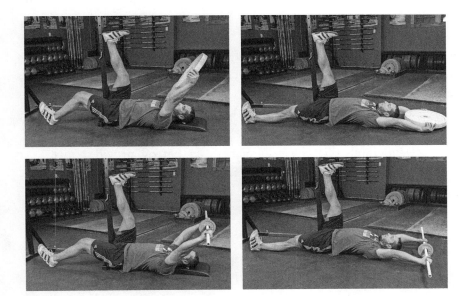

Figure 18.11 Pullover variation of the Supine Split Lower with a plate or loaded PVC pipe to add more active control to the mobilization.

(increases intensity) the knee; also by dorsiflexing (increases intensity) and plantarflexion (reduces intensity) of the ankle.

Plate Pullover Variation The athlete can also perform a plate or dowel pullover while performing the hip extension in the Supine Split Lower. Exhale, reach the plate to the ceiling and perform the heel slide. As you slide the heel, allow the weight to take your arms into shoulder flexion, staying in a comfortable range. (Figure 18.11)

Movement Cluster Option

- Alternate with 20-second bouts of SMR to the hip flexors or lats, depending on whether you are focusing on overhead or hip mobility.

Mobilization: Ribcage Locked Half Kneeling Hip Extension

We continue to build the jerk position by moving to half kneeling, which more closely resembles the split with less ground contact than supine, so the athlete requires more active stabilization. However, it obviously affords more external support than standing, so it makes a great intermediate position to learn balance and stability in the split.

We can also manipulate the half kneeling position by elevating the front foot, back foot or back knee depending on the athlete and goal.

Front Foot Elevated The front foot elevated variation of half kneeling does a great job at "locking in" the pelvis and lumbar spine, as the front foot will be in a position of deeper hip flexion. It makes for a nice preparatory tool for an athlete who may be a bit sensitive to lumbar hyperextension when going overhead, or to simply teach a stable torso. We will begin with simply holding this position, which will mobilize the hips at the same time that we are finding balance and stability in the split position.

Starting & Hold Position

- Deliberately tuck the tailbone here, as that will provide a nice mobilization of the down hip's flexor musculature without having to lunge forward and hang on the front of the hip joint unnecessarily (Figure 18.12).

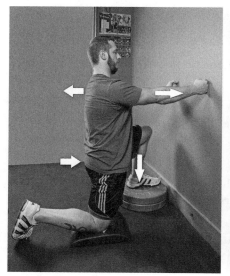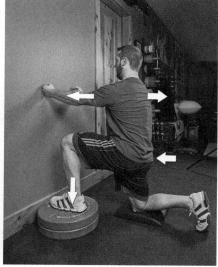

Figure 18.12 Front Foot Elevated Split Hold to mobilize the hips for the split jerk

- Breathe in this position for 4-5 full breaths. You can press on the front knee with the hands to provide added abdominal stabilization.
- You can also press both fists into a wall as you exhale forcefully. This will move the ribcage backwards and stack the hips underneath.
- Of course, this can be done without the front foot elevated.

Back Leg Lift Execution

- With the same position above, attempt to lift the back foot off of the ground (Figure 18.13). This will enhance the hip extension range of motion, while simultaneously decreasing ground contact.
- For those with decreased hip extension via the Thomas test, this will be a difficult feat to accomplish. Again, do not sacrifice pelvic or low back position in order to lift the leg.
  > This active variation is preferred for most over the more common passive version, in which the athlete props the back leg up to completely vertical. This is because the active version is self-limiting, meaning athletes will inherently only be able to move through a range that they can control. With the passive version, athletes often jam themselves into positions that they cannot sustain, which becomes a *hold your breath and watch the clock* torture-fest, leading to minimal change. The change we are looking for is an increased tolerance to full hip extension on the

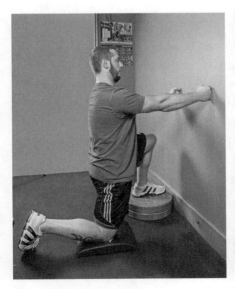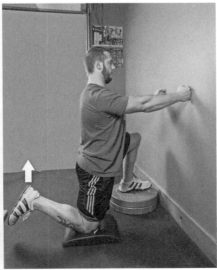

Figure 18.13 Lifting the back leg increases the mobilization, but don't force it if it's not there. If you do not have a wall, push your hands into your front knee.

down leg of the jerk, which will then be integrated into subsequent loading strategies.

> Utilize high-tension, forceful breaths here to increase core engagement.

Movement Cluster Options

- Alternate with 20-second bouts of SMR to the hip flexors or lats, depending on whether you are focusing on overhead or hip mobility.
- Alternate with Option 1 and/or Supine Split Lowers.

Stabilization: Arm Lifts & Presses

Now we begin to incorporate overhead movement into this position.

Starting Position

- Assume the same position used for the Half Kneeling Hip Extension drill above with the arms pressing into the wall.

Execution

- As we have in previous drills, simply lifting one or both arms (elbows straight) overhead without changing the position of the ribcage will be challenging for many athletes.
- We can also mimic the front rack by placing one or both hands behind the shoulders and elevating the elbows to attain upper T-spine extension.
  > Be sure to exhale through the mouth as you lift the elbows to ensure that the T/L junction is stabilized. Another cue to maximize the upright position of the torso is to "make the back of the neck long" by tucking the chin.
- And again, the front foot does not need to be elevated, it just increases the hip mobility demand and acts as a potential unilateral loading strategy for the hips.
- Perform 2-3 sets of 5-6 reps on each side. (Figure 18.14)
- Incorporating a PVC or empty barbell press here is a great progression. Since our lower body is locked into a solid split position, we can really isolate full range of motion at the shoulder joints. (Figures 18.15 & 18.16)
  > Try to recreate the overhead positions that were established with our previous wall drills.
  > Perform 1-3 sets of 4-5 reps.

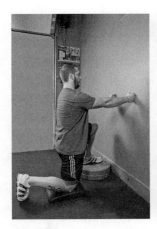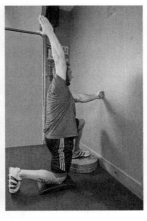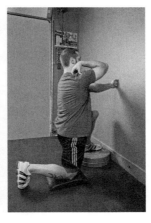

Figure 18.14 Lifting the arms like we did previously to attain overhead motion. This can also be done without the ribcage lock. Mimic the front rack position with a tall spine.

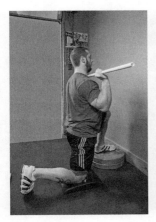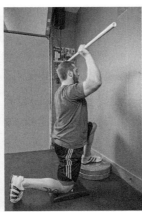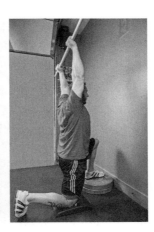

Figure 18.15 Adding presses from the front rack to the half kneeling position.

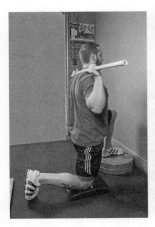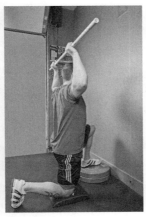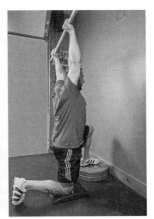

Figure 18.16 Adding presses from behind the neck to the half kneeling position.

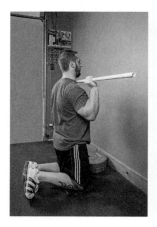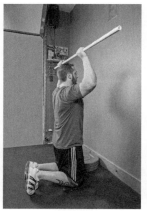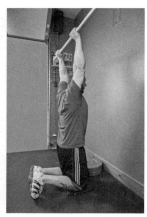

Figure 18.17 Tall kneeling as an alternative for those who use the power or squat jerk.

Single Arm Variation A Front Foot Elevated Ribcage Locked Press is an impressive isolator of the shoulder. If an athlete has side-to-side asymmetry in range of motion, this can be a great way to balance things out. If it is too difficult to achieve full elbow and shoulder lockout, regress to a Landmine Press.

Tall Kneeling Variation For those who push jerk or squat jerk, the *tall kneeling* position can be a nice alternative here. With the hip flexor musculature lengthened at both the hip and knee joints, it is challenging to sustain an overhead position. (Figure 18.17)

Be sure to maintain a slight tailbone tuck, as that will ensure pelvic neutrality. Not everyone will be able to achieve full hip extension in this position and that is OK. Work with what you have. Remember, there is no point in compensating during a corrective exercise. There are no ribbons for the athlete with the best tall kneeling position. It's simply a means to improve what really matters.

Rack Press Variation Using a rack or a doorframe can provide a nice cue here for pressing in either half kneeling or tall kneeling (Figure 18.18). Slide the dowel up the rack with the bar slightly in front of the body. The rack provides the path, while the athlete works to maintain a constant relationship between the pelvis and ribcage as he or she presses up.

Maximum range will be attained with the dowel slightly in front of the center of mass. From here, pull the dowel over your head where the barbell would be for a jerk. This movement will come from the musculature of the shoulder blades and upper back. The position of the lower back and pelvis should remain constant. Think about tipping your shoulder blades backward to attain this.

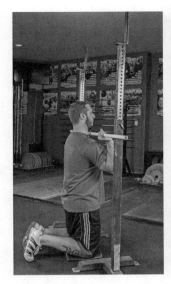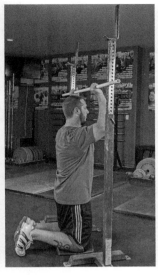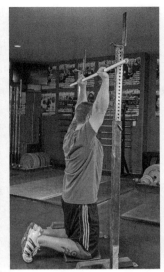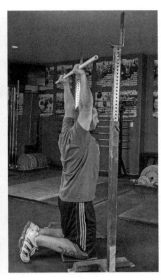

Figure 18.18 Use a rack to guide the bar path and isolate active posterior tipping of the shoulder blade to attain full range of motion. This can be done in tall kneeling (pictured) or half kneeling.

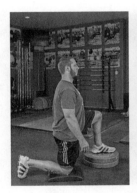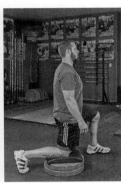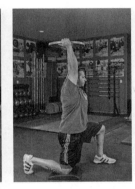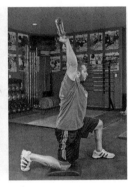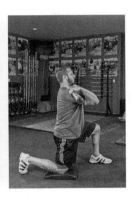

Figure 18.19 Split squat variations. Pictured: Front foot elevated, back knee elevated, overhead hold with plate, overhead hold with bar, and front rack hold.

Movement Cluster Options

- Alternate with 20-second bouts of SMR to the lats or hip flexors.
- Alternate with Option 1 and/or Front Foot Elevated Holds.
- Alternate with Supine Pullover.

Stabilization: Split Squat Variations

The split squat is a great progression from what we have been outlining, because the athlete must now support a lunge position very similar to that of the split jerk. We have several options to perform and combine, all of which are beneficial (Figure 18.19):

- Front foot elevated: to mobilize the hips as we improve stability in the split.

- Back knee elevated: beneficial to find the individual balance points of each lifter in the split, or for a novice lifter looking to gain familiarity with the split position.
- Overhead Hold: to develop overhead control.
- Front Rack Hold: especially beneficial with the front foot elevated; to develop comfort going from standing front rack to split.

Starting Position

- Half kneeling with the forward leg bent at 90 degrees at the knee and hip.
  - ❯ Create a straight line with the down leg from knee to hip to shoulder to ear.
  - ❯ Tuck the toes under the back foot, as opposed to having the top of the back foot flat on the ground. This will put the back ankle in relative dorsiflexion. Try to touch the balls of the foot to the ground.
- Establish three points of contact with the front foot.
- Pull the pelvis underneath you to restore a mild lordosis to lower back so pelvic bowl faces the ceiling.
- Place the feet hip-width apart.

Execution

- Exhale to set the ribs down, but keep the spine long and tall.
- Brace the abdominals and stand straight up while maintaining a consistent trunk position. Both knees should still be partially bent in the standing position, just like in the split jerk.
- Inhale and lower straight back down into the start position.
  - ❯ Your start and finish half kneeling position should look the same. If they do not, then you know you lost position somewhere during the movement.
- This will put the lifter in a pretty short split, which is OK as a starting point to learn the positions. The length and width of the stance can certainly be modified to mimic the split that the athlete will use when lifting. In fact, that is the point of these drills—to find the balanced split position for each individual.
- As preparation for the jerk, perform 2-4 sets of 6-8 reps of one or two variations.

One important position cue during a split squat that has carryover to the split jerk is that of pelvic position in the transverse plane. Be mindful that during the split squat, the pelvis should stay square as opposed to

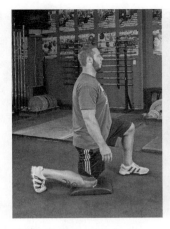 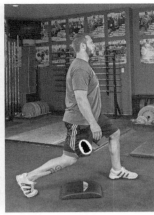 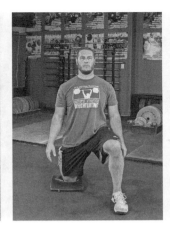 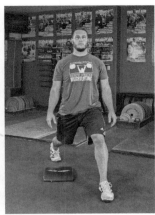

Figure 18.20 The Split Squat

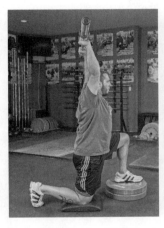 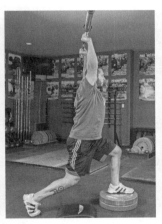 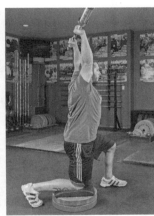 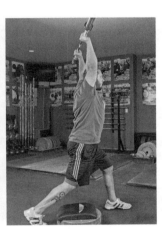

Figure 18.21 Overhead Split Squat variations. Shown: front foot elevated and rear foot elevated.

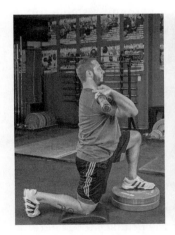 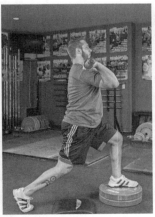 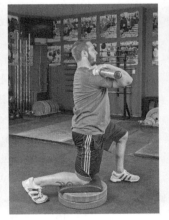 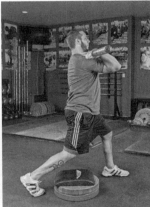

Figure 18.22 Front Rack Split Squat variations. Shown: front foot elevated and rear foot elevated.

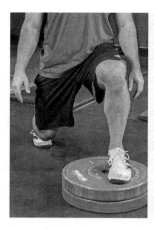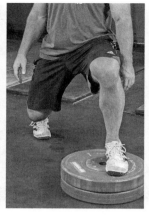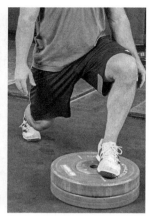

Figure 18.23 In the proper split position, the pelvis is square and the knee is over the foot (first photo). This will facilitate balance in the split. Violations of proper split positioning include the pelvis opening up to the back leg and the pelvis square, but the knee pulled out to the side.

opening up toward the back leg, and the front knee should stay lined up over the foot (Figure 18.23). This will help the athlete maintain balance.

Movement Cluster Options

- Alternate with 20-second bouts of SMR to the lats or hip flexors.
- Alternate with Option 1 and/or Front Foot Elevated Holds or Presses.

Integration: Split Press

Once the lifter has established a comfortable, balanced split position and understands how to attain full overhead mobility around a stable torso, we can reinforce and integrate it with some strict pressing from the split position (Figure 18.24).

For most, the front shin will be vertical or slightly behind vertical, with a bend in the back knee. Loading these can give the lifter a deeper understanding of his or her balance points, as the weight will require the athlete to be stacked optimally to perform the movement. Use weight in lower percentage ranges that can be controlled. What we want to avoid is the weight throwing us out of the position that will carry over to stability in the jerk. If you have to create a huge arch in your lower back to press, reduce the weight and focus on position. True top-end pressing strength will likely be done with a bilateral stance, and is not the primary focus here.

Movement Cluster Options

- Alternate with 20-second bouts of SMR to the lats or upper back.
- Alternate with Shoulder Flexion Hang.
- Alternate with Half Kneeling Press variations.

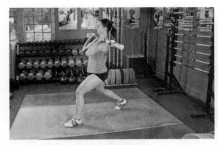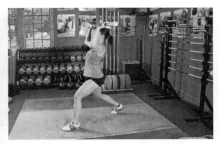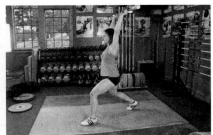

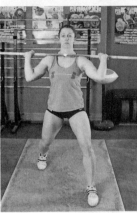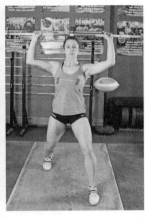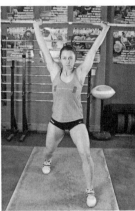

Figure 18.24 The Split Press builds stability and balance in the split position.

Integration: Jerk Balance

This drill is a progression from the more static drills above, as we add a dynamic component to cement the stability we are creating in the split jerk.

Starting Position

- Establish a balanced split position with the bar in either the front rack or on the back.

Execution

- With a small dip and drive, the lifter will pop the bar off its support into the overhead position with the legs still split (Figure 18.25).
- The point here is for one or both feet to leave the platform and be planted back down at approximately the same time the elbows are locked out overhead. This mimics the timing of the jerk and gives the lifter a chance to integrate all of the movement skills they have developed up to this point with a speed element.
  > Some will coach this movement so that the lifter actually steps forward into the split with the front foot after the dip and drive while the back foot stays in contact with the ground (Figure 18.26). The other variation is for both feet

to leave the ground, but land in the exact same spot they took off from ("Filling the footprints").

› With either variation, the ending position should resemble the lifter's split jerk position as closely as possible.

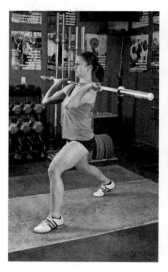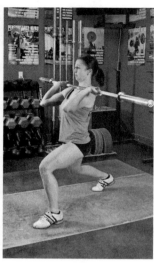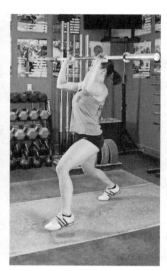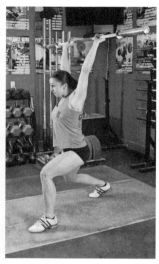

Figure 18.25 The jerk balance adds an element of speed to our previous drills.

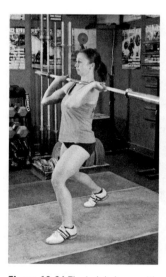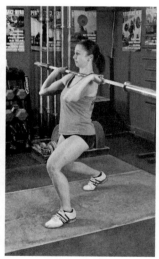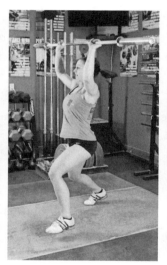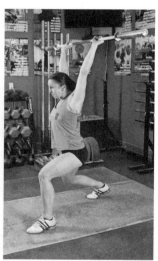

Figure 18.26 The jerk balance with a step into the final split position.

CHAPTER 19

Summary of The Jerk

A common question with regard to the jerk is *How much weight should be on either foot in the split?* The answers vary anywhere from 50/50 to 60/40 in favor of the front foot. Obviously, I have not given any such recommendations, as I find it hard for an athlete to interpret what those numbers are supposed to mean or feel like. I concede that the optimal balance is probably somewhere in that range, but if the athlete spends enough time exploring the split position in the teaching drills that we outlined, he or she will find the optimal balance naturally.

Another question I receive often is, *Should I practice split jerking on both sides so that I do not create an imbalance?* The answer to this one can be complicated, and the *it depends* caveat looms large. From a sports specificity standpoint, the answer is *no*, as we should perform as many reps as possible exactly how we will perform them in competition. Will you develop an imbalance that way? It's certainly possible.

We can't always look at the word *imbalance* in a negative light, however. If you watch high-level lifters, you will see inherent imbalances in their positioning quite often without consequence. In regard to the split, you may even see lifters put one foot slightly in front of the other (usually the foot that is forward in the jerk) instinctively as a way to prepare for the split. These nuances are things that are developed over time and should not necessarily be deliberately mimicked by less experienced lifters. For a higher-level lifter who is not having any movement or painful issues with his or her jerk, it is probably not necessary to switch up the legs, especially if a competition is anywhere near.

Having said that, if a lifter is a youth, a novice, or experiencing a noticeable twisting in the jerk that is causing pain or a decrease in performance, it can be beneficial to practice the split position the opposite way. I typically recommend simply performing the drills that we outlined previously as a means to do this, as opposed to dedicating an actual barbell session to training the other side. That doesn't mean that lifters shouldn't experiment with the opposite leg at low intensities as long as it's not interfering with the training that will make them better weightlifters overall.

As you can see, there is no clear-cut answer there, but in general, the more experienced you are as a lifter, the closer you are to competition, and the healthier you feel, the less of a need there is to have equal reps of splitting on both sides.

CHAPTER 20

Variations for Skill Transfer

In the previous chapters in the book, we outlined many barbell variations that can be used to practice positioning of the lifts, but we did so in compartmental fashion in order to implement various corrective strategies. Here, we will outline logical progressions of barbell variations with the improvement of certain aspects of performance in mind. These suggestions can also constitute the barbell warm-up that a lifter performs.

Snatch

Focus: Finishing the Second Pull with Full Extension

Snatch Pull with Balance at the Top Pausing at the top of lighter pulls or empty bar work can allow the athlete to focus on fully extending the hips and knees and finishing the push into the ground. For coaches who do not cue lifter to rise up on the toes, this may or may not be of use. However, it can be beneficial for a lifter to balance at the top of the pull for a 2-3-count in order to sustain pressure into the ground and maximize drive with the legs. It will also clue you in to whether or not a lifter possesses balance in this position. (Figure 20.01)

Muscle Snatch We take the full extension of the pull and ride the bar momentum into a muscle snatch, again with the focus on fully extending and pushing with the legs. See Chapter 10 for a demonstration.

Power Snatch The power snatch is a great way to attempt to impart maximum height on the bar through use of the fully extended position practiced with the pull and muscle snatch. Now we move the feet and add a knee rebend to receive the bar above a 90-degree squat. (Figure 20.02)

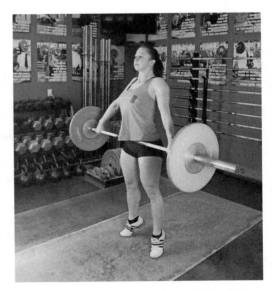

Figure 20.01 Snatch Pull with Balance at the Top: hold this position for a 2-3-count.

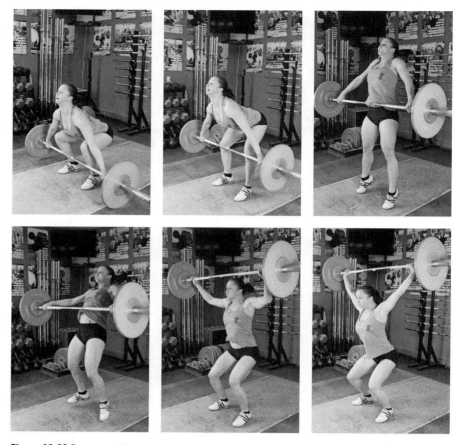

Figure 20.02 Power snatch

Focus: Speed Under the Bar from Back

When working speed in the pull under the bar (the third pull) of the snatch, it can be beneficial to practice variations with the barbell on the back as a starting point, as the variables of the pull are taken out of the equation and the lifter can simply focus on the bottom position. Here is a useful progression:

Push Press to Overhead Squat This is not a speed movement, but a starting point to develop speed under the bar. See the Snatch Grip Push Press and Overhead Squat in Chapter 11 for demonstrations.

Heaving Snatch Balance A dip and drive allows the lifter some time to get under the bar. The lifter also will start in a squatting stance; the feet may leave the ground, but they do not have to slide out, which takes more time and skill. Try to attain the same overhead squat position used in the previous exercise. See the Heaving Snatch Balance in Chapter 11 for a demonstration.

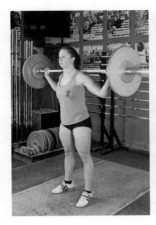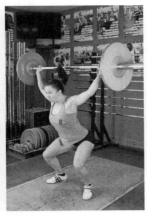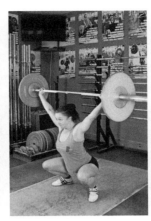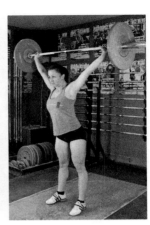

Figure 20.03 Drop Snatch. This can also be performed starting on the toes instead of flat-footed as pictured here.

Snatch Balance This is the same as the heaving snatch balance, except that we start in our pulling stance and move the feet into our receiving stance during the punch under the bar. After extending in the drive, return your feet back down to the ground quickly and punch under the bar into your bottom position. See the Standard Snatch Balance in Chapter 11 for a demonstration.

Drop Snatch This exercise uses no dip and drive, which is why it's last on our progression of behind the neck speed drills, as extra height on the bar will not be created—simply lift the feet and punch down with your arms into the bottom position. You will likely use lighter weights here. This can be performed by starting either on flat feet or from the balls of the feet, depending on coaching styles. (Figure 20.03)

Focus: Speed Under the Bar from Pull

Now we work progressions with holding the bar in front where we would for the full lift.

Dip Snatch Here we dip into the power position and perform a full snatch. The dip provides some momentum for the lifter, but not much. (Figure 20.04)

Tall Snatch Little to no upward momentum is put into the bar before pulling under. Initiate the movement with a slight shrug and then immediately begin the third pull, without a rebend or hitch of the knees. This can be done from flat feet or from the balls of the feet, depending on coaching style. See the Tall Snatch in Chapter 11 for a demonstration.

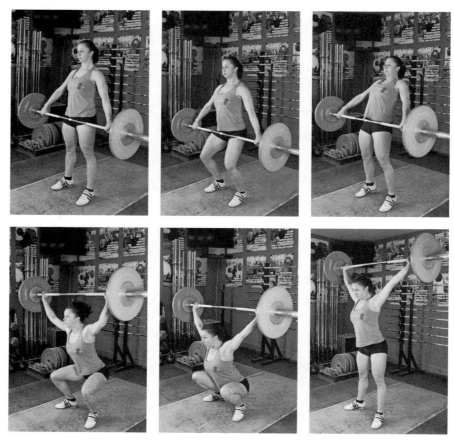

Figure 20.04 Dip Snatch

Focus: Footwork & Timing of Pulling Under the Bar

Here we lay out a progression for a lifter to improve his or her timing during the transition of full extension to pulling into a full overhead squat.

Muscle Snatch: Reset Feet & Ride it Down The muscle snatch will ingrain the motion of the finish of the pull. Once the bar is overhead, move the feet into your squat stance and perform an overhead squat to begin grooving that pattern.

Muscle Snatch: No Feet & Ride it Down Beginning the pull in your squat stance will allow you to take your muscle snatch directly into an overhead squat to practice a smoother transition. Perform this exercise as a single continuous motion.

Power Snatch: Reset Feet & Ride it Down Receiving the bar in a power snatch is more specific to the snatch, as now we must move the feet and bend the knees to move under the bar. After receiving the bar overhead, reset the feet into your correct squat stance and overhead squat to groove that pattern.

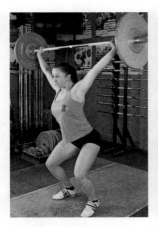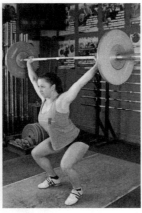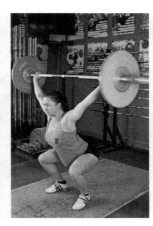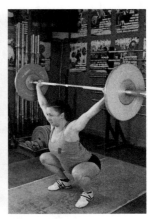

Figure 20.05 Power Snatch: Catch Progressively Lower. Receive progressively lower with power snatches until you're in a full squat.

Power Snatch: Ride it Down Now we require that the lifter receive the bar with a stance that is suitable to squat in, and there is no reset of positioning—take it right into a squat after receiving the bar overhead without changing the position of the feet.

Power Snatch: Catch Progressively Lower This drill is great for those who have difficulty with their timing when lifting lighter weights. Develop control of your third pull and connection with the barbell by dictating how low you receive the bar. Pause at the moment you receive the bar, and progressively catch lower and lower, until you are receiving the lift in a full squat. (Figure 20.05)

Clean

Focus: Finishing the Second Pull with Full Extension

Use the same progression as the snatch, but you will obviously receive the bar at the shoulders as opposed to overhead:

- Clean Pull with Balance at the Top
- Muscle Clean
- Power Clean

Focus: Speed Under the Bar

Use the same progression as the snatch from pull above, but you will obviously receive the bar at the shoulders as opposed to overhead:

- Dip Clean
- Tall Clean

One note here on the Tall Clean specifically: practice getting comfortable using a rebound out of the hole. Allow your hips, knees and ankles to hinge into the squat as much as they want, but when you feel yourself start to reverse out of the bottom, drive up fast. Spending time in the bottom of a clean can spell death for the jerk. Get used to rebounding out of there with control, but with speed.

Focus: Footwork & Timing of Pulling Under the Bar

Use the same progression as the snatch, but you will obviously receive the bar at the shoulders as opposed to overhead:

- Muscle Clean: Reset Feet & Ride it Down
- Muscle Clean: No Feet & Ride it Down
- Power Clean: Reset Feet & Ride it Down
- Power Clean: Ride it Down
- Power Clean: Catch Progressively Lower

Jerk

Focus: Finishing the Drive with Full Extension

When focusing on maximum upward drive for the jerk, it can be beneficial to perform drills with the barbell on the back in order for the variables of the front rack to be taken out of the equation. From this position, the bar can just go straight up.

Behind the Neck Push Press The focus of the lifter is a forceful push into the ground throughout the entirety of the drive phase and a strong lockout of the hips and knees as the bar is locked out overhead. The lifter can practice keeping the feet flat to maximize drive from the hips and knees. This is also beneficial for lifters who prematurely rise onto the balls of the feet in the dip. Alternatively, the lifter can rise up to the balls of the feet to mimic more of the natural action of the jerk. See the Push Press in Chapter 17 for a demonstration.

Behind the Neck Push Jerk The focus of this exercise is the same as for the push press, but now we allow a rebending of the knees to receive the bar. This will allow the athlete to lift more weight. However, the focus is upward extension, so don't shorten your drive in an effort to get under the bar—finish the drive in the same way. The lifter can practice keeping the feet flat to maximize drive from the hips and knees, or rise up to the balls of the feet to mimic more of the natural action of the jerk. (Figure 20.06)

Push Press One can perform the same two previous exercises from the front rack, with the common focus of pushing down into the ground through the duration of the drive phase until full extension of the hips and shoulders is reached. See the Push Press in Chapter 17 for a demonstration.

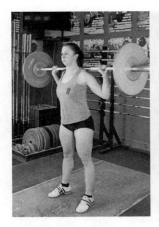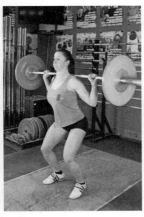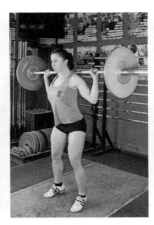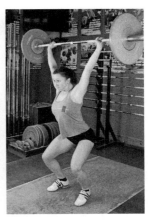

Figure 20.06 Behind the Neck Push Jerk. This exercise can be performed by staying flat-footed during the drive, or by rising to the balls of the feet as pictured.

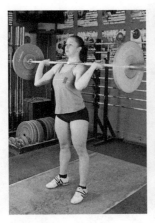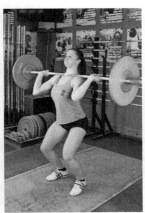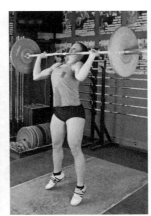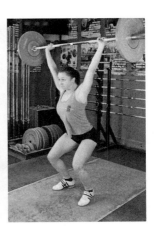

Figure 20.07 Push Jerk

Push Jerk Perform this exercise in the same way as the Behind the Neck Push Jerk, but with the bar starting in the front rack position. (Figure 20.07)

Focus: Speed Under the Bar

Once full extension of the drive phase has been established, we can work on punching under the bar with speed and precise footwork. Again, we start from behind the neck to take the variables of the front rack out of the equation.

Behind the Neck Tall Power Jerk There is no dip and drive in this exercise, similar to the Drop Snatch previously. Simply punch down under the bar, locking out the elbows and landing the feet simultaneously. This can be initiated with flat feet or from on balls of the feet. (Figure 20.08)

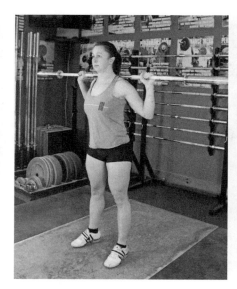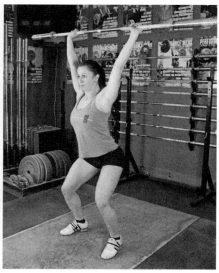

Figure 20.08 Behind The Neck Tall Power Jerk. This exercise can also be started on the balls of the feet instead of flat-footed.

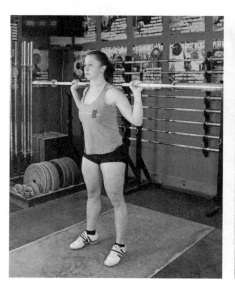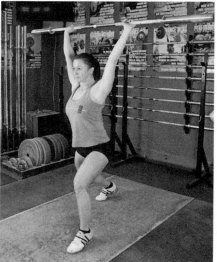

Figure 20.09 Behind The Neck Tall Split Jerk. This exercise can also be started on the balls of the feet instead of flat-footed.

Behind the Neck Tall Split Jerk This exercise is the same as Tall Power Jerk, only the lifter will receive the bar in the split position instead. Pause for a 2-3 count when you land to gauge balance. If you cannot hold for a 2-3-count, adjust your stance to improve your balance. This exercise can be initiated from flat feet or on the balls of the feet. (Figure 20.09)

Tall Power Jerk The above two lifts can also be done from the front rack to increase specificity to the jerk. Perform the Tall Power Jerk in the same way as the Behind the Neck Tall Power Jerk, but with the bar beginning in the front rack position.

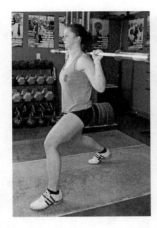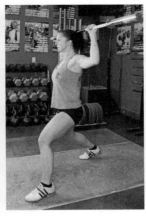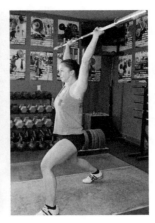

Figure 20.10 Press in Split Behind the Neck

Tall Split Jerk Perform this exercise in the same way as the Behind the Neck Tall Split Jerk, but with the bar beginning in the front rack position.

Power or Split Jerk with Pause Dip Pausing for a 3-count in the bottom of the dip takes away the advantage of both the oscillation of the bar and the stretch reflex of the legs. Driving from a static hold will require speed under the bar—and *do not cut your extension short.*

Focus: Overhead Stability & Balance

Here we focus on a progression to increase overhead stability with a balanced split position. We start from behind the neck to take the variables of the front rack position out of the equation.

Press in Split Behind the Neck Pressing in the split will give immediate feedback to the lifter as to whether the split position is balanced. You should have a solid base to press from without losing foot position. If you initiate the press and immediately lose your balance, re-establish your split and find a better position. (Figure 20.10)

Push Jerk in Split Behind the Neck Now we add a dynamic component with a dip and drive followed by a small rebend of the knees to further challenge balance, but the feet do not move. (Figure 20.11)

Split Jerk Balance Behind the Neck We add foot movement to the dip and drive to better mimic the full split jerk in this exercise. The lifter can start in a full split or in a shorter split and step forward with the front foot during the drive. (Figure 20.12)

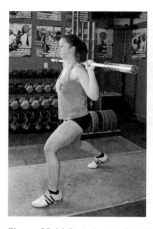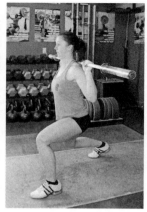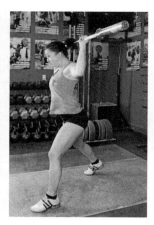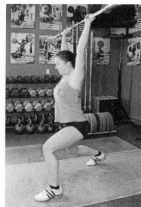

Figure 20.11 Push Jerk in Split Behind the Neck

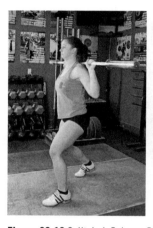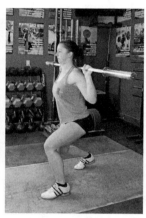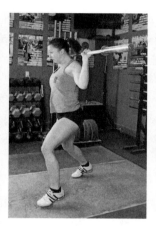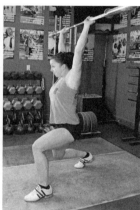

Figure 20.12 Split Jerk Balance Behind the Neck. This exercise can be done with the feet starting and landing in the full split, or started with the feet in a shorter split and stepping the front foot forward into the full split during the drive (pictured).

Press in Split The same progression can be used with the bar in the front rack as opposed to behind the neck. Perform this exercise in the same way as the Press in Split Behind the Neck, but with the bar starting in the front rack position.

Push Jerk in Split Perform this exercise the same way as the Push Jerk in Split Behind the Neck, but with the bar beginning in the front rack position.

Split Jerk Balance Perform this exercise the same way as the Split Jerk Balance, but with the bar beginning in the front rack position.

■ CHAPTER 21

Recovery

Recovery is obviously an important topic, as the exertion that we put forth in our training over time is dependent on how well our system is recovered from subsequent training bouts. One way to define recovery is the ability to reproduce a previous performance. Another way to describe recovery is the rate at which we can reduce fatigue. We also know that the nervous system is an important driver in terms of facilitating recovery—specifically the parasympathetic nervous system (rest and digest).

Sleep and nutrition are the true avenues to combating fatigue and appropriately shifting the system into a state conducive to recovery, and nothing in this book will provide an actual physiological response that comes close to those things.

For our purposes, we will simply refer to fatigue as a conscious perception of the body feeling sore or banged up after a training session or before the subsequent training session. That may not precisely represent the state of recovery our body is actually in, but it's the best that the scope of this book has to offer. Having said that, we will refer to *recovery* as the conscious perception of feeling less sore, more mobile, etc.

Inhibit/Downregulate

Deep Breathing

Breathing is one (if not the only) way to consciously attempt to drive parasympathetic signaling, slow the heart rate, decrease blood pressure, etc. There is little scientific evidence showing that performing deep breathing exercises after a training session leads to measurable amounts of recovery, but if we know that parasympathetic signaling is what we want after training, then it's not a bad way to get the ball rolling.

Refer back to Chapter 2 for our discussion on breathing mechanics. Below are two drills that you can try after an intense training session to begin ramping down: the 90-90 Recovery Position and Crocodile Breathing. Pick one and spend 2-5 minutes there, or alternate back and forth between both.

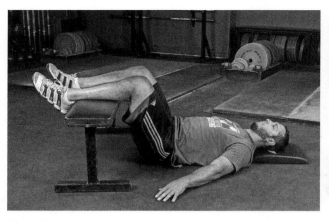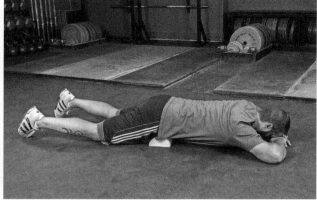

Figure 21.01 90-90 Recovery Position (left): Allow everything to unwind as you spend 2-5 minutes here taking deep breaths. This can be useful after high pulling volume to take pressure off of the erectors. Crocodile Breathing (right): Push the air into the low back. You should feel it expand. This can be useful after high squat volume to open up the front of the hips.

The focus is low tension. Calm down. Relax. Chill. Training is over. With each exhalation, you should attempt to relax more and more. Inhalations through the nose should be relatively effortless. (Figure 21.01)

Foam Rolling

There is some evidence that bouts of foam rolling can reduce perceived soreness up to 48 hours after the training session that induced the feeling, so we would be remiss to not mention it here as a way to support recovery as we have defined it for our purposes. Post-training is where 5-15 minutes of straight total body foam rolling (or at least the areas that feel the most worked) seems to have the most utility. It's a perfect opportunity to relax and make love to your roller.

Decompress

This is, again, about your perception, but it is common for lifters to end a training session and leave the gym feeling "stuck," almost like they're walking around but still stuck in the squat rack.

To remedy this feeling, we can introduce light movement or positions that put us in different planes than the ones that are constantly repeated in weightlifting. This is not to say that we need to begin training these different patterns, as we still want to adhere to the laws of specificity to the sport of weightlifting, but light implementation can send novel input to our brains that just feels good. And that's what we are after. Restoring a little perceived movement variability.

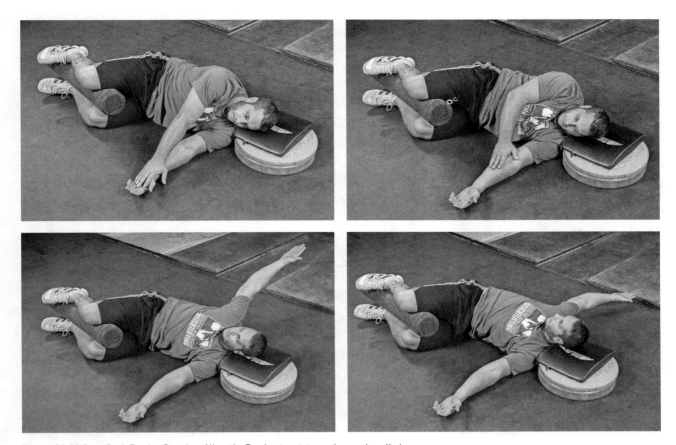

Figure 21.02 Open Book T-spine Rotation. Allow the T-spine to rotate as the arm is pulled.

Thoracic Rotation

Some light thoracic spine rotation can be a nice way to move the upper back spinal segments in different ways than they are constantly loaded. Typically an athlete will report a general feeling of increased looseness after an exercise like the Open Book T-Spine Rotation (Figure 21.02). Perform 1-2 sets of 5 reps each side.

Spinal Flexion

This can be a controversial topic, as spinal flexion (especially lumbar) has often been discussed as being injurious for the spine with repeated motions and under load. However, in our case, we will suggest a few drills to move through unloaded, bodyweight flexion as a means to counteract the largely extension-based positions of weightlifting and decrease any perceived tension in the low back.

Disclaimer: if you do not tolerate spinal flexion or experience pain with these drills, simply discontinue the exercise and get checked out. No reason that anyone should be pushing these low-level movements to pain.

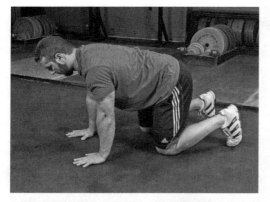

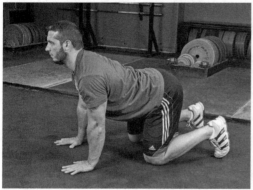

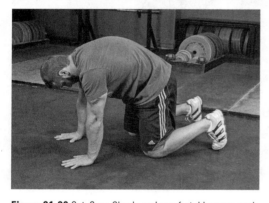

Figure 21.03 Cat-Cow: Slowly and comfortably move each spinal segment in the sagittal plane.

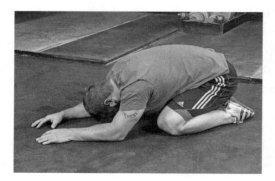

Figure 21.03 Cat-Cow: Slowly and comfortably move each spinal segment in the sagittal plane.

However, for the healthy spine, flexion is a completely normal range of motion that may provide a decompressive relief after the compressive loads of weightlifting.

Cat-Cow Cow? Camel? Who knows. I've heard both names for years. Pick whichever is your favorite. Here we work to restore control of each spinal segment *within a comfortable range*. Remember, if there is any perceived change at all after performing these drills, it should be that you stand up feeling better. Perform 2-3 sets of 8-10 total reps. (Figure 21.03)

Quadruped Rockback In this drill we are in a sustained position of spinal flexion, which may be a more relaxing position for some. From on your hands and knees, rock your hips back toward your heels, letting the lower back comfortably round and pelvis tilt posteriorly. Drop your chest so that your forearms rest on the ground, with your elbows underneath your shoulders or slightly flared out. Spread your fingers, creating as much ground contact as possible, and keep your head and neck relaxed in mid range.

Inhale through your nose with a relaxed neck while maintaining position. Exhale through your mouth, pushing lightly through your elbows and forearms, protracting your shoulder blades and rounding your upper back slightly. Maintain this position and perform 2-4 sets of 5 breath cycles. (Figure 21.04)

Summary

To reiterate, the outcome of the suggestions above can be largely individual. Try them out after a hard training session, and if they feel nice, then it's something you can revisit as you see fit.

References

Part 1

1. Shumway-Cook A, Woollacott MH. Motor Control: translating research into clinical practice. 3rd edition. Philadelphia, PA: Lippincott Williams & Wilkins; 2007

2. Neumann D. Kinesiology of the musculoskeletal system: Foundations for rehabilitation. 2nd edition. St. Louis, MO: Mosby Elsevier; 2010

3. Stergiou N., Decker L. Human movement variability, nonlinear dynamics, and pathology: Is there a connection? *Human Movement Science.* (2011), doi:10.1016/j.humov.2011.06.002

4. McQuade et al. Critical and theoretical perspective on scapular stabilization: What does it really mean, and are we on the right track? *Physical Therapy.* 2016. Vol 96(8)

5. Cholewicki et al. Delayed Trunk Muscle Reflex Responses Increase the risk of low back injuries. *SPINE.* Vol 30. No 23 pp2614-2620. 2005

6. Higgins, S. Motor Skill Acquisition. *Physical Therapy,* 71(2), (1991). 123-139.

7. Newell, KM. Motor Skill Acquisition. *Annu Rev Psychol.* 1991; 42:213-37

8. Kendall F. Muscles: Testing and Function With Posture and Pain 5th edition. Lippincott Williams & Wilkins. 2005

9. Edmondston et al. Clinical and radiological investigation of thoracic spine extension motion during bilateral arm elevation. *JOSPT.* 2012. Vol 42(10)

10. Kim et al. Overcoming the myth of proprioceptive training. *Clinical Kinesiology* 65(1); 2011

11. Lundy-Ekman L. Neuroscience: Fundamentals for Rehabilitation. 3rd edition. St. Louis, MO: Saunders Elsevier; 2007

12. Enoka R. The pull in Olympic weightlifting. *Medicine and Science in Sports.* Vol11, No2;131-137, 1979

13. Harbili E, Alptekin A. Comparative Kinematic Analysis of the Snatch Lifts in Elite Male Adolescent Weightlifters. *Journal of Sports Science & Medicine.* 2014;13(2):417-422.

14. Kalichova et al. Optimalisation of the snatch technique in weightlifting based on kinematic measurements.

15. Viorel et al. Biomechanical characteristics of movement phases of clean & jerk style in weightlifting performance. *Social and Behavioral Sciences.* 2014. 64-69

16. Gourgoulis et al. Snatch lift kinematics and bar energetics in male adolescent and adult weightlifters. *J Sports Med Phy Fitness.* 2004;44:126-31

17. Kipp et al. Weightlifting performance is related to kinematic and kinetic patterns of the hip and knee joints. *JSCR.* 2012. Vol 26(7)

18. Glasgow P et al. Being able to adapt to variable stimuli: the key driver in injury and illness prevention? *BJSM.* Jan 213 Vol 74(2)

19. Hamill et al. Coordinative variability and overuse injury. *Sports Medicine, Arthroscopy, Rehabiliation, Therapy & Technology* 2012

20. Harbourne R. Sergiou N. Movement variability and the use of nonlinear tools: Principles to guide physical therapist practice. *Phys Ther.* 2009. Mar; 98(3):267-282

21. Finucane et al. Efficiency of the normal human diaphragm with hyperinflation. *J Appl Physiol.* 2005. 99:1402-1411

22. Reid W Darlene, Dechman Gail. Considerations When Testing and Training the Respiratory Muscles. *Physical Therapy.* 1995; 75:971-982

23. Hodges W. Paul, Gandevia C. Simon, Richardson A. Carolyn. Contractions of specific abdominal muscles in postural tasks are affected by respiratory maneuvers. *Journal of Applied Physiology.* Sept 1997 Vol. 83 753-760

24. Hodges, P. W., Butler, J. E., McKenzie, D. K., & Gandevia, S. C. (1997). Contraction of the human diaphragm during rapid postural adjustments. *The Journal of physiology,505*(Pt 2), 539-548

25. Hodges PW, Gandevia SC. Activation of the human diaphragm during a repetitive postural task. *Journal of Physiology.* (2000) pp.165-175

26. McKenzie DK1, Gandevia SC, Gorman RB, Southon FC.. Dynamic changes in the zone of apposition and diaphragm length during maximal respiratory efforts. *Thorax.* 1994 Jul;49(7):634-8.

27. Cluzel et al. Diaphragm and chest wall: assessment of the inspiratory pump with MR imaging-preliminary observations. *Radiology.* 2000; 215:574-583

28. Bradley H., Esformes J. Breathing Pattern Disorders & Functional Movement. *The International Journal of Sports Physical Therapy.* Vol 9, (1) Feb 2014. P28

29. De Palo Va, Parker Al, Al-Bilbeisi F, McCool Fd: Respiratory muscle strength training with nonrespiratory maneuvers. *J Appl Physiol.* 96: 731-734, 2004.

30. J Vera-Garcia; J Elvira; S Brown; S McGill. Effects of abdominal stabilization manoeuvres on the control of spine motion and stability against sudden trunk perturbations. *Journal of Electromyography and Kinesiology.* 17 (2007) 556-567

31. Grenier S., McGill S., Quantification of lumbar stability by using 2 different abdominal activation strategies. *Arch Phys Med Rehabil.* Vol 88. Jan 2007

32. Kolar P. Analysis of diaphragm movement during tidal breathing and during its activation while breath holding using MRI synchronized with spirometry. *Physiol Res.* 58: 383-392, 2009

33. Hodges et al. Postural activity of the diaphragm is reduced in humans when respiratory demand increases. *Journal of Physiology*(2001), pp999-1008

34. Hodges PW, Gandevia SC. Changes in intra-abdominal pressure during postural and respiratory activation of the human diaphragm. *J Appl Physiol.* 2000. 89:967-976

35. Hodges et al. Postural and Respiratory Functions of the Pelvic Floor Muscles. *Neuroourology and Urodynamic* 26:362-371(2007)

36. Takazakura et al. Diaphragmatic motion in the sitting and supine positions: Healthy subject study using a vertically open magnetic resonance system. *Journal of Magnetic Resonance Imaging.* 19:605-609(2004).

37. Kawabata et al. Changes in intra-abdominal pressure and spontaneous breath volume by magnitude of lifting effort: highly trained athletes versus healthy men. *Eur J Appl Physiol.* 2010 109(2):279-86

38. Al-Bilbeisi F, McCool FD. Diaphragm recruitment during nonrespiratory activities. *Am J Respir Crit Care Med.* 2000. Vol 162. Pp456-459

39. Shirley et al. Spinal Stiffness changes throughout the respiratory cycle. *J Appl Physiol*. Vol 96. Oct 2008

40. Cholewicki J. Can increased intra-abdominal pressure in humans be decoupled from trunk muscle co-contraction during steady state isometric exertions? *Eur J Appl Physiol*. 2002 Jun;87(2):127-33

41. Lee B. McGill S. The effect of short-term isometric training on core/torso stiffness. *Journal of Sports Sciences*. 2016.

42. Ross et al. Effect of changes in pelvic tilt on range of motion to impingement and radiographic parameters of acetabular morphologic characteristics. *The American Journal of Sports Medicine*. July 2014, 43 (1).

43. Azevedo et al. Pelvic rotation in femoroacetabular impingement is decreased compared to other symptomatic hip conditions. *JOSPT*. 2016.

44. Bagwell et al. Hip kinematics and kinetics in persons with and without cam femoroacetabular impingement during a deep squat task. *Clinical Biomechanics*

45. Lander et al. The effectiveness of weight-belts during multiple repetitions of the squat exercise. *Medicine and Science*. 1992. Vol 24(5)

46. Miyamoto et al. Fast MRI used to evaluate the effect of abdominal belts during contraction of trunk muscles. *Spine*. 2002. Vol27(16)

47. Kingma et al. Effect of a stiff lifting belt on spine compression during lifting. *Spine*. 2006. Vol 31(22)

48. McGill SM. On the use weight belts. *Review for NSCA*. March 2005.

49. Zink et al. The effects of a weight belt on trunk and leg muscle activity and joint kinematics during the squat exercise. *JSCR*. 2001. Vol 15(2)

Part 2

1. Ferreira et al. Quantitative assessment of postural alignment in young adults based on photographs of anterior, posterior, and lateral views. *Journal of Manipulative and Physiological Therapeutics*. 2011

2. Cleland JA, Koppenhaver S. Orthopaedic Clinical Examination: an evidence-based approach. 2nd edition. Philadelphia, PA: Saunders Elsevier; 2011

3. Frost DM. FMS scores change with performers' knowledge of the grading criteria – Are general whole-body movement screens capturing "dysfunction"? *J Strength Cond Res*. 2013 Nov 20

4. Beardsley C. The Functional Movement Screen: a review. Strength & Cond Journal. Oct 2014

5. Anthony G Schache, Peter D Blanch, Anna T Murphy. Relation of anterior pelvic tilt during running to clinical and kinematic measures of hip extension. *Br J Sports Med* 2000;34:279–283

6. Vigotsky et al. (2016), The modified Thomas test is not a valid measure of hip extension unless pelvic tilt is controlled. PeerJ 4:e2325; DOI 10.7717/peerj.2325

7. Kibler et al. Clinical implications of scapular dyskinesis in shoulder injury: the 2013 consensus statement from the 'scapular summit'. *Br J Sports Med*. 2013;47:877-885

8. Macrum E, Bell DR, Boling M, Lewek M, Padua D. Effect of limiting ankle-dorsiflexion range of motion on lower extremity kinematics and muscle-activation patterns during a squat. J Sport Rehabil. 2012 May;21(2):144-50.

9. Rabin et al. The Association of Ankle dorsiflexion range of motion with hip and knee kinematics during the lateral step down test. *JOSPT*. 2016

10. Grafton K, O'shea, S. The intra and inter-rater reliability of a modified weight-bearing lunge measure of ankle dorsiflexion. *Sheffield Hallam University Research Archive*. 2013

11. Bennell et al. Intra-rater and inter-rate reliability of a weight-bearing lunge measure of ankle dorsiflexion. *Australian Physiotherapy*. 1998. Vol 44(3)

12. Venturini C, Ituassu NT, Teixeira LM, Deus CVO. Intrarater and interrater reliability of two methods for measuring the active range of motion for ankle dorsiflexion in healthy subjects. *BJPT*. Oct./Dec. 2006 (10) 4, p. 377-381

13. Konor et al. Reliability of three measures of ankle dorsiflexion range of motion. *IJSPT*. 2012. Vol 7(3)

14. Chisholm et al. Reliability and validity of a weight-bearing measure of ankle dorsiflexion range of motion. *Physiotherapy Canada*. 2012. Vol 64(4)

15. Mauntel et al. The effects of lower extremity muscle activation and passive range of motion on single leg squat performance. *J Strength Cond Res*. 2013 Jul;27(7):1813-23

16. Hicks JH. The mechanics of the foot, II: the plantar aponeurosis and the arch. J Anat. 1954;88:25–30.

Part 3

1. Glasgow P. Optimal loading: key variables and mechanisms. *Br J Sports Med*. 2015;49:278-279

2. Wallden M. Designing effective corrective exercise programs: the importance of dosage. *Journal of Bodywork & Movement Therapies*. 2015. 19, 352-356

3. Hedrick, Allen. Physiological Responses to Warm-Up. *Exercise Physiology*. Oct 1992. Vol 14 (5): 25-27

4. Chaudhry H, Schleip R, Ji Z, Bukiet B, Maney M, Findley T. Three-dimensional mathematical model for deformation of human fasciae in manual therapy. J Am Osteopath Assoc. 2008 Aug;108(8):379-90.

5. Chaudhry, H., Bukiet, B., Ji, Z., Stecco, A., & Findley, T. W. (2014). Deformations Experienced in the Human Skin, Adipose Tissue, and Fascia in Osteopathic Manipulative Medicine. JAOA: Journal of the American Osteopathic Association, 114(10), 780787

6. MacDonald GZ, Penney MD, Mullaley ME, Cuconato AL, Drake CD, Behm DG, Button DC. An acute bout of self-myofascial release increases range of motion without a subsequent decrease in muscle activation or force. J Strength Cond Res. 2013 Mar;27(3):812-21.

7. Kathleen M. Sullivan, Bachelor of Kinesiology, Dustin B.J. Silvey, Bachelor of Kinesiology, Duane C. Button, PhD, and David G. Behm. Roller-massager application to the hamstrings increases sit-and-reach range of motion within five to ten seconds without performance impairments. Int J Sports Phys Ther. Jun 2013; 8(3): 228–236.

8. Halperin I, Aboodarda SJ, Button DC, Andersen LL, Behm DG. Roller massager improves range of motion of plantar flexor muscles without subsequent decreases in force parameters. Int J Sports Phys Ther. 2014 Feb;9(1):92-102.

9. Jay K, Sundstrup E, Søndergaard SD, Behm D, Brandt M, Særvoll CA, Jakobsen MD, Andersen LL. Specific and cross over effects of massage for muscle soreness: randomized controlled trial. Int J Sports Phys Ther. 2014 Feb;9(1):82-91.

10. Jeffrey Janot, Brittany Malin, Ryan Cook, Jacob Hagenbucher, Andrew Draeger, Melissa Jordan, Esther Quinn. Effects of Self Myofascial Release and Static

Stretching on Anaerobic Power Output. Journal of Fitness Research. Issue: Vol. 2, No. 1 2013

11. Healey KC, Hatfield DL, Blanpied P, Dorfman LR, Riebe D. The effects of myofascial release with foam rolling on performance.J Strength Cond Res. 2014 Jan;28(1):61-8.

12. Okamoto T1, Masuhara M, Ikuta K. Acute effects of self-myofascial release using a foam roller on arterial function. J Strength Cond Res. 2014 Jan;28(1):69-73.

13. Jacklyn K. Miller, Ashley M. Rockey. UW-L Journal of Undergraduate Research IX Foam Rollers Show No Increase in the Flexibility of the Hamstring Muscle Group. (2006)

14. Mohr RA, Long BC, Goad CL Foam rolling and static stretching on passive hip flexion range of motion. Human Performance, Oklahoma State University. Jan 2014

15. Fama BJ, Bueti DR, The acute effect of self-myofascial release on lower extremity plyometric performance. Sacred Heart University Theses and Dissertations. Apr 2011.

16. Effects of long-term self-massage at the musculotendinous junction on hamstring extensibility, stiffness, stretch tolerance, and structural indices: a randomized controlled trial. *Physical Therapy in Sport*. 2016. 21: 38-45

17. Kim, K., Park, S., Goo, B. O., & Choi, S. C. (2014). Effect of Selfmyofascial Release on Reduction of Physical Stress: A Pilot Study. Journal of physical therapy science, 26(11), 1779

18. Fama, Brian J. and Bueti, David R., "The Acute Effect Of Self-Myofascial Release On Lower Extremity Plyometric Performance"(2011). Theses and Dissertations. Paper 2.

19. Vigotsky et al. Acute effects of anterior thigh foam rolling on hip angle, knee angle, and rectus femoris length in the modified Thomas test. *PeerJ*. 2015

20. McHugh MP, Tallent J, Johnson CD. The role of neural tension in stretch-induced strength loss. J Strength Cond Res. 2013 May;27(5):1327-32.

21. Behm et al. Acute bouts of upper and lower body static and dynamics stretching increase non-local joint range of motion_2015. *Eur J Appl Physiol*. 2015

22. Andersen J.C. Stretching before and after exercise: effect on muscle soreness and injury risk. *Journal of Athletic Training*. 2005; 40(3): 218-220

23. Thacker et al. Effect of Stretching on Sport Injury Risk: a Review *Clinical Journal of Sport Medicine*: March 2005 - Volume 15 - Issue 2 - p 113

24. Konrad A. Increased range of motion after static stretching is not due to changes in muscle and tendon structures. *Clin Biomech*. 2014 Jun;29(6):636-42

25. Andersen JC. Stretching Before and After Exercise: Effect on Muscle soreness and injury risk. Journ of Ath Tr. 2005

26. Lima et al. Assessment of muscle architecture of the biceps femoris and vastus lateralis by ultrasound after a chronic stretching program. *Clinical Journal of sport medicine*. 2014. Vol 0(0)

27. Nakamura et al. Time course of changes in passive properties of the gastrocnemius muscle-tendon unit during 5 min of static stretching. *Manual Therapy*. 2013. 211-215

28. Nakamura, M, Ikezoe, T, Takeno, Y, and Ichihashi, N. Effects of a 4-week static stretch training program on passive stiffness of human gastrocnemius muscle-tendon unit in vivo. Eur J Appl Physiol 112: 2749–2755, 2012.

29. Magnusson SP, Simonsen EB, Aagaard P, Sørensen H, Kjaer M. A mechanism for altered flexibility in human skeletal muscle. J Physiol. 1996 Nov 15;497

30. Weppler CH1, Magnusson SP. Increasing muscle extensibility: a matter of increasing length or modifying sensation? Phys Ther. 2010 Mar;90(3):438-49

31. Mitchell et al. Neurophysiological reflex mechanisms' lack of contribution to the success of PNF stretches. *J Sport Rehabil.* 2009 Aug; 18(3):343-57

32. Decoster, L. C., Cleland, J., Altieri, C., & Russell, P. (2005). The effects of hamstring stretching on range of motion: a systematic literature review. Journal of Orthopaedic & Sports Physical Therapy, 35(6), 377387

33. Russell et al. A comparison of the immediate effects of eccentric training vs. static stretch on hamstring flexibility in high school and college athletes. *North Am Journal of Sports Phy Ther.* 2006. Vol 1(2)

34. Radford, J. A., Burns, J., Buchbinder, R., Landorf, K. B., & Cook, C. (2006). Does stretching increase ankle dorsiflexion range of motion? A systematic review. British Journal of Sports Medicine, 40(10), 870875

35. Andersen J.C. Stretching Before & After Exercise: Effect on Muscle Soreness and Injury Risk. *Journal of Athletic Training.* 2005;40(3)218-230

36. Kjaer M. Eccentric exercise: acute and chronic effects on healthy and diseased tendons. J Appl Physiol. 2014

37. Nelson et al. A comparison of the immediate effects of eccentric training vs. static stretch on hamstring flexibility in high school and college athletes. *North American Journal of Sports Physical Therapy.* May 2006. Vol 1(2).

38. Behm et al. Acute effects of muscle stretching on physical performance, range of motion, and injury incidence in healthy active individuals: a systematic review. *Appl. Physiol. Nutr. Metab.* 41: 1-11(2016)

39. Cramer et al. Acute effects of static stretching on characteristics of the isokinetic angle-torque relationship, surface electromyography, and mechanomyography. *Journal of Sports Sciences.* 2007;25(6):687-698

40. Pope et al. A randomized trial of preexercise stretching for prevention of lower-limb injury. *Journal of the American College of Sports Medicine.* 2000.

41. Shrier I. Does stretching improve performance? A systematic and critical review of the literature. *Clin J Sport Med.* Vol 14(5)Sept2004

42. Laursen et al. The effectiveness of exercise interventions to prevent sports injuries: a systematic review and meta-analysis of randomized controlled trials. *Br J Sports Med.* 2014;48:87

43. Osawa Y, Oguma, Y. Effects of vibration on flexibility: a meta-analysis. *J Musculoskelet Neuronal Interact.* 2013; 13(4): 442-453

44. Piek J. The role of variability in early motor development. *Infant Behavior & Development.* 25 (2002) 452-465

45. Calatayud J. Importance of mind-muscle connection during progressive resistance training. *Eur J Appl Physiol.* 2016. 116:527-533

46. Gray C. *Movement.* Lotus Publishing; 2011

47. Bishop D. Warm up I: Potential mechanisms and the effects of passive warm up on exercise performance. *Sports Med.* 2003: 33(6):439-454

48. Heinemeier K. In vivo investigation of tendon responses to mechanical loading. *J Musculoskelet Neuronal Interact* 2011; 11(2):115-123

49. Arampatzis et al. Adaptational responses of the human Achilles tendon by modulation of the applied cyclic strain magnitude. *The Journal of Experimental Biology.* 2007

50. Kongsgaard et al. Corticosteroid injections, eccentric decline squat training and heavy slow resistance training in patellar tendinopathy. *Scand J Med Sci Sports*. 2009. 19:790-802

51. Khan K. Mechanotherapy: how physical therapists' prescription of exercise promotes tissue repair. *Br J Sports Med*. 2009;43:247-251

52. Bohm et al. Human tendon adaptation in response to mechanical loading: a systematic review and meta-analysis of exercise intervention studies on healthy adults. *Sports Medicine*. (2015).

53. Naugle et al. A meta-analytic review of the hypoalgesic effects of exercise. *J Pain*. 2012; 13(12)

54. Rio et al. Isometric exercise induces analgesia and reduces inhibition in patellar tendinopathy. *Br J Sports Med*. 2015; 49:1277-1283

55. Wirth et al. Core stability in athletes: a critical analysis of current guidelines. *Sports Med*. 2016. Review Article

56. Hagen Hartmann, Klaus Wirth, Markus Klusemann. Analysis of the Load on the Knee Joint and Vertebral Column with Changes in Squatting Depth and Weight Load. *Sports Med* (2013) 43:993–1008

57. Schenau VI. From Rotation to translation: constraints on multi-joint movements and the unique action of bi-articular muscles. *Human Movement Science*. 1989. 301-337

58. Chiu et al. Net joint moments and muscle activation in barbell squats without and with restricted anterior leg rotation. *Journal of Sports Sciences*. 2016.

59. Vigotsky AD, Harper EN, Ryan DR, Contreras B. (2015) Effects of load on good morning kinematics and EMG activity. *PeerJ* 3:e708

60. McKean et al. The Lumbar and sacrum movement pattern during the back squat exercise. *JSCR*. Vol 24(10) Oct 2010

61. Potvin JR[1], McGill SM, Norman RW. Trunk muscle and lumbar ligament contributions to dynamic lifts with varying degrees of trunk flexion. *Spine* 1991 Sep;16(9):1099-107.

62. McGill SM[1], Marshall LW. Kettlebell swing, snatch, and bottoms-up carry: back and hip muscle activation, motion, and low back loads. *J Strength Cond Res*. 2012 Jan;26(1):16-27

63. Castelein et al. Superficial and deep scapulothoracic muscle electromyographic activity during elevation exercises in the scapular plane. *JOSPT*. 2016; Vol 46(3)

Part 4

1. Jerath et al. Physiology of long pranayamic breathing: neural respiratory elements may provide a mechanism that explains how slow deep breathing shifts the autonomic nervous system. *Med Hypotheses*. 2006;67(3):566-71. Apr 2006

2. Pramanik et al. Immediate effect of slow pace bhastrika pranayama on blood pressure and heart rate. *J Altern Complement Med*. 2009 Mar; 15(3):293-5

3. Radaelli et al. Effects of slow, controlled breathing on baroreceptor control of heart rate and blood pressure in healthy men. *J Hypertens*. 2004 Jul;22(7):1361-70

4. Seals et al. Influence of lung volume on sympathetic nerve discharge in normal humans. *Circulation Research*. Vol 67, No1, July 1990

5. MacDonald GZ, Button DC, Drinkwater EJ, Behm DG. Foam Rolling as a Recovery Tool after an Intense Bout of Physical Activity. Medicine & Science in Sports & Exercise: January 2014 - Volume 46 - Issue 1 - p 131–142

6. Pearcey, G. E., BradburySquires,D. J., Kawamoto, J. E., Drinkwater, E. J., Behm, D. G., & Button, D. C. (2015). Foam Rolling for Delayed Onset Muscle Soreness and Recovery of Dynamic Performance Measures. Journal of athletic training, 50(1), 513

7. Callaghan JP, McGill SM. Intervertebral disc herniation: studies on a porcine model exposed to highly repetitive flexion/extension motion with compressive force. *Clin Biomech*. 2001 Jan;16(1):28-37.

8. Adams et al. Healing of a painful intervertebral disc should not be confused with reversing disc degeneration: Implications for physical therapies for discogenic back pain. *Clinical Biomechanics*. 25 (2010) 961–971 963

9. Kokmeyer et al. Gait considerations in patients with femoroacetabular impingement. *IJSPT*. 2014. Vol 9(6)